promoting normal birth

— research, reflections & guidelines —

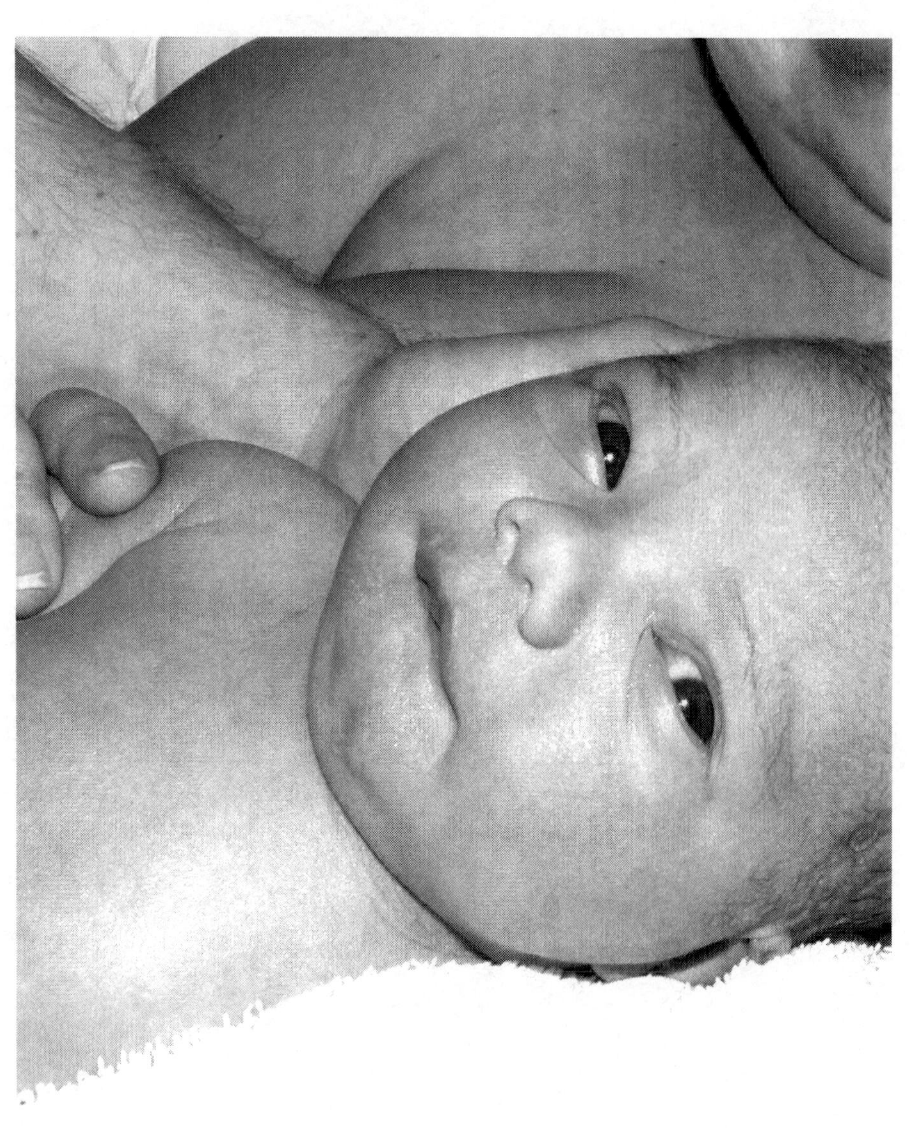

promoting normal birth

— research, reflections & guidelines —

an international collaboration of caregivers,
lecturers and researchers

edited by Sylvie Donna

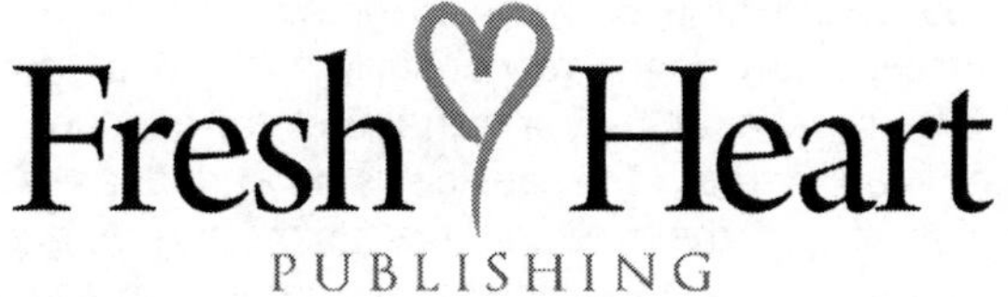

1st British edition

Published in 2011 by
FRESH HEART PUBLISHING
a division of Fresh Heart Ltd
PO Box 225, Chester le Street, DH3 9BQ, United Kingdom
www.freshheartpublishing.co.uk

A CIP catalogue record for this publication is available from the British Library

ISBN: 978 1 906619 06 0

Set in Franklin Gothic Book, Eras ITC and Bradley Hand ITC
Designed and typeset by Fresh Heart Publishing
Printed in the UK by Lightning Source UK Ltd
Cover design by Fresh Heart Publishing
Cover photo of Pithiviers Maternity Hospital, near Paris by Sylvie Donna

Dedication

Dedicated to anyone who has ever wondered what makes birth good... and what makes it traumatic or less safe... and what makes it inspirational...

Contents

Reflections... 111

Guidelines... 239

Contributors

Jette Aaroe Clausen, PhD
Senior Lecturer in Midwifery. Centre for Science and Technology Studies, Aarhus University, Denmark.

Suzanne Arms
Suzanne Arms, mother and grandmother, is an author/photojournalist with seven published books, an international speaker, advocate and activist. She is also founder-director of the international charity, Birthing The Future, located in Colorado USA. Website: www.BirthingTheFuture.org

Valerie Bader, MN, CNM
Instructor of Clinical Nursing, University of Missouri, Columbia Missouri.

Sarah Davies, BSc (hons), RM, Cert Ed, Cert Counselling, MPhil
Senior Lecturer in Midwifery, University of Salford, UK.

Robbie Davis-Floyd, PhD
Senior Research Fellow, Dept. of Anthropology, University of Texas Austin, Fellow of the Society for Applied Anthropology, Board Member, International Mother-Baby Childbirth Organization (MBCO).

Sylvie Donna, MA, BEd, RSA Dip, RSA Cert
Founder of Fresh Heart Publishing and author of books about birth, language and teaching; MA lecturer, dissertation supervisor and marker for Durham University and Birmingham University; also provides academic writing support for Durham University's home and international students (particularly at postgraduate level).

Soo Downe, PhD, MSc, RM, BA (hons)
Professor of Midwifery Studies at the University of Central Lancashire (UCLan) in England, UK. Set up the UCLan Midwifery Studies Research Unit in Oct 2002. Now leads the Research in Childbirth and Health (ReaCH) group and is chair of the UK Royal College of Midwives Campaign of Normal Birth steering committee and the ICM Research Standing Committee. Also a member of various other midwifery committees, nationally and around the world. Has held various visiting professorships in Belgium, Hong Kong, Sweden and Australia.

Ngai Fen Cheung, PhD, MSc, RM, RGN
Professor and Head of the first Chinese Midwifery Research Unit of the Nursing College of Hangzhou Normal University in China.

Kathleen Fahy, RM, RN, BN, Med, PhD.
FACM Professor of Midwifery, University of Newcastle, NSW, Australia.

Mandy Forrester, MA, RN, RM, ADM, PCGEA
Midwifery Adviser, Nursing and Midwifery Council, London

Dianne Garland, SRN, RM, ADM, PGCEA, MSc
Lecturer in midwifery, expert witness, trustee to APEC (Action on Pre-Eclampsia) and freelance midwifery consultant (www.midwifeexpert.com). A midwife since 1983 and waterbirth teacher since 1989. Author of *Revisiting Waterbirth—an Attitude of Care* (Palgrave, 2010).

Ami Goldstein, CNM, FNP, MSN
Assistant Clinical Professor. Department of Family Medicine. University of North Carolina at Chapel Hill. Chapel Hill, North Carolina, USA.

Carolyn Hastie, RM, IBCLC, Dip Teach, Grad Dip PHC, MPhil
Midwife, educator, facilitator, birth activist, blogger and writer; PhD student

Els Hendrix, CM, MSc
Midwife; Master in Health Sciences; Senior Lecturer, PHL University College, Belgium.

Asheya Hennessey, BEd
Founder & Executive Director, Mothers of Change for Maternity Care, Canada. Founder, Yukoners for Funded Midwifery, Yukon Territory, Canada. Certified Teacher, British Columbia, Canada. Mother of three.

Ricardo Herbert Jones, MD
Obstetrician, gynecologist and homeopath. Member of ReHuNa—Humanization of Childbirth Network (Brazil), the Association for Humanization of Childbirth (Portugal) and the IMBCO—International Motherbaby Childbirth Organization. Medical Advisor of ANDO—National Association of Doulas (Brazil). Professor of national and international courses for doulas and perinatal educators.

Michael Klein, MD, CCFP, FAAP (Neonatal-Perinatal), FCFP, ABFP, FCPS
Emeritus Professor Family Practice & Pediatrics, University British Columbia; Senior Scientist Emeritus, Centre Developmental Neurosciences & Child Health Child and Family Research Institute, Vancouver British Columbia, Canada . Founder and Listmaster of the multidisciplinary MCDG (Maternity Care Discussion Group).

Céline Lemay, PhD, MA, Midwife
Midwife and lecturer on the midwifery practice programme at the university in Quebec, Canada (Université du Québec à Trois-Rivières).

Karen McDonald, MN, RM, MTD.
Senior Lecturer , Faculty of Education, Health and Midwifery. School of Health, Nursing and Midwifery. The University of the West of Scotland, Scotland, UK.

Evelyn Mohammed, MSc, BSc (Hons) Dip N (Glas) RM, RGN, PGCert (TLHE)
Midwifery Lecturer, Faculty of Education, Health and Midwifery. School of Health, Nursing and Midwifery. The University of the West of Scotland, Scotland, UK

Ole Olsen, Msc
Statistician; Senior Researcher, National Research Center for the Working Environment, Copenhagen, Denmark; Senior Researcher, The Research Unit for General Practice in Copenhagen.

Lesley Page, PhD, MSC, BA, RM, RN, FRCM (honorary)
Professor Lesley Page PhD, MSC, BA, RM, RN, FRCM (honorary) is visiting professor of midwifery at King's College London (UK), University of Technology Sydney and University of Sydney (Australia).

Anshi Pan, PhD, MSc, MPhil
Researcher in social anthropology and other subjects in social sciences.

Verena Schmid
Verena Schmid, certified midwife; teacher of physiology and salutogenesis; founder and director of the international school of The Art of Midwifery in Florence, Italy and the professional magazine D&D, *Donna e Donna*; author of professional books for midwives and promoter of self-determined, conscious childbirth.

Shannon Senefeld, MA
Senior Technical Advisor, Catholic Relief Services, Baltimore, MD; Therapist, Mt. Washington Pediatric Hospital, Baltimore, MD; doctoral candidate in clinical psychology, Argosy University, Washington, DC.

Alex Smith, BA, PGCE
Childbirth Educator and Antenatal Tutor with the NCT

Jenny Smith, RN, RM, ADM, PGCEA
Registered nurse and registered midwife; Senior midwife, Imperial college London UK. Founder of Jentle Childbirth Foundation administered by Genesis research trust (Registered charity 292518). Lectures widely on normalising birth.

Madge Russell, MM, B.Sc.,PGCE (PSE), RMT, RM, RGN
Lecturer and Supervisor of midwives. Faculty of Education, Health and Midwifery. School of Health, Nursing and Midwifery. The University of the West of Scotland. Scotland, UK.

Susan Rutledge Stapleton, DNP, CNM, FACNM
Certified Nurse-Midwife; Research Committee Chairperson, American Association of Birth Centers; President, Commission for the Accreditation of Birth Centers.

Trudy Stevens, RM, RN, MA (Cantab), MSc, PhD, PGDip L&T
Midwife, Senior Lecturer, Faculty of Health and Social Care, Anglia Ruskin University, Chelmsford, England.

Adela Stockton, MA
Trained midwife and homeopath. Doula UK recognised doula; doula educator/course leader, Mindful Doulas (Birth Consultancy, Scotland). Childbirth writer/author. Joint Assessor/Mentor Co-ordinator, Doula UK.

Jan Tritten, BA, CCM
Jan Tritten is the founder, editor-in-chief and mother of *Midwifery Today* magazine. She became a midwife in 1976 after the amazing home birth of her second daughter. Her mission is to make loving midwifery care the norm for birthing women and their babies throughout the world.

Hélène Vadeboncoeur, PhD, MSc
Childbirth researcher. Member of the Board of Directors of the International MotherBaby Childbirth Organization.

Naoli Vinaver, CPM, BA
Mexican Traditional and Professional Midwife. Founded Luz de Luna HomeBirth Services in 1990. Birth Activist, Mexican Representative of Midwives Alliance of North America (MANA) from 1994-1998. Author of birth books, video productions and conference speaker and organiser as well as teacher. Member of the Board of Nueve Lunas Midwifery School in Oaxaca.

Marsden Wagner, MD, MS
Former Director of Women's and Children's Health at the World Health Organization (for 15 years), after several years at UCLA and the California State Dept of Public Health. Consultant to governments and NGOs and author of many scientific papers and books.

Susan Way, PhD MSc PGCEA ADM RM
Lead Midwife for Education, Bournemouth University, UK

Linda Wylie, BA (Open), MM, PGCert (TLHE), PGCert (Research Methods), RGN, RM, RMT
Programme Leader BSc Midwifery, Faculty of Education, Health and Midwifery. School of Health, Nursing and Midwifery. The University of the West of Scotland, Scotland, UK.

Heba Zaphiriou-Zarifi, MA-DEA

An analytical psychotherapist, based in London, in her final stages of qualifying in analytical psychology with GAPS-UKCP. Also a leader in BodySoul Rhythms at the Marion Woodman Foundation.

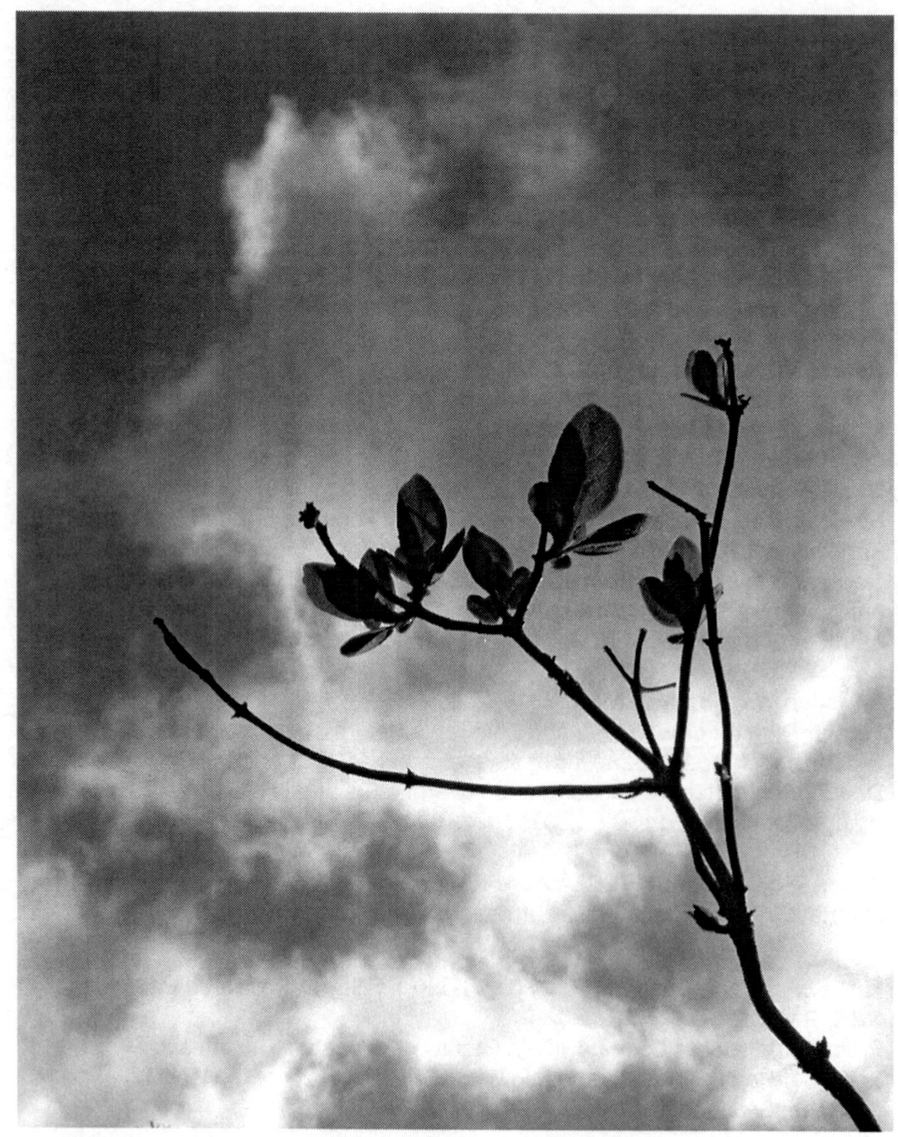

Introduction

Sylvie Donna

You may have wondered, on first seeing this book, why the title includes the word 'promoting'. Why should normal birth be promoted particularly? The answer is simple: other forms of birth—those involving plenty of intervention, especially caesareans—get plenty of promotion, simply because they may often appear to be the easiest options for caregivers, or the least frightening ones for pregnant women. After all, a ward full of women with an epidural may be easier to cope with emotionally for many caregivers, and forceps or ventouse may seem a quick solution to a long second stage, particularly if they have never given birth themselves, or if they have not done so physiologically; caesareans may seem the easier option for many consultant obstetricians, particularly if they are afraid of lawsuits, or are tired of having a constantly disrupted social life. And women may prefer these options, particularly if they have never given birth before... simply out of fear. The pain of birth is widely reported to be outrageous, beyond anything which is normally experienced, so why would any woman want to subject herself to it and also risk damaging her pelvic floor (so the fallacy goes) and stretching her vagina? In addition, one apparently small intervention (such as ARM) may lead to a cascade of interventions; pregnancy magazines often seem to encourage these 'trivial' interventions, while implicitly encouraging women to submit to the protocols of an institution, despite the fact that—let's face it—protocols are outdated in many cases or inappropriate for a particular woman. Beyond these factors, there is also the ubiquity of advertising from pharmaceutical companies or from manufacturers of obstetric or midwifery equipment... And after a hospital manager has invested in a 'beautiful' new (and helpfully impressive-looking) electronic fetal monitor and an ultrasound machine, won't he or she want to justify the purchases by billing clients for their use, or at least *showing* through their 'usefulness' in everyday practice that the decisions to purchase were wise ones?

You may also question the use of the word 'normal'. What could it mean? If it's used to refer to physiological birth, then how can this possibly be justified, given that caesareans have become the 'new norm' in urban hospitals in countries such as China and Brazil, where caesarean rates have reportedly reached 90% or even 95% in many hospitals? And if the meaning of 'normal' in this book is indeed 'entirely physiological' how can this possibly be justified in the light of the definitions used at conferences in the UK and US and much of the relevant literature, where births with opioid analgesia are also included? The answer, again, is simple: physiological birth with no drugs or interventions is the natural default. In other words, if we do nothing else, a pregnant woman will in most cases produce a baby without any 'help' in the form of pain relief or interventions. (She may appreciate some moral support, but this is not necessary for her to give birth.) This is not to say that pain relief or interventions are bad *per se.* It is just that they do not need to be promoted—for the reasons mentioned above and also, and more importantly, because a) women should always have the right to *choose* how they give birth (and that includes whether or not they use pain relief of any kind, and b) in a tiny minority of cases interventions will always be necessary because there is always likely to be a small number of women or babies who need help to get born safely.

If you, therefore, accept the basic premise of this book—that normal birth really does need to be promoted—I hope this book will help you to do that. Inspired by your own personal experience of giving birth normally, or by witnessing other women do so—let's call them 'clients', not 'patients'—you may well agree that there is a real need to work towards reversing the tide of recent development.

If, on the other hand, you are not at all inspired by 'normal' birth—defining it as physiological birth with no drugs or interventions—and if you are only reading this book because you have been asked to do so (as part of a professional development exercise or because it's one of the books on your recommended reading list), I at least hope you will be open to hearing about other people's views. The 37 people who have contributed to this book have an enormous amount of shared experience, which must encompass many, many years and many, many clients. As you will see, all the writing is well-referenced to the relevant academic literature (with the exception of a couple of personal pieces or texts outlining professional suggestions, based on experience). And as well as being well-referenced, the texts also include suggestions for many practical solutions to well-known problems. Many of them also prompt us to reconsider assumptions which are often not questioned, but which result in practices with which we might not actually agree... if we take the time to reconsider them. In any case, the material in this book should help you to decide where you are now and how your views change as your work progresses into the future...

But how can you use this book ? Here are a few ideas and suggestions:

- First, you may just want to read through the whole book, or dip in according to your interests, so that you can reflect alone.
- If you are a working midwife, obstetrician, maternity care assistant, nurse or doula you may well want to share some of the content with some of your colleagues, perhaps during a meeting or an in-service training session.
- You can use the Index to consider any issue which crops up in your day-to-day studies or work. As you may expect, certain topics are considered by various authors and each one has a different perspective, all of which are useful.
- If you are a lecturer of midwifery or obstetrics, or even of general medicine (or a related field) you may find plenty of material in this book for seminars and assignments. At the end of each of the book's three sections you will find some quotations from the chapters in the previous section, some questions to prompt reflection or discussion and/or some extracts from birth stories or commentary (from professionals of various kinds). You could perhaps ask students to read some of these (selecting which ones, according to your focus of study) in preparation for a seminar. In the seminar itself you could ask students to choose two of the quotes/questions/extracts for discussion within pairs or smaller groups, before opening the discussion up to the whole class. (All the material has been specially written to prompt discussion and the exchange of ideas and the way in which it is written and presented is based on my own long years of experience teaching adults. I am, in fact, the author of most of the material for reflection and discussion.) In many cases, as you will see, it is helpful to check the research on a particular topic before discussing the material—so of course students could also check this out in advance. Finally, students could write assignments based on any of the topics included.

That brings me to another issue... which is how perspectives on birth relate to the research. As I am sure you know, there has been an impressive and useful drive in recent years to make practice in the fields of midwifery and obstetrics evidence-based. This is wonderful, given that many practices which were widespread in the past (e.g. amniotomy, episiotomy and routine EFM on admission) were not based on a single shred of evidence. In fact, studies have since shown that many practices are more likely to be harmful than helpful—and amniotomy, episiotomy and routine EFM are included in this list, as you probably know. However—and this is a big 'however'—there are disadvantages to this strong focus on everything being evidenced based, as follows:

- Some areas have not yet been researched and this should not mean we simply use the 'old way' as the default option. There are many other ways in which practices can be judged, including a consideration of physiology, philosophies (of birth) and pain management. Therefore, we should be prepared to embrace certain unresearched, or under-researched practices if we can find other justifications for them. (For example, encouraging a woman to be upright and leaning forward during the second stage can be justified on the basis of *physiology,* while a preference to wait and not have forceps or ventouse used can be justified by a sense of aesthetics or philosophy, provided of course there is no fetal distress or other indications for intervention.)
- Maternal choice makes it impossible for research to be carried out in many cases, either because women do not want to be randomised or because they might want to opt for procedures which research has clearly shown are not evidence-based. (Caesarean section which is not indicated for medical reasons is a case in point here. Other examples would include cases where caregivers feel a particular risk is very high, but where the mother *still* wants to go ahead with her preferred option.) It is essential that women have the right to choose how and where they give birth—and also with whom!
- In many cases research has limitations and is unlikely to reveal clear 'answers'. Randomised controlled trials (RCTs) are a particular problem in this respect because they simply cannot be used in so many cases, where birth is concerned. As well as there being too many potentially confounding factors for even the best statistician to cope with, there are also the issues of maternal choice and the unpredictability and individuality of birth—which make prospective studies impossible in many cases.

In other words, although research findings already support the promotion of physiological birth, we must be aware of the limitations of this basis for decision-making, particularly if the focus is only on randomised controlled trials.

Finally, before I sign off and let you get on with the important business of reading and exploring further, let me leave you with an invitation... This book will come out in a second edition at some point in the near future and you may well want to contribute to that. Do you have experience or thoughts which you would like to share? Do you disagree with or want to add to anything you read here? Do you have any suggestions for other topics or elements which should be included? If you have any ideas or material to contribute, please email Fresh Heart at: info@freshheartpublishing.co.uk. In the meantime, happy reading.

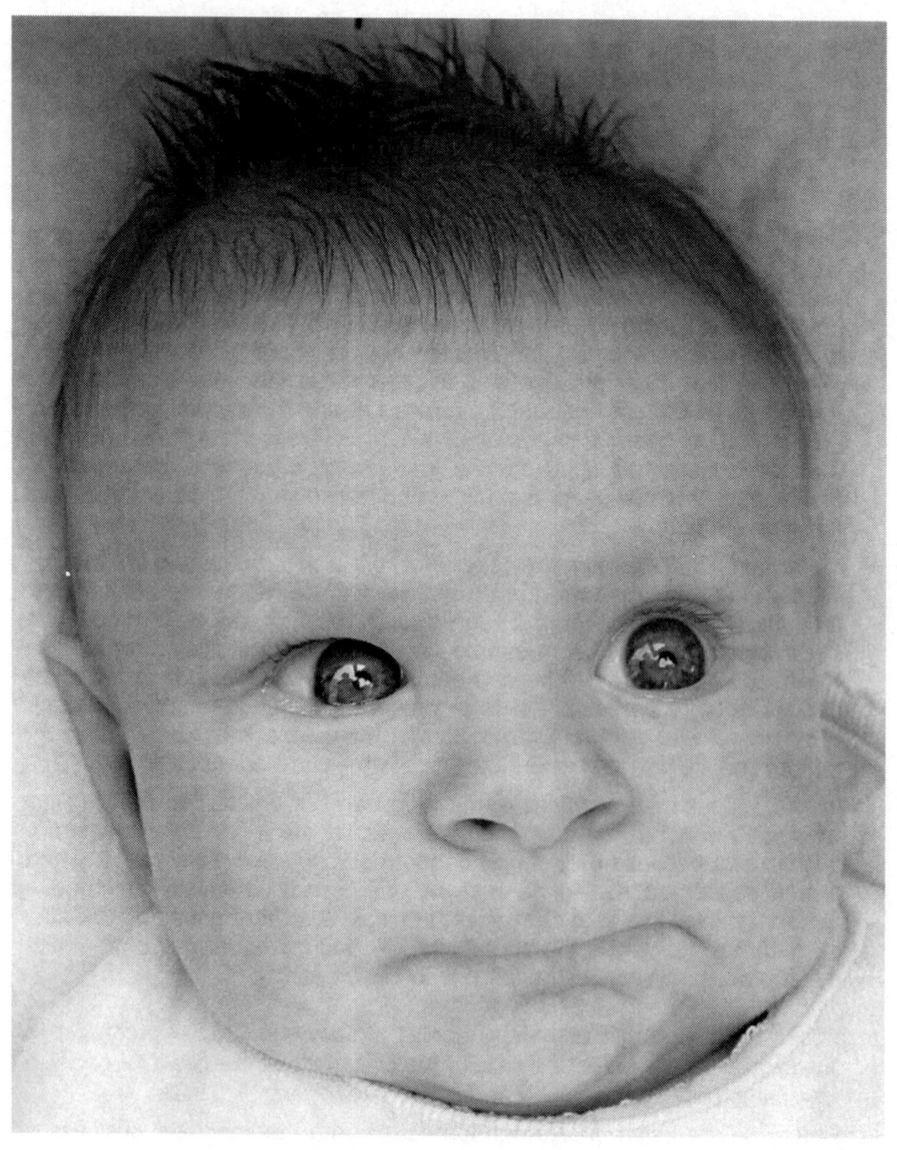

part one:
research

- routine interventions
- epidurals—benefits and liabilities
- physiological third and fourth stage
- supporting longer labours and births
- most effective models of care
- birth centres as a site for normal birth
- home birth and statistics
- maternal mental health
- the value of doulas

Routine interventions during normal labour and birth... are they really necessary?

Els Hendrix

Historically women gave birth at home with the assistance of a midwife. Throughout the past century society has become industrialised and childbirth has moved into hospitals. This trend has led to a greater use of interventions. Midwives have often been replaced by obstetricians, mostly men, and so the birthing culture has become a male-dominated. This has involved a shift from a more social model of care towards a more technocratic model of care. According to Robbie Davis-Floyd,[1] this model is characterised by, amongst other things, a high appreciation of technology, seeing the patient as an object and a machine, and carrying out aggressive interventions with an emphasis on short-term results.

Routine interventions such as perineal shaving and enemas before vaginal delivery, continuous electronic fetal monitoring (EFM) intrapartum, induction and augmentation, epidural analgesia, directed pushing and supine birthing positions, episiotomy and early cord clamping are interventions that have become prevalent in many areas of the industrialised world.

However, alongside this trend towards more interventionist birthing practices, a movement has also sprung up which supports natural childbirth. Supporters emphasise the emotional aspects of labour and delivery and they see the mother as an active participant, rather than a birthing machine. As Hunter says:[2] "Women give birth and pizzas are delivered." (Of course, here Hunter was emphasising that they way people talk about birth reflects our way of thinking about it and the model of care we offer. The word 'deliver' implicitly suggests that women have rather a passive role and the practitioner an active one, while the words 'give birth', by contrast, emphasise the woman's active role and imply that the caregiver is just a facilitator.) For a long time, scientific evidence has been available showing clearly that these routine interventions might not be so beneficial for either the physical or psychological health of mother and baby. Sadly, however, when we look at the statistics (Table 1),[3] we find that a large proportion of women still undergo these interventions. It is therefore the task of midwives to make the research available to those who work with women and babies. This chapter gives an overview of the most common routine interventions (with the exception of epidural analgesia, which will be discussed in the next chapter). The most recent scientific evidence is considered in each case, while also contemplating the outlook for the future.

Evidence shows routine interventions are not beneficial for either mother or baby

Next page: **Childbirth in US Hospitals, 2005: Listening to Mothers II Survey**[3]

Medical induction and self-induction

♥ Any attempt to induce labour with drugs and/or techniques	50%
♥ Professional attempted to induce labour	41%
♥ Mother attempted to induce labour	22%
♥ Labour was actually induced	39%
♥ Professional's actions started labour	34%
♥ Mother's actions started labour	4%

Fetal monitoring (experienced labour)

♥ Any electronic fetal monitoring (EFM)	94%
♥ EFM continuously throughout labour	71%
♥ EFM most of the time during labour	16%
♥ Handheld device alone for monitoring	3%

Other labour and birth interventions

♥ Synthetic oxytocin to induce and/or speed labour	57%
♥ Rupture of membranes to induce or speed labour	65%
♥ Epidural or spinal analgesia	76%
♥ Narcotic analgesia	22%
♥ Intravenous drip	3%
♥ Bladder catheter	56%

Restrictions

♥ No mobility after well-established contractions (experienced labour)	76%
♥ No oral fluids (experienced labour)	59%
♥ No oral solids (experienced labour)	85%
♥ Back-lying position for giving birth (vaginal births)	57%

Mode of birth

♥ Total vaginal	68%
♥ Vaginal, spontaneous	60%
♥ Vaginal, vacuum extraction/forceps	7%
♥ Vaginal birth after caesarean (VBAC)	2%
♥ Total caesarean	32%
♥ Primary (first-time) caesarean	16%
♥ Repeat caesarean	16%

Hospital practices that can interfere with breastfeeding (mother intended to exclusively breastfeed at the end of pregnancy)

♥ Baby primarily with staff for routine care first hour after birth	39%
♥ Mother given free formula samples / offers	66%
♥ Baby given formula or water 'supplement'	38%
♥ Baby given dummy	44%

Breastfeeding

♥ Intended exclusive breastfeeding at end of pregnancy	61%
♥ Exclusively breastfeeding one week after birth	51%

Perineal shaving

Routine shaving, a procedure which has ceased to exist in the UK, still continues in some other countries. It is a practice which arose during the transition from midwifery-led birth under a social model of care to births which are controlled by obstetricians, under a surgical model of care. During this period, the most common position for birthing changed from an upright posture to a supine position; this occurred so as to make the perineum more visible to caregivers. The change also implied that a woman's genital area changed from being private, and became public. This had further consequences: it also became a surgical part instead of a physiological part. In this context, perineal shaving was introduced so as to prepare the perineum for possible surgery. In this way, the perineum was pathologised.[4]

Perineal shaving used to be carried out so as to reduce the risk of infection and facilitate suturing or an operative delivery.[5,6] Basevi and Lavender[7] reviewed three trials including in total 1,039 women. They found no microbiological evidence to suggest differences in maternal infection between different groups of women. There is therefore, sufficient evidence to justify stopping the routine use of perineal shaving prior to labour.[7]

Enemas

In some places enemas are frequently given for similar purposes to perineal shaving, name(y to reduce the risk of infection (maternal as well as neonatal), in this case through contamination with faeces.[8,9] Opponents of this procedure argue that it is widely accepted that this intervention generates discomfort for women and increases the workload of health workers and the costs of care.[10] Reveiz, Gaitán and Cuervo[11] included four randomised controlled trials in their Cochrane review which looked at a total of 1,917 women. This review found that enemas did not reduce puerperal or neonatal infection rates, episiotomy dehiscence rates or maternal satisfaction. Therefore, their use is unlikely to benefit women or newborn children, and there is no reliable scientific basis for recommending their routine use. These findings should, in fact, discourage the routine use of enemas during labour.[11]

Continuous electronic fetal monitoring intrapartum

Continuous electronic fetal monitoring (EFM) intrapartum became available in 1968. EFM initially seems to have the advantage of providing continuous tracking of the fetal heart rate, which appears to facilitate evaluation of fetal response to uterine contractions so that fetal distress can be detected immediately. However, although EFM provides a sensitive trace, it is unreliable as a method for detecting fetal distress. In other words it has a high false-positive rate in predicting adverse neonatal outcomes.[12] A very important side-effect of the use of EFM is that many (if not most) labouring women are confined to a bed. In a Canadian survey nearly 91% of women reported having EFM at some time during their labour.[13] This probably reflects routines in other

Western labour wards. As one woman reported, as well as the EFM being unhelpful (in terms of detecting fetal distress and also in terms of immobilising the labouring woman), it also had an impact in terms of the care received: "As soon as I got hooked up to the monitor, all everyone did was stare at it. The nurses didn't even look at me any more when they came into the room—they went straight to the monitor. I got the weirdest feeling that 'it' was having the baby, not me."[14]

Alfirevic, Devane and Gyte[15] published a Cochrane Review where they included 12 trials (looking at 37,000 women) (although only two were high quality). Compared to intermittent auscultation, continuous cardiotocography showed no significant difference in the overall perinatal death rate. Except for a reduction in neonatal seizures they did not find any benefit for the newborn in terms of mortality or substantial long-term morbidity, such as cerebral palsy. There was, however, a significant increase in caesarean sections (RR 1.66) and instrumental vaginal births (RR 1.16), especially around normal labour, when women had had EFM. Given these results, we can conclude that there is no evidence available to support the routine use of EFM. Intermittent auscultation for 60 seconds every 15 minutes using a Sonicaid or Pinard for monitoring the fetal heart is the preferred method according to WHO guidelines.[16]

Induction and augmentation

Rates of induction of labour are increasing in almost all parts of the world. Rates have risen to 39% in the United States[3] and 20% in other Western countries. Indications for labour induction can be either maternal or fetal but there is a growing percentage of elective inductions. In these cases there is no medical reason for the induction. An elective induction is not always due to a pregnant woman's whim but may be prompted by discomfort, the availability of her partner after the birth, or because of professional reasons. Medical practitioners also sometimes recommend an induction for non-medical reasons, because of their availability, their holiday leave, or for economical reasons. NICE agrees that a large part of this growing percentage is due to 'soft' medical indications, i.e. indications lacking good research evidence, such as suspected macrosomia.[17]

Glantz studied 11,849 records of women having a normal labour.[18] He found that induction was associated with higher rates of women having caesarean sections, greater use of epidural anaesthesia and higher numbers of non-reassuring fetal heart rate patterns. There were no improvements in neonatal outcomes. A large Australian study (involving 753,895 women) confirmed these results.[19] These Australian researchers found that approximately 20% of all labours are induced. Low-risk primiparous women with induced or augmented labours were twice as likely to have a caesarean delivery and one and a half times as likely to have an instrumental birth.

Low-risk primips with induced or augmented labours were twice as likely to have a caesarean

Oxytocin, the 'hormone of love', can only express itself fully in a safe and intimate environment

Oxytocin, which Michel Odent calls the 'hormone of love',[20] can only express itself fully in a safe and intimate environment. When obstetric interventions are used, it is produced in lower amounts, if at all. Synthetic (exogenous) oxytocin (syntocinon or pitocin) is then often used to 'solve the problem'. However, there are basic differences between synthetic oxytocin and natural (endogenous) oxytocin. Oxytocin released by the pituitary gland has the ability to cross the blood-brain barrier, but synthetic oxytocin cannot cross this barrier. This means that certain positive effects of natural oxytocin will not appear when synthetic oxytocin is used, including calmness, relaxation and social interaction.[21] Synthetic oxytocin is, therefore, not comparable to the hormone of love. A second difference is that natural oxytocin works in a pulsatile way, while intravenous or injected oxytocin is released continuously and much higher doses are necessary in order for a comparable effect to be achieved in terms of stimulating uterine contractions.[22]

Another disadvantage of using synthetic versions of oxytocin is that Kerstin Uvnäs-Möberg found a negative correlation between the use of synthetic oxytocin during labour and the prevalence of natural oxytocin during breastfeeding postpartum.[21] The more synthetic oxytocin was used during labour, the less oxytocin was released during breastfeeding, which explains why women who have had an induced labour experience problems with breastfeeding.[23] This can be further explained through several mechanisms: disruption of the natural, pulsatile secretion (meaning that natural oxytocin levels fluctuate), augmentation of the mother's stress response, and perhaps also infant and mother behaviour, which are negatively affected when there are inadequate amounts of natural oxytocin.[23] Our conclusion must be that it is not advisable for inductions to be carried out for non-medical reasons or for medical reasons which are not supported by evidence, and that inductions should certainly not be carried out before 41 weeks of gestation.[17,24]

This is because of the well-known problem of induction due to supposed prolonged pregnancy. In the absence of an induction policy, only 7% of pregnancies progress beyond 41 weeks and only 1.4% beyond 42 weeks.[25] A retrospective cohort-study in Ireland showed that nearly one-third of the women of their studied cohort of 3,262 women were induced. 60,2% of women were induced according to hospital policy 10 days after the expected date of delivery but also over 33% of women were induced earlier with 'prolonged pregnancy' as indication.[26] Questions can be raised about the medical necessity of these inductions. In a large prospective randomised controlled trial in Sweden there was no significant difference in neonatal outcome between routine induction (according to policy) and fetal assessment every three days.[27] In a time where not only physical parameters are taken into account this provides evidence for a policy of expectant management where the mother should be offered the chance to make an informed decision and thus also the chance for a spontaneous labour and birth.

Cascade of interventions

Research results relating to EFM, induction and augmentation reveal many cases of what is called a cascade of interventions. This is because many intrapartum interventions have unintended effects, which need to be 'solved' through the use of subsequent interventions, which have new unintended effects, which may in turn create yet more problems...[28] For example, when labour is not allowed to start spontaneously, the first technological intervention is induction. Then, since induced labour is often experienced as more painful than spontaneous labour, in traditional hospital settings this leads to more frequent use of epidural analgesia. Once a woman has an induced labour and epidural analgesia, the chances of her having an unassisted vaginal birth are very low. (Tracy found that there was an eight times higher risk of having an instrumental delivery and a 50 times higher risk of having a caesarean section.[19]) The figure below provides an overview of how things can go wrong and illustrates why it is advisable to avoid routine interventions.

Cascade of interventions

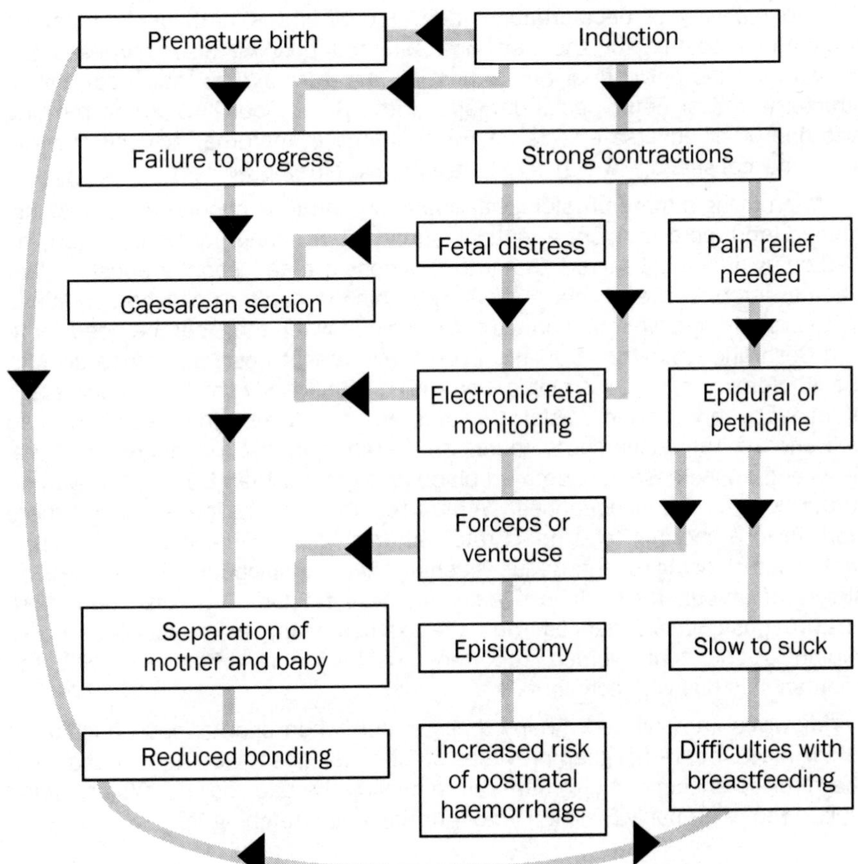

Directed pushing and supine birthing positions

There are basically two ways of managing the second stage of labour: either spontaneous pushing can take place, or it is directed by caregivers. Spontaneous pushing implies that the woman can follow her own physical sensations. This means that her glottis is open (i.e. her mouth) and that she usually makes sounds. She will usually push three to four times and the duration of each pushing period will typically be around four to six seconds. The second method is the well-known Valsalva method (forced pushing), where the caregiver leads and the birthing woman follows instructions. The mother is instructed to hold her breath for 10 seconds and push downwards at the same time.[29] This method is almost always combined with a supine birthing position. Roberts and Hanson reviewed the recent literature[30] and found that the Valsalva method, which is routinely used, has negative effects on both the fetus and mother. Sustained bearing down efforts result in more frequent occurrence of non-reassuring fetal heart rate (FHR) patterns, delayed recovery of FHR decelerations, lower umbilical cord pH and PO_2 levels and subsequent newborn acidaemia and lower Apgar scores. (Worryingly, Yildrim[31] found that the first two consequences (non-reassuring fetal heart rate patterns and delayed recovery of decelerations) persisted after the birth itself, meaning continued problems for the newborn. Directed pushing also increases the pressure on the pelvic floor and almost all literature agrees that it can cause structural and/or neurological damage to the pelvic floor.[30] Directed pushing also has other adverse effects for the mother, i.e. maternal acidosis, fatigue and maternal stress,[30] which is to be avoided in birthing women.

When using a more physiological approach and thus spontaneous pushing, women tend more to adopt a vertical, squatting or sitting position. As early as 1882 Engelmann observed that the positions women spontaneously adopt when giving birth are upright.[32] Women birthing in non-medicalised conditions try to avoid lying down and change their position when they feel the need for it. In a Cochrane review of 2009 the use of any upright position, compared with the lithotomy position, was associated with a significantly shorter second stage of labour, a reduction in episiotomy rates and a reduction in rates of assisted deliveries.[33] The researchers found an increase in second degree perineal tears and an increase in estimated blood loss greater than 500ml, but with no further long-term consequences. Women reported less severe pain and there were fewer abnormal fetal heart rate patterns. Yildirim[31] and Chang[34] found that women doing spontaneous pushing had significantly shorter second stages of labour, they felt less pain and less fatigue. They also had more positive pushing experiences than the women using the Valsalva method. Yildirim found that women reported pushing more effectively with the spontaneous pushing technique.[31]

Midwives can still accompany their women when spontaneous pushing is taking place, but rather than providing strict guidelines for women's behaviour, they provide encouraging words: "You're moving the baby down," "You're doing well," "You're probably feeling a lot of burning and stretching."[35]

Taking all factors into account and the research data, it is therefore advisable to give birthing women the space and freedom they need to find an optimal position and to let them autonomously and thus spontaneously push during the second stage of labour.

Episiotomy

Episiotomy is the most common form of obstetric surgery[36] and there are many indications to suggest its use. Maternal indications for routinely performing an episiotomy are the prevention of perineal tears, more specifically the prevention of anal sphincter laceration and the protection of the pelvic floor.[37] Routine episiotomy is also often used to shorten the second stage of labour so as to prevent maternal exhaustion or fetal distress, and even because the practitioner has financial reasons for carrying out the procedure–i.e. he or she can charge for it. However, the routine use of episiotomy has been questioned. In their Cochrane review published in 2009[38] Carolli and Mignini found that restrictive use of episiotomy was associated with less severe perineal trauma (RR 0.67), less suturing (RR 0.71) and fewer healing complications (RR 0.69), compared to routine use. The restrictive use of episiotomy was, however, associated with more anterior perineal trauma. This was confirmed recently by Räisänen.[39] There were more first- and second-degree perineal injuries as well as injuries to the vagina, labia minora and urethra in births performed without episiotomies among primiparous women, but these lacerations are less severe than the third-degree perineal lacerations which were more common when episiotomy was performed. There was no significant difference in dyspareunia or urinary incontinence in the two groups.[38]

Perineal injuries create a lot of discomfort to women in a period when they have to take care of their new baby. Sheila Kitzinger[40] asked women whether the pain resulting from their perineal repair distracted them when breastfeeding. It seems that 17% of the women with an episiotomy and 21% of the women with an episiotomy *and tear* were troubled by perineal pain while breastfeeding, compared to 9% of women with a perineal tear and 3% of women with no injury to their perineum. The reason women reported less pain with a tear than with an episiotomy is explained by the fact that an episiotomy usually causes more damage than a spontaneous tear. Furthermore, the deepest tears occurring are often exclusively extensions of episiotomies. This makes sense, since everyone knows that when you try to tear a cloth it is markedly resistant until it is cut, after which point it rips... Verena Schmid confirmed this when she studied the physiology of the pelvic floor and especially its dynamics during childbirth.[41] She found that the muscles of the pelvic floor retract one by one when the head of the baby is moving down the birth canal. They form a kind of telescope around the fetal head and while the mother is pushing they perform peristaltic movements so as to move the baby out. When performing an episiotomy, these muscles may well be cut before they are retracted and this creates damage to the innermost pelvic floor muscles, such as the levator ani. Any episiotomy also damages oxytocin receptors and thus reduces the strength of contractions.

Given this research and the physiology of the perineal muscles, it is not surprising that NICE advises restricting the use of episiotomy, since routine use has harmful effects.[42]

Early cord clamping

Clamping and cutting the umbilical cord is a routine procedure, which is often carried out without any concern about its timing. In many hospital settings this procedure is completed seconds after the birth as part of active management of the third stage. However, in the last few years the timing of cord clamping has been increasingly discussed and researched.[43]

In their 2008 Cochrane review[44] McDonald and Middleton included 11 trials of 2,989 mothers and their babies. They found no significant difference in rates of maternal haemorrhage between babies who had experienced early and late cord clamping. Newborns whose cord had been clamped late experienced significant benefits, with higher haemoglobin levels and higher ferritin levels. Levels of ferritin remained high even at six months of age in cases where babies had had the cord clamped late. McDonald and Middleton have reported finding a significant increase in infants needing phototherapy for jaundice (RR 0.59) in the late cord-clamping group in their research.[44] [For an explanation of 'RR', see page 32.] Hutton and Hassan also failed to find any increased risk of developing neonatal jaundice within the first 24-48 hours of life, after analysing the pooled data of eight trials (1,009 children), in the case of late cord clamping.[44] In addition they found no significant differences in the proportion of newborns needing phototherapy. They also found a clinically important reduced risk of anaemia within the late cord clamping group, which is obviously helpful.

When we look at definitions of late cord clamping, most of the research defines this as after two to four minutes, although Odent suggests that such early clamping still constitutes an obstetric intervention.[45] Therefore, it would perhaps be better to speak about late cord-clamping as meaning clamping the umbilical cord after the blood flow has stopped, i.e. when the cord can no longer be observed pulsating. In this way, the baby becomes familiar with the germs and bacteria of his or her mother and thus increases his or her natural resistance; in other words, the baby obtains maximum benefit from the mother's natural immunity. (This is because he or she has to be placed on the mother when clamping is delayed, i.e. the baby cannot be whisked away for various immediate procedures.) Without the disturbance of early clamping mother and baby are also able to bond without interference from caregivers. Not only is this likely to lead to a better start for breastfeeding, it is also likely to facilitate the flow of natural oxytocin (the hormone of love) straight after birth.[45]

For all the reasons outlined, delaying clamping of the umbilical cord in full-term neonates seems to confer benefits on the newborn which also extend into infancy.[43]

Delaying clamping seems to confer benefits

Conclusion and discussion

Research clearly shows that interfering with the normal physiological processes of labour and birth increases risk factors and complications for both mother and baby. This review of the literature has aimed to provide a research-based answer to questions raised about many interventions which are performed routinely during many normal labours and births. While this review cannot claim to be complete, it certainly does lead us to conclude that interventions should only be used cautiously, when benefits clearly outweigh risks. Other interventions, which have not been discussed–such as the restriction of food intake, the routine use of IV drips, or the use of elective caesareans–should prompt further research and reflection... After all, it is important to understand that these routine interventions can have consequences not only for a woman's labour and birth, but also for the mother and baby immediately after birth and/or some time later, even up to adulthood. For example, Jacobson and Bygdeman found that a traumatic birth was associated with a five-fold increase in the likelihood of violent suicide in men and a doubled risk in women in adulthood.[46] Although more research is necessary to explore these possible correlations further, it is clearly important to respect nature and the normal, physiological processes and reserve interventions for those situations where they really are required. If this is not the case, caregivers will do more harm than good when they routinely use these interventions.

On a positive note, attitudes are changing around the world as regards the use of interventions. For example, I visited several midwifery-led birthing units, such as 'La Margherita' in Florence (Italy), 'Het Geboortecentrum' in Amsterdam (The Netherlands), 'Das Geburtshaus' in Vienna (Austria), 'Bolle Buik' in Leuven (Belgium), and 'The Edgware Birth Centre' in London (UK)... In these and numerous other birth centres caregivers are making great efforts to reduce rates of routine interventions.

Following the lead of Sheila Kitzinger several decades ago, the New European Surgical Academy (NESA), founded in 2007 and led by Michael Stark, [47] has launched an anti-episiotomy campaign so as to inform colleagues about the disadvantages of the routine use of episiotomy. The Royal College of Midwives is also running a major UK-wide initiative called the 'Campaign for Normal Birth' which aims to inspire and promote normal birthing practices around Britain. In addition, many conferences have been organised for birth professionals around the world to promote normal birth, such as the *Midwifery Today* conferences (in the USA, in Europe and in other countries around the world) and there have been conferences on the 'humanisation of birth' in South America. Womb Ecology (set up by Michel Odent) also started a new initiative by organising the Mid-Atlantic Conference on Birth and Primal Health Research in Las Palmas (Gran Canaria in 2010), and by planning a follow-up conference (the Mid-Pacific Conference on Birth and Primal Health Research) in Honolulu in 2012.

There are also local initiatives, such as the International Conference on the Art of Midwifery in Castiglioncello (Italy) in 2007 and the courses which teach 'the art of midwifery', all organised by Verena Schmid and colleagues, which take place in Italy (in Florence) and Austria. The courses in evidence-based medicine run by Denis Walsh around the UK are further evidence of initiatives to promote normality in birth.

Both conferences and courses bring together people, they disseminate relevant research, and they inspire and encourage birth professionals who are keen to promote paths towards more natural births. Even women are standing up for their birthing rights and, when searching the Internet, it is possible to find several women's movements that focus on natural birth, such as www.mybirth.com.au (Australia).

Publishers are also helping these women to gain information about research, so that they can more easily refuse interventions which are not medically necessary and gain the confidence to consciously choose a more normal birth.

Finally, using all the resources at their disposal, midwives are informing women during pregnancy about more evidence-based care (as regards interventions), so that women can make informed choices during labour and birth—and this is clearly a very important part of the process.

As health professionals, we certainly have a responsibility to encourage our colleagues and the women we care for in this work. We need to support all these initiatives for normalising birth so as to help create a better world!

Els Hendrix teaches on the midwifery programme at the PHL University College in Belgium. She is particularly interested in researching issues of normal birth and midwifery models. She puts great emphasis on evidence-based midwifery and adjusting midwifery care to the specific needs and values of the individual mother, baby and family. Previously she worked as a midwife in a private practice in the Netherlands and is very familiar with home births. She is married to Pieter and has two boys, Wannes and Toon, whom she had at home and breastfed through toddlerhood. She is now pregnant with their third little one.

References

1 Davis-Floyd R (2001). The technocratic, humanistic, and holistic paradigms of childbirth. *International Journal of Gynecology & Obstetrics, 75,* S5-S23.

2 Hunter LP 2006. Women give birth and pizzas are delivered: language and Western childbirth paradigms. *Journal of Midwifery and Womens Health, 51,* 119-124.

3 Declercq ER, Sakala C, Corry MP, Applebaum S 2006. *Listening to Mothers II: Report of the second national US survey of women's childbearing experiences.* New York: Childbirth Connection. Available at www.childbirthconnection.org/listeningtomothers

4 Dahlen HG, Homer CSE, Leap N, Tracy SK (2010). From social to surgical: Historical perspectives on perineal care during labour and birth. *Women and birth,* in press.

5 Kantor HI, Rember R, Tabio P, Buchaon R 1965. Value of shaving the pudendal-perineal area in delivery preparation. *Obsterics & Gynecology, 25,* 509-512.

6 Kovavisarach E, Jirasettasiri P 2005. Randomised controlled trial of perineal shaving versus hair cutting in parturients on admission in labor. *Journal of the medical association of Thailand, 88,* 1167-1171.

7 Basevi V, Lavender T 2009. Routine perineal shaving on admission in labour. *Cochrane Database of Systematic Reviews, 2.*

8 Lopes MHB, Silva MAS, Christoforo FFM, Andrade DCJ, Bellini NR, Cervi RC 2001. The use of intertestinal cleansers to prepare for labour: analysis of advantages and disadvantages (O uso do enteroclisma no prepare para o parto: análise de suas antagens e desvantagens). *Revista Latino-Americana de Enfermagem, 9*(6), 49-55.

9 Romney ML, Gordon H 1981. Is your enema really necessary? *The British Medical Journal, 282*(6272), 1269-1271.

10 Cuervo LG, Bernal MP, Menoza N 2006. Effects of high volume saline enemas versus no enema during labour—the N-Ma randomised controlled trial. *Biomedcentral Pregnancy and Childbirth, 6* (8).

11 Reveiz L, Gaitán HG, Curevo LG 2010. Enemas during labour. *Cochrane Database of Systematic Reviews, 7.*

12 Chen C-Y, Wang K-G 2006. Are routine interventions necessary in normal birth? *Taiwanese Journal of Obstetrics and Gynecology, 45,* 4, 302-306.

13 Chalmers B, Kaczorowki J, Levitt C, Dzakpasu S, O'Brien B, Lee L, Boscoe M, Young D 2009. Use of routine interventions in vaginal labour and birth: Findings from the Maternity Experiences Survey. *Birth, 36* (1), 12-25.

14 Davis-Floyd R (1992). *Birth as an American rite of passage.* Berkeley, Los Angeles, London: University of California Press.

15 Alfirevic Z, Devane D, Gyte DM 2006. Continuous cardiotocography (CTG) as a form of electronic fetal monitoring (EFM) for fetal assessment during labour. *Cochrane Database of Systematic Review, 19,* 3.

16 World Health Organization 1997. *Care in normal birth: a practical guide.* Geneva: WHO.

17 National Collaborating Centre for Women's and Children's Health, Commissioned by the National Institute for Health and Clinical Excellence (NICE) 2008. Induction of labour–Clinical guideline 2nd edition. London: RCOG Press.

18 Glantz JC 2005. Elective induction versus spontaneous labor: associations and outcomes. *Journal of Reproductive Medicine, 50* (4), 235-240.

19 Tracy SK, Sullivan E, Wang YA, Black D, Tracy M 2007. Birth outcomes associated with interventions in labour amongst low risk women: A population-based study. *Women and Birth, 20,* 41-48.

20 Odent M (1999). *The scientification of love.* London: Free Association Books Limited.

21 Uvnäs-Möberg K (2010). How do ward routines influence behaviour/health of mother, infant and the coming generations? Wombecology, The Mid-Pacific Conference on Birth and Primal Health Research, 26-28 February. Las Palmas: Alfredo Krauss Auditorium.

22 Odent M (2010). In-labour intrauterine life—Drips of synthetic oxytocin. Available at: www.wombecology.com [Accessed 31 October 2010].

23 Jordan S, Emery S, Watkins A, Evans D, Storey M, Morgan C (2009). Associations of drugs routinely given in labour with breastfeeding at 48 hours analysis of the Cardiff Births Survey. British Journal of Obstetrics and Gynecology, 116 (12), 1622-1632.

24 McCarthy FP, Kenny LC (2010). Induction of labour. *Obstetrics, Gynaecology and Reproductive Medicine,* article in press.

25 Mandruzatto, G, Alfirevic Z, Chervenak, F, Gruenebaum, A, Heimstad, R, Heinonen, S, Levene, M, Salvesen, K, Saugstad, O, Skupski, D, Thilaganathan, B (2010). Guidelines for the management of postterm pregnancy. *Journal of Perinatal Medicine, 38,* 111-119.

26 Duff, C, Sinclair, M (2000). Exploring the risks associated with induction of labour: a retrospective study using the NIMATS database. *Journal of Advanced Nursing, 31(2),* 410-417.

27 Heimstad, R, Skogvull, E, Mattson, L-A, Johansen, O L, Eik-Nes, S, Salvesen, K A (2007). Induction of labor or serial antenatal fetal monitoring in postterm pregnancy: a randomized controlled trial. Obstetrics *& Gynecology, 109*(3), 609-617.

28 Davis-Floyd R, Barclay L, Tritten J 2009. *Birth models that work.* Berkely and Los Angeles, California: University of California Press

29 Roberts JE 2003. A new understanding of the second stage of labour: implications for nursing care. *Journal of Obstetric, Gynecologic and Neonatal Nursing 32,* 794–801.

30 Roberts J, Hanson L 2007. Best practices in second stage labor care: maternal bearing down and positioning. Journal of Midwifery & Women's Health, 52 (3), 238-245.

31 Yildirim G, Beji NK 2008. Effects of pushing techniques in birth on mother and fetus: a randomized study. *Birth, 35* (1), 25-30.

32 Engelmann GJ (1882). *Labor among primitive peoples*. St. Louis: JH Chambers.

33 Gupta JK, Hofmeyr GJ, Smyth RMD (2009). Position in the second stage of labour for women without epidural anaesthesia. *Cochrane Database of Systematic Reviews, 4.*

34 Chang S-C, Chou M-M, Lin K-C, Lin L-C, Lin Y-L, Kuo S-C 2010. Effects of a pushing intervention on pain, fatigue and birthing experiences among Taiwanese women during the second stage of labour. *Midwifery,* article in press.

35 Sampselle CM, Miller JM, Luecha Y, Fischer K, Rosten L (2005). Provider support of spontaneous pushing during the second-stage of labor. *Journal of Obstetrical and Gynecological and Neonatal Nursing, 34,* 695–702.

36 Stepp KJ, Siddiqui NY, Emery SP, Barber MD 2006. Textbook recommendations for preventing and treating perineal injury at vaginal delivery. *Obstetrics & Gynecology 107,* 361–365.

37 Cleary-Goldman J, Robinson J 2003. The role of episiotomy in current obstetric practice. *Seminars in Perinatology 27,* 3–12.

38 Carolli G, Mignini L 2009. Episiotomy for vaginal birth. *Cochrane Database of Systematic Reviews, 1.*

39 Räisänen S, Vehviläinen-Julkunen K, Heinonen S 2010. Need for and consequences of episiotomy in vaginal birth: a critical approach. *Midwifery, 26,* 348-356.

40 Kitzinger, S (1981). Some women's experiences of episiotomy. In: National Childbirth Trust, ed. Pamplet NLM #05304054-6. London: National Childbirth Trust.

41 Schmid V (2005). About physiology in pregnancy and childbirth. Florence: Scuola elementale di arte ostetrica.

42 National Collaborating Centre for Women's and Children's Health, Commissioned by the National Institute for Health and Clinical Excellence (NICE) 2007. Intrapartum care: care of healthy women and their babies during childbirth—Clinical guideline. London: RCOG Press.

43 Hutton EK, Hassen ES 2007. Late versus early clamping of the umbilical cord in full-term neonates: Systematic review and meta-analysis of controlled trials. *Journal of American Medical Association, 297* (11), 1241-1252.

44 McDonald SJ, Middleton P 2008. Effect of timing of umbilical cord clamping of term infants on maternal and neonatal outcomes. *Cochrane Database of Systematic Reviews, 3.*

45 Odent M (2010). To cut or not the cut: That's another question? Wombecology, The Mid-Pacific Conference on Birth and Primal Health Research, 26-28 February. Las Palmas: Alfredo Krauss Auditorium.

46 Jacobson B, Bygdeman M (1998). Obstetric care and proneness of off-spring to suicide as adults: case-control study. *British Medical Journal, 317* (7169), 1346-1349.

47 Stark M (2009). Episiotomy—destructive traditions: The anti-episiotomy campaign, in: Proceedings of the 8th Turkish-German Gynecology Congress. TAJEV Turkish-German Gynecological Education and Research Foundation, 45(6)

Epidural analgesia for pain management: the positive and the negative

Michael Klein

Varying attitudes toward epidurals amongst women

In current practice, most women seem to fall into two general categories when they think of labour pain management–initial preference for epidural analgesia versus initial preference for other ways of dealing with the pain of labour. For many women, the issue of how they will be assisted with the pain of labour is the central focus of their upcoming experience. For some, the decision to request epidural analgesia is driven by their previous experiences of pain or by their anticipatory fear of the pain of labour. Women electing home birth know that epidural analgesia will not be available unless a transfer occurs for specific fetal or maternal indications or for pain management

A short history of epidural analgesia

It was not until the 1960s and 1970s that epidural analgesia became widely available. Prior to that, anaesthesia services dedicated to the provision of epidural analgesia were generally unavailable. Anaesthetists had to take care of a wide variety of surgical and emergency services, such that in most hospitals providing a woman with an epidural for labour and birth was a low priority. Furthermore, it was not until the 1990s that obstetric anaesthesia services dedicated to maternity care became common in developed countries.

At first it appeared that the advent of epidurals made the midwife's job easier: when women were quiet and comfortable, obstetricians felt better as well. The woman could then be alone with her partner, and seemingly did not need much attention.

At first it appeared that advent of epidurals made the midwife's job easier: women were quiet and comfortable

During an era when, in many services, there was one-to-one midwifery and epidural analgesia was relatively unavailable, the midwife could use her skills to reassure, massage, breathe with the woman through contractions, and she employed a range of methods to handle labour pain. But today, the shortage of staff and the institutional demands on midwives make these more time-consuming skills difficult to provide. In addition, the education of midwives has taken a more technical turn, and the 'old-fashioned' skills of hands-on midwifery have been replaced, in many educational programs, by teaching technical skills relating to the use of equipment and the increasing number of interventions on offer.

The implications of epidural use

Although it first seemed that epidural analgesia freed up midwives to care for more than one woman at a time, in fact, it soon became clear that the midwife's time was consumed by the technical requirements of safely managing the epidural and the rest of the technical requirements of her job, leaving little time for hands-on midwifery support.[1] A woman who has an epidural requires an intravenous line and continuous electronic fetal monitoring to measure the fetal heartbeat and the contraction pattern. Because labour usually slows after an epidural, usually the woman then requires synthetic oxytocin (syntocinon) augmentation to replace her natural oxytocin production, which is inhibited by the epidural itself. Syntocinon can cause painful contractions, and its use requires detailed charting and monitoring for the potential complications of the epidural itself.

It soon became clear that time was consumed by the technical requirements of safely managing the epidural... leaving little time for hands-on support

In most cases with an epidural, a woman has to remain in bed because she cannot feel her legs and she is attached to many wires and lines, so this limits her ability to walk or change position. 'Walking epidurals' and telemetry are available only in rare settings and by particular anaesthetists. Tethered to intravenous lines and other lines (e.g. a urinary catheter and a blood pressure cuff, the fetal monitor and the contraction transducer) and unable to walk, it is almost impossible for the woman to use gravity and different positions to help her labour.

In most cases a woman has to remain in bed...

It became clear that to make epidural analgesia reliably available, a dedicated anaesthetic staff had to develop. Once such staff were in place, there was great pressure to keep them busy. In some settings anaesthetists were on the labour floor on a regular basis, determining if women needed an epidural. And in some cases the anaesthetic staff were on a salary, so they needed to justify their activity to the business managers of the organisations in which they worked. Therefore, rather than being pain-management consultants, most anaesthetists mainly provided an epidural service following requests either from the medical/nursing staff or from labouring women.

To make epidural analgesia reliably available, a dedicated anaesthetic staff had to develop. Once such staff was in place, there was great pressure to keep them busy.

Early on, after epidurals became more available, a debate ensued, and goes on to this day, about whether withholding an epidural was interfering with a woman's autonomy. This discussion did not seem to take into consideration that women might not select an epidural if they knew more precisely how long severe pain would last, or if they understood the benefits and problems associated with epidural use, or if staff had a variety of other effective techniques to assist with the pain of labour. In fact, many women are directly or indirectly pressured to accept an epidural.

The development of new pain management techniques

Prior to the availability of epidural analgesia, the childbirth education movement used a variety of techniques that were physiologically helpful to reduce pain, such as breathing and imaging. These methods began to take hold in the culture in the 1950s and 1960s but today are less prominent in childbirth education classes. Some classes are more focused on teaching women compliance with particular hospital technological methods and approaches, routines and policies, rather than on teaching women coping skills.

In the late 1970s and early 1980s, the first studies appeared, showing the value of continuous emotional and physical support by a caring, trained and knowledgeable woman, whose responsibility was to focus solely on the woman rather than on the institution or equipment—the *doula*. Backed by randomised studies,[2-4] it has become apparent that this emotional and physical continuous support from a doula gives women more confidence and ability to work with their labour. All studies to date have demonstrated that hospital-based midwives cannot function as doulas,[5,6] even if they are direct-entry midwives. It is not the fact of being either a midwife that matters, but the fact that when she (or he) is *employed* by the hospital, the midwife's primary allegiance is to the institution and she is *professionally* responsible for the conduct of the labour and the safety of both mother and fetus. A doula who is employed by the woman is responsible only to her. Autonomous midwives (e.g. in Canada) are strongly supportive of doulas, with whom they frequently work in collaboration.

Pain moderation by transcutaneous nerve stimulation (TENS) or intradermal water injections can be very helpful, especially in the earlier stages of labour. Other non-pharmacological methods like baths or showers or birthing balls are also helpful for many women who find that partial pain relief is sufficient to help them through contractions. Doula care provides another or complementary approach which can reduce the need for an epidural or delay epidural usage until the active phase of labour, when some of the negative effects of epidural analgesia are reduced. In particular, during her labour, it allows the mother more opportunity to produce oxytocin naturally (production being orchestrated by her own brain). Natural oxytocin has some important effects: it is the anti-stress hormone, and helps contractions to be more productive; it is also the 'love hormone' that enhances bonding, an effect suppressed by synthetic oxytocin, little of which enters the brain of either mother or fetus.

Is epidural analgesia the best form of pain relief?

Epidural analgesia is a very effective form of pain relief. If there were no problems associated with epidural analgesia, almost everybody would want it.

Epidural analgesia is a very effective form of pain relief, meaning that compared to a variety of other pharmacological and non-pharmacological methods, it provides generally consistent pain reduction. If there were no problems associated with epidural analgesia, almost everybody would want it. Unfortunately, though, associated with its use there are various unwanted side effects, including:

- longer first stage labours
- longer second stage labours
- increased incidence of maternal fever directly caused by the epidural, which often leads to the use of antibiotics in both the labouring woman and her newborn
- increased rates of operative vaginal delivery (forceps and ventouse)
- increased perineal trauma with and without instrumental births—including severe tears into the rectum (third degree tears).
- a variety of complications such as a placement of an epidural too high on the spine (leading to breathing problems).
- failure of the epidural to provide any pain relief, or insufficient pain relief—requiring the continued use of other methods of pain relief
- increased need for a bladder catheter
- maternal hypotension leading to worrying fetal heart rate changes
- an increase in the likelihood of the need for a caesarean section—this last complication being the subject of great debate, which will be discussed further

Of course, some of these problems may occur whether the epidural was or was not truly needed. And when an epidural is truly needed for pain relief or to solve a specific problem, it can dramatically change a situation for the better and can *improve* outcome. It is only when epidurals are used routinely, and especially very early in labour that these complications are very much more likely to occur.

Unfortunately, various unwanted side-effects are associated with the use of epidurals

Research into the consequences of epidural use

Whether the benefits outweigh the potential risks has been the subject of many controversies over recent decades. In my department we have studied these controversies extensively. On a regular basis we looked at our own performance in caring for labouring women. The Department of Family Practice at British Columbia Women's Hospital in Canada (familiarly known as 'BC Women's') is made up of over 100 family doctors, who all attend births. BC Women's is the largest maternity hospital in Canada, with more than 7,000 births per year, and family doctors are responsible for almost half of these births, despite the hospital also being the tertiary care referral centre for the province. This makes us the largest group of family doctors attending births in Canada.

We knew from the literature that epidural analgesia use early in labour, before the fetus was well down in the pelvis, could cause malpositions (occiput posterior or transverse)[7] due to extension of the fetal head. If the fetal head is extended, it cannot rotate or descend. We found that obstetricians who were frequent and early epidural users in our department had more clients with malpositions.[8] They also had more clients who required more synthetic oxytocin stimulation or augmentation of labour. They had fewer spontaneous births and more caesarean sections than those in the department who used epidurals less often. Also, surprisingly, high epidural users had more newborns with low 5-minute Apgar scores and more babies admitted to the newborn intensive care unit.

We found that obstetricians with mean epidural use rates under 40% for women having their first baby, had caesarean section rates of about 10%. In contrast, those family doctors with mean epidural usage rates of 71-100% had caesarean section rates of 23.4%, the others having rates between the two extremes. The women cared for by the three groups were similar. Thus it appeared that only obstetrician practice difference could have accounted for such large differences in outcome. Interestingly, the caesarean rates of women who were having their second or more births were unaffected by the way in which their obstetricians used epidurals.

Our departmental experience was similar to results from an observational study in which we compared outcomes at a nearby community hospital with our tertiary care centre.[9] In the community care setting, mean epidural analgesia rates were 15.4% compared with 67.2% in the tertiary care centre, for comparable women. The odds of having a caesarean section was 3.4 times greater at the tertiary care centre than in the community hospital. The increased and earlier use of epidural analgesia in the tertiary care setting almost completely explained this difference. The community hospital also gave epidurals later, when they used them, than the tertiary care setting. We were also interested to note that those obstetricians who used epidurals less often, actually spent *more* time with their clients, even though on average their clients spent *less* time in hospital. The time they spent with their clients involved more intimate, hands-on, supportive care.

It is because of these studies that we had trouble accepting the results of the 2004 Cochrane meta-analysis that concluded that epidural analgesia did not raise the caesarean section rate.[10] This conclusion was the same in the most recent Cochrane meta-analysis,[11] this new one deeply flawed by the inclusion of many studies of women who suffered from complex medical conditions, and many studies that randomised women late, particularly since conventional practice is to use epidurals earlier. Clearly, any meta-analysis is only as good as the individual studies included in the meta-analysis—illustrating the well-known principle: rubbish in, rubbish out.

In fact, it appeared to us that the increasing use of epidural analgesia was *transforming birth*. This observation was confirmed by a report from the Canadian Institute for Hospital Information, which indicated that 4 in 5 Canadian women received one or more major obstetric interventions, with epidurals high on the list at rates of 40-50% of births in various Canadian settings.[12]

We then decided to look more closely at the earlier Cochrane's[10] individual studies that made up the meta-analysis addressing the effect of epidural analgesia. These studies revealed that, epidural analgesia increased the length of the first stage of labour by 4.3 hours. Similarly, the second stage of labour was increase by 1.4 hours. Malpositions were found in 15% of cases where epidurals were used but in only 7% of cases where narcotics were used. Synthetic oxytocin augmentation of labour was found in 52% of women with epidurals and in 7% of women who had narcotic analgesia. Instrumentation (forceps and ventouse) was found in 27% of epidural cases compared with a rate of 16% among women not getting an epidural. Maternal fever was dramatically higher in the epidural versus narcotic groups, i.e. 24% vs 6%. (Fever is increased because epidural analgesia interferes with the normal methods that the body uses to eliminate heat. And since it is hard to know if the fever is due to infection or simply an epidural effect of little consequence, a full infection evaluation is usually carried out for the mother and often a caesarean section is performed due to concerns for fetal well-being. These concerns are usually unfounded, but it is hard to know if infection is present or not. And because the mother was evaluated for infection, regardless of what might be found, the newborn will often be exposed to a full infection study and will often receive antibiotics.) In other studies, perineal trauma increased two-fold in women who had had an epidural, due in part to an increased use of forceps and ventouse, which are associated with more perineal trauma, with or without epidurals.[13,14]

Given all the other increases in intervention rates, we found it hard to understand why caesarean section rates were not also higher in the Cochrane meta-analysis. In fact, when we separated out the studies that made up the 2004 Cochrane meta-analysis, we found that, in those studies that showed no difference in caesarean section rates, epidurals had been administered *after* labour was well established (in the active phase at 4-5cm or more of cervical dilation). In the studies where epidurals were given early on in labour, before the active phase or before 4-5cm of cervical dilation—the caesarean section rate increased *more than 2.5 times*.[15, 16]

Inadvertently, the Cochrane meta-analysis of epidural analgesia has caused more frequent use of epidural analgesia, and thence more continuous electronic fetal monitoring, keeping women in bed [usually with an intravenous line] and this has led to more instrumentation, perineal trauma, and an increase in the caesarean section rate. Because more women will have received a caesarean section, another consequence will be an increase in problems in the next pregnancies relating to placentation issues (previa, accrete, percreta, abruption), infertility, and ectopic pregnancy.[17-20] In most maternity care settings, these downstream consequences ('collateral damage') from epidural use are not discussed.

Dealing with the reality of the labour ward

For some women it will not be possible to delay epidural analgesia until 4-5cm, until the active phase of labour. The particular circumstances of a particular woman's particular labour pattern, pain severity, and her pain tolerance, may make it necessary for her to receive an early epidural. But for her, *if she really needs it*, the paradox is that an epidural may help to normalise her labour and improve her birth process and experience, and lead to *less* use of other interventions. But if a woman or her provider merely decide to use an early epidural without trying other less invasive approaches first, the woman may be exposed to a range of other interventions that may culminate in various negative outcomes and a caesarean section (which could cause further problems, either immediately or later on).

Given this paradox and the severity of some of the side-effects of epidural analgesia, it is time to be honest about the full effects of this excellent technology. Actually there is no such thing as a side-effect. There are only effects, some of which we like and some of which we don't. When epidurals are used specifically to problem-solve, the risks of complications and other interventions are in fact reduced. When used routinely and mindlessly, epidural analgesia increases problems and adverse outcomes. Women need to be fully informed of this before agreeing to an epidural. Today women are usually only informed of the *direct* consequences of epidural analgesia, such as a headache or even very *rare* neurological complications, but they are *rarely* told *common* side-effects or the problems that can occur if epidurals are given too early. They are rarely told how an epidural can interfere with the woman's labour and lead to a cascade of unnecessary interventions, and they are rarely informed about how the midwifery care that an epidural requires for the sake of safety, will divert midwives from hands-on attention to the labouring woman towards technological and mechanical concerns.

In conclusion, epidural analgesia is clearly a very valuable form of pain relief but it can also have less desirable consequences. Women need to know the full picture of all procedures and approaches that they can use to help them with their pain and with their labour and birth. No matter how well intended, epidural analgesia increases the likelihood that women will have a variety of other interventions, especially if the epidural is given without specific medical indication (e.g. to lower dangerously high blood pressure or to help a woman exhausted from a long prodromal labour, i.e. latent phase), and even if it is administered for good pain relief reasons. Women need to know that when epidural analgesia is given before the active phase of labour, it more than doubles the probability of a caesarean section.

The importance of timing and setting

Women also need to be reassured that when epidural analgesia is given in the active phase of labour, it *does not* increase the caesarean section rate. This may motivate women to use other pain relief modalities and methods to help them, if possible, to get to the active phase before requesting an epidural.

Readers of the literature also need to remember the importance of setting when reading about the research on epidural analgesia and any other interventions. All the statistics and outcomes that have been here discussed are in fact specific to the setting or environment from which the individual study or meta-analysis emanate. It is important to remember that adverse effects of epidural analgesia can be mitigated, especially if the setting generally limits the use of interventions. It appears, for example that in settings with low caesarean section rates (below 10%), even early epidurals *do not increase* the caesarean section rate,[21] but in more typical settings where caesarean section rates are higher than 20%, it does. This is a general principle. For all studies, randomised or not, the reader needs to ask the question: do the caregivers in the studies practise the way that I do? If they do, the study may apply but if not, they may not.

The bottom line is that epidural analgesia has completely transformed birth. This massive change in the way that many women receive care in labour and birth has been based on a technique that, when used selectively and as a second line approach, provides an important and valuable tool among the many other ways to assist women with labour and birth. However, when used routinely as a first line agent, epidural analgesia can create problems that could have been avoided. Most Canadian younger obstetricians[22] and women approaching their first birth[24] do not even know that epidural analgesia interferes with labour. The older generation of obstetricians knows that it does. They have experienced the changes described above during their many years in practice before and after the common use of epidural analgesia. It is time we told the truth about epidural analgesia—to colleagues and women—and engaged in a truly informed decision-making discussion with women about its optimal use.

Michael Klein is a pediatrician/neonatologist and family physician who has been researching optimal birth issues for 30 years. He is best known for his North American randomised controlled trial, which shows that routine episiotomy causes the very trauma that it was supposed to prevent. His current Canadian National research is about the attitudes and beliefs of all maternity providers and women and how non-evidence-based attitudes interfere with informed consent. He is also the founder and Listmaster of the multidisciplinary MCDG (Maternity Care Discussion Group).

References

1 McNiven P, Hodnett E, O'Brien-Pallas LL. Supporting women in labour: a work sampling study of the activities of labour and delivery nurses. Birth 1992;19(1):3-8; discussion 8-9.

2 Kennell J, Klaus M, McGrath S, Robertson S, Hinkley C. Continuous emotional support during labour in a US hospital. A randomized controlled trial. Journal of the American Medical Association.1991;265(17):2197-201.

3 Sosa R, Kennell J, Klaus M, Robertson S, Urrutia J. The effect of a supportive companion on perinatal problems, length of labor, and mother-infant interaction. New England Journal of Medicine 1980;303(11):597-600.

4 McGrath SK, Kennell JH. A randomized controlled trial of continuous labor support for middle-class couples: effect on cesarean delivery rates. Birth 2008;35(2):92-7.

5 Gagnon AJ, Waghorn K, Covell C. A randomized trial of one-to-one nurse support of women in labor. Birth 1997;24(2):71-7.

6 Hodnett ED, Lowe NK, Hannah ME, Willan AR, Stevens B, Weston JA, et al. Effectiveness of nurses as providers of birth labor support in North American hospitals: a randomized controlled trial. Journal of the American Medical Association. 2002;288(11):1373-81.

7 Hoult I, MacLennan A, Carrie L. Lumbar epidural analgesia in labour: relation to fetal malposition and instrumental delivery. British Medical Journal. 1977;1:14-16.

8 Klein MC, Grzybowski S, Harris S, Liston R, Spence A, Le G, et al. Epidural analgesia use as a marker for physician approach to birth: implications for maternal and newborn outcomes. Birth 2001;28(4):243-8.

9 Janssen PA, Klein MC, Soolsma JH. Differences in institutional cesarean delivery rates-the role of pain management. Journal of Family Practice 2001;50(3):217-23.

10 Howell C. Epidural versus non-epidural analgesia for pain relief in labour. In: The Cochrane Library, Copyright 2004, The Cochrane Collaboration; 2004.

11 Anim-Somuah M, Smyth R, Howell C. Epidural versus non-epidural or no analgesia in labour [Systematic Review]: Cochrane Database of Systematic Reviews 2005; (4); 2005.

12 CIHI. Giving Birth in Canada: Providers of Maternity and Infant Care. Ottawa: Canadian Institute for Health Information (CIHI); 2004 2004.

13 Carroll TG, Engelken M, Mosier MC, Nazir N. Epidural analgesia and severe perineal laceration in a community-based obstetric practice. Journal of the American Board of Family Practice 2003;16(1):1-6.

14 Lieberman E, O'Donoghue C. Unintended effects of epidural analgesia during labor: a systematic review.[see comment]. American Journal of Obstetrics & Gynecology 2002;186(5 Suppl Nature):S31-68.

15 Klein MC. Epidural analgesia: does it or doesn't it? Birth 2006;33(1):74-6.

16 Klein MC. Does epidural analgesia increase the rate of cesarean section? Canadian Family Physician.2006;52:419-421.

17 Hemminki E, Merilainen J. Long-term effects of cesarean sections: ectopic pregnancies and placental problems. American Journal of Obstetrics & Gynecology. 1996;174(5):1569-74.

18 Getahun D, Oyelese Y, Salihu HM, Ananth CVP. Previous Cesarean Delivery and Risks of Placenta Previa and Placental Abruption. Obstetrics & Gynecology 2006.

19 Gilliam M, Rosenberg D, Davis F. The likelihood of placenta previa with greater number of cesarean deliveries and higher parity. Obstetrics & Gynecology 2002;99 (6):976.

20 Miller DA, Chollet JA, Goodwin TM. Clinical risk factors for placenta previa-placenta accreta. American Journal of Obstetrics & Gynecology. 1997;177(1):210-4.

21 Ohel G, Gonen R, Vaida S, Barak S, Gaitini L. Early versus late initiation of epidural analgesia in labor: Does it increase the risk of cesarean section? A randomized trial. American Journal of Obstetrics and Gynecology 2006;194(3):600.

22 Klein MC, Kaczorowski J, Hall W, Fraser W, Liston R, Eftekhary S, Brant R, Mâsse LC, Rosinski J, Mehrabadi A, Baradaran N, Tomkinson J, Dore S, McNiven P, Saxell L, Lindstrom K, Grant J, Chamberlaine A. The attitudes of Canadian maternity care practitioners towards labour and birth: many differences but important similarities. Journal Obstetrics & Gynaecology Canada. 2009;31(9):827-840.

23 Klein MC, Liston R, Fraser WD, Baradaran N, Hearps SJC, Tomkinson J, Kaczorowski J, Brant R. The attitudes of the new generation of Canadian obstetricians: how do they differ from their predecessors? Birth (in press June 2011)

24 Klein MC, Kaczorowsk J, Hearps SJC, Tomkinson J, Baradaran N, Hall W, McNiven P, Brant R, Grant J, Dore S, Fraser WD. What are the attitudes of Canadian women approaching their first birth towards birth technology and their roles in birth? Journal Obstetrics & Gynecology Canada. (In press 2011).

Physiological care in the third and fourth stages of labour... When is it safe?

Kathleen Fahy and Carolyn Hastie

Our interest in pursuing this topic peaked when we saw the excellent outcomes women were experiencing at the stand-alone, midwife-led birthing Belmont Birthing Services which Carolyn developed and led. The Belmont Birthing Services (BBS) are part of the same health service and has seamless referral to the John Hunter Hospital (JHH) (a tertiary referral service located 20 minutes away). As we have described previously[1] we were aware that undisturbed labour and birth facilitates the release of a woman's reproductive hormones in an exquisite cascade that optimises birth physiology and healthy psychological functioning for both mother and baby. At the BBS the majority of women choose to give birth naturally and decline unnecessary medication including a prophylactic synthetic oxytocic (syntometrine or ergometrine) in the third stage of labour; the postpartum haemorrhage (PPH) rate at BBS was 3%. By contrast, at the nearby maternity unit, the JHH which is part of the same health service, the PPH rate at the time was 20%. We wondered if the differences in PPH rates would be explained by the differences in risk status of the women at the two different maternity units or if the lack of interference in labour and birth at the birth centre was a better explanation.

Within the standard maternity care environment physiological third stage labour care is automatically assumed to be unsafe because most caregivers believe women whose third stage is not actively managed are more likely to experience PPH. Research in support of the active management of third stage labour is believed to be so strong that no room for doubt or debate exists.[2] We disagree and we have good, strong, evidence-informed reasons to support our claim.

In this chapter we will demonstrate that for women at low risk of PPH who birth healthy babies within peaceful environments with skilled maternity caregivers in attendance, PPH rates are lower than in a matched group of low risk women who have obstetrically managed labour with active management of the third stage. This chapter draws on and summarises three of our previous publications. (The most important one to read is 'Optimising psychophysiology in the third stage of labour' if you would like to follow up on what we summarise here[1] because it provides details about reproductive physiology and a detailed theoretical account of how to optimise third stage outcomes.) We shall begin by defining key terms relevant to third stage care in Table 1 (opposite). Some key statistical terms are defined in Table 2 and these will enable a novice to interpret the statistics associated with the research that is described and critiqued in this chapter. The research related to the safety of active versus physiological third stage of labour care is then described and critiqued. As part of our critique we present an evidence-informed midwifery practice guideline which will assist you to a) identify when a woman is a good candidate for physiological care, and b) provide the essential elements of the Midwifery Guardianship Model of third stage care.

Table 1:
Definition of key terms related to third and fourth stages of labour

KEY TERMS	DEFINITIONS
third stage of labour	the period from the birth of the baby until the birth of the placenta—note that 'placenta' in our definition includes the membranes
fourth stage of labour	the period from the birth of the placenta until the baby is one hour old; the concept of the fourth stage labour is critical to maintaining the woman and baby in a state of optimal psychophysiological functioning and reducing PPH rates
psychophysiology	the branches of psychology and biological sciences that study mind-body interactions and effect; *reproductive* psychophysiology concerns the ways in which thinking and feeling affect the physiological processes associated with sexual response, pregnancy, labour, birth, breastfeeding and nurturing[3,4]
physiological third stage labour (also referred to as the Midwifery Guardianship Model)	the healthy woman and baby have uninterrupted skin-to-skin contact with unrestricted access to the woman's breast in quite a warm environment; the uterus contracts spontaneously and, with the woman in an upright position, the placenta is birthed by maternal effort alone—note that more detail is provided in the text
postpartum haemorrhage	until fairly recently blood loss up to 599ml in the first 24 hours after birth was considered to be within the normal range[5-7]; the current WHO definition is that a PPH is any amount of blood loss greater than 499ml in the first 24 hours after birth[8]
active management of the third stage of labour	using an artificial oxytocic combined with controlled cord traction and supra pubic guarding so that the birth attendant delivers the placenta in the shortest possible time

The research

In order to make the claim that postpartum haemorrhage rates are lower for women who have physiological third stage care it is essential to first review the existing scientific literature to see if it is valid and applicable to this specific group of women who are at low risk of PPH. To that end, we conducted a systematic search of randomised trials conducted within the last 20 years on the effectiveness of third stage labour care where a synthetic oxytocic injection was compared with expectant or physiological care. Studies which were included in our review used syntocinon, syntometrine or ergometrine in the 'active management arm' and compared that with 'expectant' or 'physiological management' in the other arm. Studies involving misoprostol (a synthetic prostaglandin used to manage third stage and/or PPH in some settings) were excluded. Four randomised trials of the effectiveness of third stage of labour care were retrieved.[9-12] The Cochrane review of active management versus expectant management of the third stage of labour, which was based on these four trials, was also considered.[13] No new trials were found.

If one were to read only the abstract of the Cochrane review it would seem completely true that active management reduces the risk of PPH, but...

In brief, the Cochrane meta-analysis reported on the combined health outcomes for 6,284 women who were randomly assigned to receive either active or expectant management in the third stage of labour. The major finding was that active management of the third stage of labour was associated with a lower PPH rate of 5.2% compared to 13.5% for expectant management; (relative risk 0.38, 95% confidence interval 0.32-0.46).[13] The meanings of the words 'relative risk' (RR) and 'confidence intervals' (CI) are discussed opposite. If one were to read only the abstract of this Cochrane Review then it would seem completely 'true' that active management of the third stage of labour reduces PPH and by extension, one would believe that active management saves women's lives.

Critique of the Cochrane review of third stage management

An extensive critique of the Cochrane review of active versus expectant management of the third stage of labour has been published.[15] A summary of some of the most important critiques is provided here. Firstly, in all four trials underpinning the Cochrane review, randomisation of subjects occurred early, i.e. before their risk status for PPH could be known. This early randomisation was is in spite of the claim in their research protocols that only women who are at low risk of PPH would be enrolled and therefore able to be randomised to receive 'expectant management'. As the table overleaf shows, many of the risk factors develop later on in pregnancy or during labour and birth.

Physiological third stage care is most beneficial to women when their pregnancies, labours and births have been normal

In the studies under consideration, the percentage of subjects who were actually at high risk of PPH varied between 15-76% of all subjects.[9-12] In another paper[1] we argue that physiological third stage care is most beneficial to women when their pregnancies, labours and births have been normal because if anything upsets the delicate balance of reproductive hormones, there is an increased risk of serious haemorrhage, as Table 3 attests. Thus, generalising findings from these trials[9-12] to a population of women who are at low risk of PPH, (such as women who have been accepted for birth at home or at a birth centre) is not valid.

Another important critique of the Cochrane review is that they used the terms 'physiological management' and 'expectant management' synonymously when they are not, in fact, synonymous. The Cochrane review had a minimal definition of the concept of 'expectant management in the third stage of labour' i.e.

- a 'hands off' policy
- signs of separation are awaited
- the placenta is allowed to delivery spontaneously[11,13]

This definition is not accepted by midwives because the 'expectant management' definition leaves out so much that is important to protecting the woman from PPH during the third stage of labour.[1,17,18] This definition needs to be considered in contrast to the theory which describes and explains how to optimise physiological third stage labour so as to minimise PPH.[1]

The Midwifery Guardianship Model of care: a clinical practice guideline

This model depends upon the midwife and the woman adopting a psychophysiological approach to third stage of labour care which we term 'holistic psychophysiological care in the third stage of labour'. The concept of 'holistic psychophysiological care' is much more sophisticated and physiologically sound than the definition of 'expectant management' used by the Cochrane review (above). The essential element of the concept 'holistic psychophysiological care in the third stage of labour' can be summarised to provide a clinical practice guideline for Midwifery Guardianship in the third stage of labour as follows...

If anything upsets the delicate balance of reproductive hormones, there is an increased risk of haemorrhage

Table 2:

What is the meaning of Relative Risk and Confidence Intervals?

These two statistics are used to provide evidence about whether an outcome of interest (e.g. PPH) is significantly different between two groups (cohorts) of subjects who have had two different treatments; usually a new treatment is compared with standard care. In the case of the Cochrane review the two treatments in the third stage of labour were 'active management' versus their definition of 'physiological management'.

- **Relative risk (RR)** reports on whether one treatment decreases the risk of the outcome of interest occurring (e.g. does the treatment 'active management' decrease the risk of PPH when compared with the treatment 'physiological management'). If there is no difference in outcomes between the two groups then the RR would be 1:1 (i.e. the same). In the Cochrane review, the RR was 0.38, which means that the risk of PPH for a woman in the actively managed group was 0.38/1. Expressed differently, we can say that for every 100 women who had a PPH in the physiologically managed group, only 38 women in the actively managed group had a PPH.
- In order to know whether the RR is statistically significant we need a number that will tell us (so that we can be 95% confident) that this finding did not occur by chance and is therefore likely to be true. **Confidence interval (CI)** functions like a 'p' value. In other words, the absence of the number 1 within the confidence interval range means that we are 95% confident that this finding did not occur by chance. If the number 1 was included in the confidence interval then it would include the possibility that the risk ratio was really the same i.e. 1:1. However, in the Cochrane review the difference in outcomes between the two groups showed a relative risk of 0.38, and a 95% confidence interval of 0.32-0.46 (NB for this CI, the interval between 0.32 and 0.46 does not include the number 1) and therefore (assuming the research was scientifically valid) we can be confident that there is a real risk of experiencing higher rates of the outcome of interest: in this case PPH for the women who were enrolled in the 'physiological management' group.[14] [Note that the scientific quality of the original trials is criticised in this chapter.]
- You will also come across the term; **odds ratio (OR)**. The OR is the ratio of the odds of an event occurring in one group compared to another. It is similar to RR in that it measures the same thing; it is just a different statistical test.

Table 3: Obstetric risk factors for PPH

- previous history of primary PPH
- abnormal uterine anatomy: e.g. fibroids, uterine septum, previous uterine surgery including caesarean
- over-distended uterus: e.g. due to multiple gestation, carrying a big baby or polyhydramnios.
- parity of six or greater
- abnormalities of the placenta: e.g. low lying placenta (placenta praevia)
- antepartum haemorrhage
- haemoglobin (Hb) of less than 110gm per litre
- abnormalities of coagulation: e.g. due to fetal death in utero, hypertension, clotting diseases, anti-coagulant therapy, antepartum haemorrhage, general infections
- obstetric or anaesthetic interventions: e.g. induction, augmentation, epidurals, forceps, ventouse, shoulder dystocia, episiotomy or tear requiring suturing
- intrapartum haemorrhage
- uterine muscle exhaustion: e.g. due to induction, augmentation, labour longer than 15 hours, or maternal exhaustion
- intra amniotic infection: as indicted by pyrexia and/or prolonged ruptured membranes (<24 hrs)
- drug-induced uterine hypotonia: e.g. magnesium sulphate, nifedipine and salbutamol[16]

The context

- The environmental conditions need to be 'right 'in order for the woman's physiology to function optimally, usually warm, comfortable, dimly lit and private, with no strangers present.
- There are no distractions, e.g. phone calls or texting, or talking between caregivers within the room
- The woman needs to feel safe, secure, cared about and confident that her privacy will be maintained.[1]
- The woman is well hydrated, well nourished and has a relatively empty bladder.
- The attending midwife must be knowledgeable and feel confident working with normal reproductive psychophysiology.
- The woman and support people know in advance that labour is continuing until the placenta is born and the uterus is firmly contracted.
- The woman's chest is easily accessible to the baby immediately at birth.

The procedure

- Ensure immediate and sustained skin-to-skin contact between the woman and baby.
- Keep the cord intact throughout. (It can be clamped and cut as soon as it has stopped pulsing, or later if the woman prefers.)
- Keep the woman and baby warm.
- Support and/or encourage the woman to focus on her baby.
- Assist the woman to an upright or semi-upright position.
- Ensure that all interactions in the room remain focused on mother and baby.
- Observe that there is 'self-attachment' breastfeeding (i.e. that the newborn is facilitated to latch on spontaneously).
- Unobtrusively observe for signs of separation of the placenta.
- Keep hands off the fundus, do not meddle at all and do not carry out any massage.
- Ensure that the placenta is birthed entirely by maternal effort and gravity.
- As long as there is no excessive blood loss, impose no arbitrary time limits.
- After 30 minutes, if the placenta has not birthed, encourage the woman to sit on the toilet (lined with a bin liner) as the placenta is probably in the vagina and just needs a push from the woman; this is also a good time to encourage the woman to pass urine so as to keep the bladder empty.
- After the birth of the placenta frequently check the fundus to ensure that it is firm and central. (In some cases, before the birth you or another caregiver may have decided to teach the woman how to do this herself.)
- Observe blood loss and monitor blood pressure and pulse rate directly after the birth, then after 30 minutes, then after another 30 minutes, unless otherwise indicated.
- Only massage the fundus if it is not firm and contracted.

If any part of this 'package of care' is missing or discordant then holistic 'psychophysiological care' has not been provided and active management of labour is advisable.[1] None of the trials underpinning the Cochrane review defined or controlled the 'expectant management' strategy in the manner we have described as the psychophysiological approach. None of the trials reported on any quality assurance undertaken to ensure that the care was delivered as planned.[13] None of the trials paid attention to environmental conditions and, with the exception of the Hinchinbrook trial,[12] the midwives who provided 'physiological care' had no, or little, training or experience in providing any version of physiological third stage care. This comparison of 'expectant management' and 'holistic psychophysiological care' shows that 'holistic psychophysiological care' was not tested by the Cochrane review or the randomised trials it reviewed.

The Cochrane review[13] has now been withdrawn, but from our perspective its influence is undiminished. Kathleen was so convinced of the invalidity of this Cochrane review that she led a research team to compare active and physiological care, including in the study only women at low risk of PPH.

A cohort study of women at low risk of PPH in two settings

Two maternity units, which were part of the same area health service, both with excellent consultation and referral relationships, contributed data to this study (n = 3,495). The tertiary maternity unit at John Hunter Hospital contributed data on 3,075 low risk women. This unit is a major obstetric and neonatal referral centre for the state with about 4,000 babies being born there annually. The tertiary unit contains a birth centre, which at the time of this study, was mostly staffed by midwives working shifts and overseen by the medical staff on duty in the delivery suite. Active management of the third stage of labour is the policy and routine practice at the tertiary maternity unit, including the birth centre. According to the policy, an intramuscular injection (IMI) of 10 units of syntocinon is given within one minute of the birth of the baby, the umbilical cord is clamped and cut immediately, and then controlled cord traction and supra pubic guarding is used until the placenta emerges. Fundal massage is given immediately after the placenta is born.

The midwifery-led unit, Belmont Birthing Services (BBS), was the comparison for the cohort study and provided data on 361 low risk women. BBS is located about 20 minutes by road from the tertiary unit within a community hospital where there is no obstetric, anaesthetic or paediatric medical officers. This unit is reserved for women who are deemed to be 'low risk' and therefore able to give birth away from immediate medical services. Approximately 300 babies are born there annually. All the midwives at BBS at the time of the study were experienced and have been credentialled in Advanced Life Support for women and babies and their training included neonatal intubation, intravenous cannulation and the administration of drugs using an agreed protocol. At BBS each midwife works in a modified caseload model of care and is the primary midwife for 40 women a year and the second midwife for another 40 women. Women who choose to birth at this unit do so because they want a natural birth, they want to know their midwife, they like the philosophy of the unit and they want to give birth in an uninterrupted way. The women usually give informed refusal to all drugs in labour, including the third stage. The midwives at the midwifery-led unit have been taught and practise holistic psychophysiological care as described above and elsewhere.[1]

Data was drawn from a computer-based 'Midwives Data Set' which forms the basis of all New South Wales maternity service outcome reports to Departments of Health.

Three analyses were conducted using SPSS [software for statistical analysis]. The first involved working with the whole data set to exclude women who were at known risk of PPH because the differences in PPH rates between the two units might be explained by the higher risk status at the tertiary unit. The Australian

College of Midwives' National Guidelines for Consultation and Referral[13] were used to assist two midwife-researchers to make individual decisions about factors that might pose a risk for PPH such as 'surgery this pregnancy' based on the type of surgery performed. The second and third analyses were conducted on the data for women who were at low risk of PPH. The second analysis was based on the planned form of treatment (i.e. 'intention-to-treat') at each unit. 'Active management' was the intention at the tertiary referral unit and 'holistic psychophysiological care' was the intention at the midwifery-led unit. The third analysis was based on 'treatment received', depending on whether 'active management' or 'holistic psychophysiological care' was provided during third stage of labour; regardless of site. We present the association between the interventions used to manage the third stage of labour as odds ratios with 95% confidence intervals.

Results

The total number of women who gave birth during the study period was 9,744. This number was comprised of 431 women at the midwifery-led unit and 9,313 women at the tertiary maternity unit. The crude PPH rate for the tertiary unit was 20% and for the midwifery-led unit it was 3%. We excluded 6,240 out of the 9,313 women (67.0%) at the tertiary unit and 70 out of the 431 women (16.2%) at the midwifery-led unit due to possible increased risk of PPH. The intention-to-treat analysis is presented in Table 4 and a PPH rate of 11.2% is shown for active management of the third stage of labour at the tertiary unit, compared with 2.8% for holistic, psychophysiological care at the midwife-led unit, where OR = 4.4, 95% CI [2.3, 8.4].

Table 4: Postpartum blood loss by intention-to-treat: low risk women

Treatment groups and numbers		**Postpartum blood loss**				
		<500 ml	^{3}500 <1000 ml	^{3}1000 £1500 ml	> 1500 ml	Total PPH
Psycho-physiological; midwifery-led group n = 361	Count	351	7	2	1	10
	% within groups	97.2%	1.9%	.6%	.3%	**2.8%**
Active; tertiary hospital group n = 3075	Count	2731	257	53	34	344
	% within groups	88.8%	8.4%	1.7%	1.1%	**11.2%**

Regardless of the policies and standard practices for third stage care at both units, the intention-to-treat was not always consistent with the treatment actually received. The analysis of treatment received is presented in Table 5 and this data shows the effect on postpartum blood loss of receiving 'active' and 'holistic psychophysiological' interventions both by individual unit and in both units combined.

Table 5: Postpartum blood loss by treatment received: low risk women

Third stage care	Unit	Number and %	<500 ml	>=500 <1000ml	>=1000<=1500ml	> 1500 ml	Total PPH
HOLISTIC PSYCHOPHYSIOLOGICAL GROUP	Midwife-led n = 313	Count	309	2	1	1	4
		% within unit	98.7%	.6%	.3%	.3%	1.3%
	Tertiary n = 107	Count	104	3	0	0	3
		% within unit	97.2%	2.8%	.0%	.0%	2.8%
	Number in both units combined		413	5	1	1	7
	% in both units combined		98.3%	1.2%	.2%	.2%	**1.7%**
ACTIVE MANAGEMENT GROUP	Midwife-led n = 48	Count	42	5	1	0	6
		% within unit	87.5%	10.4%	2.1%	.0%	12.3%
	Tertiary n = 2968	Count	2627	254	53	34	341
		% within unit	88.5%	8.6%	1.8%	1.1%	11.5%
	Number in both units combined		2669	259	54	34	341
	% in both units combined		88.5%	8.6%	1.8%	1.1%	**11.5%**

Considering both units together, active management of the third stage of labour was received by 3,016 women and was associated with 347 postpartum haemorrhages (11.5%). This compares with holistic psychophysiological care which was received by 420 woman and associated with 7 (1.7%) postpartum haemorrhages OR = 7.7, 95% CI [3.6, 16.3]. The benefit of 'holistic psychophysiological third stage care' compared with 'active management' is apparent at all levels of PPH but most particularly at the $\geq$500 but <1000 ml level (1.2% versus 8.6%). Within the tertiary unit alone 'holistic psychophysiological care' was associated with 3 out of 107 (2.8%) postpartum haemorrhages, compared with 341 out of 2,968 (11.5%) postpartum haemorrhages for those women who received 'active management' of third stage labour, so OR = 4.5, 95% CI [1.4, 14.3]. In other words; regardless of the context, when women are at low risk for PPH 'holistic psychophysiological care' was safer than active management.

Discussion

This cohort study involved only women who were assessed as being at low risk of PPH. For this group of women the risk of having a PPH was seven to eight times higher if 'active management' of third stage labour was used, compared with 'holistic psychophysiological care'. This finding is in stark contrast to previous research and the Cochrane review of third stage care.[2-6] Some readers may be tempted to dismiss our findings because the data was collected by a non-randomised research design. However, the tendency to limit knowledge to only that which can be tested via randomised trials would undoubtedly bias the evidence toward interventions that seem simple and easy to define and measure; in the case of the third stage of labour trials this apparent simplicity is illusory. Maternity care practices, and the contexts of care, are highly complex and not easily amenable to reduction to single cause and effect relationships. Interventions that can be studied under randomised conditions are not necessarily the safest and most effective interventions and they are not necessarily cost-effective.[15] The challenge in cohort studies is to make valid inferences about cause and effect in the presence of known and unknown confounders. Our aim in reporting this cohort study has been to be open and transparent so that possible confounders can be identified and discussed.

What does seem clear is that for women who are at low risk of postpartum haemorrhage and who want to have holistic psychophysiological third stage care, the results of the present study are more trustworthy than those of previous studies. This trustworthiness is because, as argued above, the randomised trials concerning 'active' versus 'expectant' management of the third stage of labour cannot satisfactorily be generalised to this specific group of women who are at low risk of PPH. There have been no randomised trials which have tested holistic psychophysiological care in the third stage of labour. If the Cochrane review is as scientifically robust as assumed, then the findings should accurately predict the effect on PPH rates of both active and physiological management the third stage of labour. Yet the PPH rates at both maternity units in this study are very different from what was predicted by the

Cochrane review.[3] The 3% rate at the midwifery-led unit is much lower than the 13.5% predicted and the 20% rate at the tertiary unit is much higher than the predicted 5.2%.[3] Furthermore, the direction of PPH rates is opposite to the prediction of the Cochrane review, i.e. active management seems to be 'causing' more PPHs than holistic psychophysiological care in third stage.

When is a particular level of blood loss after birth life-threatening?

The word 'haemorrhage' is synonymous with the word 'bleeding'[19] so it is not possible to have a baby without a 'haemorrhage'. Nevertheless, for most people the word 'haemorrhage' conjures up an event which is quite serious and life-threatening. We therefore need to ask the question: when is bleeding after birth 'bad'? According to current definitions [using the key terms as defined in Table 1] 500ml is thought to be 'bad' even though this figure is an arbitrary one. William's Obstetrics[20] argues that the 500ml limit "is unreasonable because nearly half of all women who are delivered vaginally shed that amount of blood or more when measured quantitatively". The reason that healthy women are not haemodynamically compromised by a haemorrhage of 500ml or more is that pregnancy induces a normal state of hypervolaemia (increase in normal blood volume) which amounts to 1500-2000ml for average-sized women. The average, healthy woman can lose most of this extra blood volume during the first 24 hours after birth without experiencing hemodynamic compromise or anaemia.[1] At the other end of the continuum, in the case of women who are not healthy or who already have anaemia, a haemorrhage of even 250ml can cause shock.

We need to ask: when is bleeding after birth 'bad'?

Conclusion

We have presented an evidence-informed midwifery practice guideline which will assist you to a) identify when a woman is a good candidate for physiological care, and b) provide the essential elements of the Midwifery Guardianship Model of third stage care. Physiological third stage care, as described in this chapter, is the safest and best way to provide care to women at low risk of PPH. What is essential is that a holistic, psychophysiological approach means that the woman and baby are both healthy at the end of the second stage, there is immediate and sustained skin-to-skin contact after the birth, the cord remains intact at least until it stops pulsing, if not through the fourth stage too, the environment remains peaceful, the focus is on the woman and baby and the woman's condition is unobtrusively observed for an hour after the birth of the placenta. Of course, if you are the maternity caregiver, you also need to be skilled, alert and calm throughout the third stage and fourth stages of labour.

Physiological care, as described here, is the safest and best way to provide care to women at low risk of PPH

Kathleen Fahy began her midwifery career in 1971 at the Women's Hospital, Crown St, Sydney. She has a long experience as an academic and continues to stay up-to-date with practice. Kathleen is currently appointed as Professor of Midwifery at Newcastle University: she also practises as a midwife at the Maternity Unit at the John Hunter Hospital. She is an active scholar, researcher and theorist and an editor of the book *Birth Territory and Midwifery Guardianship*. Her research is aimed at understanding and, if indicated, changing the way maternity care is provided in order to optimise the health and well-being of women and babies.

Carolyn Hastie has had a lifelong fascination with human development, growth and experience and the role of emotions and perceptions in human behaviour and relationships. In particular her interest and writing has focused on childbearing and the baby's perinatal experience. For over 30 years Carolyn has provided and promoted relationship-based, one-to-one midwifery care for childbearing women and their families. She has recently established a publically funded midwifery service for healthy childbearing women in NSW. Despite widespread initial opposition, that service is very successful and includes the option for women to birth at home or at the stand-alone birth centre. Carolyn's PhD is a historical, sociological case study of her influential and ground-breaking, private midwifery practice conducted with several midwifery colleagues in the 1980s and early 1990s.

References

1 Hastie C, Fahy KM. Optimising Psychophysiology in the third stage of labour: theory applied to practice. Women and Birth 2009;22(3):89-96.

2 Lumley J. Any room left for disagreement about assisting breech births at term? The Lancet. 2000;356:1368-9.

3 Soanes C, Stevenson A. Psychophysiology (noun). Oxford English Dictionary Online [serial on the Internet]. 2005 12 December, 2010]: Available from: <http://0-www.oxfordreference.com.library.newcastle.edu. au/views/ENTRY.html?subview=Main&entry=t140.e62440>

4 Cacioppo J, Tassinary L, Berntson G, editors. Handbook of psychophysiology. third ed. New York: Cambridge University Press; 2007.

5 Mayes B. Practical Obstetrics. Sydney: Agnus and Robertson; 1954.

6 Myles M. A textbook for midwives. Edinburgh: E & S Livingstone; 1953.

7 Williams J. Obstetrics: a textbook for the use of students and practitioners. 6th ed. New York: D. Appleton & Co; 1930.

8 Organisation WH. The prevention and management of postpartum haemorrhage. WHO report of technical working group Geneva1090.

9 Begley C. A comparison of `active' and `physiological' management of the third stage of labour. . Midwifery. 1990;6(1):3-17.

10 Khan G, John I, Wani S, Doherty T, Sibai M. Controlled cord traction versus minimal intervention techniques in delivery of the placenta: a randomised controlled trial. American Journal of Obstetrics and Gynaecology. 1997;177(4):770-4.

11 Prendiville W, Harding J, Elbourne D, Stirrat G. The Bristol third stage trial: Active versus physiological management of third stage of labour. British Medical Journal. 1988;297(6659):1295-300.

12 Rogers J, Wood J, McCandlish R, Ayers S, Truesdale A, Elbourne D. Active versus expectant management of third stage of labour: the Hinchingbrooke randomised controlled trial. The Lancet. 1998;351(9104):693-9.

13 Prendiville D, Elbourne D, McDonald S. Active versus expectant management in the third stage of labour. The Cochrane Database of Systematic Reviews. 2000;3 (Article number CD000007.DOI:10.1002/14651858.CD000007):http://www.mrw.interscience.wiley.com/cochrane/clsysrev/articles/CD000007/frame.html [accessed Jan 10th 2011].

14 Levine D, Stephan D. Even you can learn statistics. A guide for everyone who has ever been afraid of statistics (2nd ed.). New Jersey: F.T. Press; 2010.

15 Fahy K. Third stage of labour care for women at low risk of postpartum haemorrhage. Midwifery and Women's Health. 2009;54(5):380-6.

16 Director General. Policy Directive. Postpartum haemorrhage (PPH) framework for prevention, early recogniton and management. New South Wales Health. 2005;Sydney.

17 Fry J. Physiological third stage of labour: support it or lose it. . British Journal of Midwifery 2007;15(11):893-5.

18 Gyte G. Evaluation of the meta-analyse on the effects, on both mother and baby, of the various components of 'active managment of the third stage of labour. Midwifery. 1994;10(4):183-99.

19 Martin E, editor. Colour Medical Dictionary. Oxford: Oxford University Press; 2010.

20 Cunningham G. William's Obstetrics. 22nd ed. New York: McGraw-Hill; 2005, pages 823-4.

A longer labour and birth... one size does not fit all!

Sarah Davies

The longer labour is a topic very close to my heart, as I myself had a long labour with my first baby. According to the midwives in attendance, my cervix stayed at 6cm for about 12 hours and the whole labour lasted well over 48 hours. However, I found the experience hugely empowering and started out on my motherhood journey feeling confident and strong. This chapter will not address the diagnosis of obstructed labour (an essential part of midwifery education) but will explore ideas and research relating to the 'normal' length of labour and suggest some ways in which women experiencing a longer labour can be enabled to have more positive outcomes by a change in approach.

A key to reducing rates of morbidity and mortality

'Failure to progress' in labour, or dystocia, is one of the most common reasons for caesarean section. High caesarean rates are an issue of international public health concern because not only is caesarean birth more resource-intensive, it is also associated with higher morbidity and mortality rates for mothers and babies.[1,2] Furthermore, caesarean section performed during labour is associated with higher maternal morbidity rates than elective caesarean.[3] It is therefore essential to re-examine approaches to dealing with slow labours.

Time and its impact on practice

Attitudes to time vary between cultures and have changed throughout history. Christine McCourt and Fiona Dykes analyse the historical shift from pre-modern/traditional to industrial and post-modern concepts of time.[4] They cite EP Thompson's landmark essay,[5] which examined how in pre-industrial society, tasks were decided according to what needed to be done, and were closely intertwined with the natural cycles of night/day, tides and seasons. In contrast, capitalist societies espouse a rhetoric of 'time thrift', where "all time must be consumed, marketed, put to use."[6] When people have this attitude, work becomes fragmented, and tasks are made to fit the production line. In the 1980s Robbie Davis-Floyd critiqued the 'technological paradigm' of birth, describing the hospital as 'a highly sophisticated technological factory' where "a woman's reproductive tract is treated like a birthing machine by skilled technicians working under semi-flexible timetables to meet production and quality control demands."[7] Emily Martin has pointed out the irony that since the 15th century, the same English word (*labour*), from the same root, has been used to describe what women do in bringing forth children, and what men and women do in making things for use and exchange in the home and market.[8]

High caesarean rates are an issue of public health concern

Changing notions of normal lengths of labour

The notion of 'how long is normal?' has shifted over time. Before 1900, even though the old adage 'Never let the sun set twice on a labour' shows that prolonged labour was a matter for concern, and opposing attitudes to its management were certainly evident in the 19th century (as Jo Murphy-Lawless has pointed out),[9] labours longer than 24 hours were commonplace.[10] In the 20th century, the length considered 'normal' for labour has become increasingly contracted although longer labours were well tolerated even in the 1950s and 60s. In the 1950s labour was termed 'prolonged' only when it exceeded 24 hours;[11] and as late as 1963 the ex-Master (lead obstetrician) of the Rotunda hospital in Dublin showed an understanding of the individual variation in labour when he stated: "It has always been the clinical policy in the Rotunda hospital not to set an arbitrary time limit such as 30, 36 or 48 hours... each case is treated on its own merits and mere prolongation of labour is not necessarily regarded as an unjustifiable hazard."[12]

Justifications for intervention

Intervention to speed up labour was totally bound up with rising levels of hospital birth, which brought a need for efficient use of space and human resources. In the 1970s O'Driscoll and colleagues in Dublin, Ireland developed the 'active management of labour' approach. This gave women expecting their first baby the 'assurance' that the baby would be born within 12 hours.[13] O'Driscoll argued: "The passive concept of labour has been replaced by an intensive care situation in which every patient has a personal nurse and every labour is controlled." He described the labours of 1,000 primigravidae, all of whom, apart from seven, had labours of 12 hours or less under the new regime. He saw this as an unalloyed good that would reduce women's anxiety about labour... although his work did not include research into women's experiences. (O'Driscoll's 'active management' package consisted of customised antenatal preparation, strict criteria for the diagnosis of labour, standardised management of labour including early amniotomy and synthetic oxytocin if cervical dilation was less than 1cm/hour, and one-to-one care). Obstetric units were quick to adopt O'Driscoll's approach but few adopted all elements; most omitted the only element that has since been shown to demonstrably improve outcomes—continuous labour support.[14]

A new approach to care and its justification

The origins of the 'progress paradigm'[15] lie in the work of Friedman in the 1950s and 60s,[16] who depicted the progress of labour in a sigmoid curve for first and subsequent births. The Friedman curve was hugely influential in understanding and assessing labour progress and was incorporated into obstetric and midwifery textbooks over the next 50 years.[17] This was despite the fact that Friedman used statistical calculations to separate 95% of all women in clinical practice from the slowest 5% so, as Leah Albers notes, "this statistical concept of 'normal' [was] translated into a clinical practice definition of normal labour."[18] In 1972 Philpott and Castle[19] developed Friedman's concept into a tool for monitoring labour (the cervicograph) by adding 'alert' and 'action' lines to the graph. Their study was conducted in an isolated area in Rhodesia (now Zimbabwe) and was concerned with access to healthcare in a resource-poor setting. The alert line was set at a rate of 1cm per hour, and suggested to the attendants a need to keep careful watch. A transfer line was set two hours behind that, indicating transfer was needed to a major hospital, and the action line itself was an indication to rupture the membranes and administer syntocinon.

The partogram was adopted very quickly around the world

In 1973 Studd, who conducted further research in the UK and modified Philpott's graphic record, argued that the partogram, as it became known, would "identify an 'at risk' group of patients requiring acceleration of labour, intensive monitoring and probable second-stage instrumentation."[20] The partogram was then adopted very quickly around the world and endorsed by the World Health Organisation. In 2008, however, Lavender and colleagues conducted a systematic review of research evidence which found no evidence of improved outcomes due to use of the partogram.[21]

An updated assessment of best approaches, based on recent data

The knowledge base is changing and so, therefore, must attitudes to labour duration. As long ago as the year 2000 Enkin and Kierse[22] were arguing for a more relaxed approach to labour duration, and research data over the past decade or so suggests that normal labour can last far longer than has previously been appreciated.

In 2001 Leah Albers, who has conducted extensive research on the duration of normal labour, reported on midwifery data from the University of New Mexico which indicated that the normal values for first stage labour were twice that of Friedman's norms.[23] Follow-up studies in nine hospital-based midwifery practices came to the same conclusion: "Normal labour may last far longer than many clinicians assume and excess time in labour is not necessarily associated with untoward outcomes for mother or infant."[24]

In 2010 Neal et al conducted a systematic review of 25 studies and concluded that "nulliparous women with spontaneous labour onset have longer 'active' labours and therefore slower dilation rates than are traditionally associated with active labour."[25] They argue that "faster dilation expectations (e.g. 1 cm/hour) are likely to contribute to an overdiagnosis of dystocia in contemporary practice and, subsequently, to an overuse of interventions aimed at accelerating labour progress."[26]

The knowledge base is changing and so, therefore, must attitudes to labour duration

Also in 2010, Jun Zhang et al[27] examined data from the National Collaborative Perinatal Project, a large, multicentre, prospective, observational study conducted between 1959 and 1966, when obstetric interventions were less common. The rationale for using this dataset (26,838 labours) was that it is now impossible to study the progression of natural labour in a large group of women, due to the frequency of medical intervention and the high rate of caesarean delivery. The researchers concluded that multiparas may not enter the active phase of labour until 5cm, while nulliparas may start the active phase even later.

Contemporary guidelines

In the UK, evidence-based guidelines for intrapartum care[28] now state that a diagnosis of delay in the established first stage of labour needs to consider all aspects of progress in labour, including:

- cervical dilation of less than 2 cm in four hours for first labours
- cervical dilation of less than 2 cm in four hours or a slowing in the progress of labour for second or subsequent labours
- descent and rotation of the fetal head
- changes in the strength, duration and frequency of uterine contractions

The All Wales Clinical Pathway for Normal Labour[29] also uses the 2cm-in-four-hours criterion, but allows for more flexibility still and does not indicate immediate intervention if progress is slower than this, but recommends evaluation by the midwife, considering issues such as whether the woman is indeed in active labour, whether she is mobile, how far the head has descended, and also whether she needs positive encouragement and recommends another vaginal examination within two hours if there are no signs of full dilation after all these factors have been taken into account.

Clearly, although linear notions of labour progress are still prevalent, they are being modified both in terms of the strictness of time criteria and also according to an understanding that labour progress should not be defined by cervical dilation alone.

More advanced understanding of the physiology of labour

Even more importantly, there is now far greater understanding of the complex hormonal balance of physiological labour[30,31] and of the delicate interactions of hormones which create the rhythms of labour. These rhythms include natural 'plateaux' when contractions cease for a while, which do not have to be seen as problematic if there are no other signs of problems.[32] Midwives Clare Winter and Margie Duff point out from their qualitative research with independent midwives that labour is not a linear, orderly process. Midwives interviewed were comfortable with uncertainty and did not use vaginal examinations to measure progress as advocated by the medically defined 'cervical dilation' approach.

Instead, they used vaginal examinations diagnostically only if they needed to, and used other ways of assessing the progress of labour: connecting with the woman and 'listening to the labour', as one midwife phrased it. They saw vaginal examinations as intrusive and felt they possibly interrupted the physiological process. Duff proposed a set of phrases based on audible and visual physiological cues that better reflect the process of labour: 'starting out'; 'getting into it'; 'getting on with it', 'nearly there' and 'the end is in sight'.[33]

New methods for assessing labour progress

It seems eminently sensible for midwives to learn other ways of assessing progress and to keep assessments, especially vaginal examinations, to a minimum, given that it is now understood that privacy and a dark peaceful environment optimise the hormones of labour. Indeed, our current efforts to monitor and measure the progress of labour may have hitherto unrecognised detrimental effects. For example, if there is excessive production of catecholamines due to maternal stress there will be reduced blood flow to the uterus, which will in turn reduce the efficiency of uterine contractions and diminish blood flow to the fetus, which will then lead to a delay in labour and fetal distress.[34] Therefore, attendants, far from ensuring safety by monitoring the well-being of mother and baby may unwittingly be jeopardising the safety of the mother-baby dyad. Chandra and Browne,[35] in a plea for 'slow midwifery', write of the extent to which midwives spend their time counting, timekeeping and measuring, saying that this potentially disrupts the mother-midwife relationship and contributes to the idea prevalent in society that fast is always better than slow.

New ways of tracking labour progress

Indeed the mechanistic, 'first, second and third stage' approach to understanding labour is now being challenged. Cervical dilation is not a predictable, constant process either within or between individuals, as Clare Winter and Joan Cameron point out.[36] Furthermore, the concept of the latent phase of labour is extremely important, as labour is considered to be much longer if this phase is included; yet its diagnosis is extremely problematic.[37,38]

Time management, as experienced by labouring women

Christine McCourt,[39] drawing on data from a larger study in 1998, examines narrative accounts of how the management of time in labour was experienced by women in a unit with a medicalised ethos, where midwives did not usually practise with a high degree of autonomy. Time was clearly important to the women, but McCourt observed a disjuncture between women's embodied experiences and the judgement of the midwives, which could lead to women feeling undermined. There were particular difficulties around the 'latent phase' of labour (sometimes called 'false labour' by the midwives) where women felt they were made to feel rather foolish and unable to trust their own bodily experiences if they arrived at the hospital 'too early'. In active labour, women felt that 'the clock was ticking against them'. One woman said: "[the midwife] emphasised that I only had an hour in which to push the baby out. After that time if I hadn't managed to produce a baby then they'd have to consider some sort of intervention. So she laid out the rules quite clearly to me."[40] Time was seen as limited so that it must be used and spent properly. (The commonly heard refrain of the midwife exhorting a woman not to 'waste your pain' also comes to mind.) The practice of coached, unphysiological or 'purple pushing' persists despite evidence that it is detrimental to mother and fetus.[41]

Ways round 'old' systems

In an atmosphere where times are judged and used as a basis for clinical decision-making it is also widely recognised that midwives will adapt their recording of time in labour simply in order to protect women from the effects of the 'ticking clock' of obstetric timekeeping. They may do this by delaying the 'starting of the clock'[42] at different stages, for example by not starting the partogram in early labour, or by not recording full dilation, or by misrecording it as 'a rim' (8 to 9cm) when the cervix is in fact fully dilated. This may also protect the midwife herself from censure by those wishing to speed up the process either because of institutional pressures or through a misunderstanding of physiology, or both. The phenomenon of 'doing good by stealth'[43] applies perhaps most particularly to midwives' relationship to time in labour and suggests that the technocratic model[44] is still dominant and considered authoritative. However, as Brigitte Jordan observed, for any particular domain several knowledge systems exist. Some become dominant either because they explain a phenomenon better or because they are associated with a stronger power base.[45] Although imbalances of power will no doubt continue to exist, current research evidence underlines the importance of treating every labouring woman individually rather than relying on a rigid timeframe.

Practical approaches when a labour appears long

It is down to midwives and birth activists to embrace these new understandings in order to support and protect physiological birth. Midwives and women therefore need to understand how best to support a longer labour. I suggest the most important element is the maintenance of a positive attitude and a belief in the woman's ability to give birth. This is hugely enhanced by continuity of care where the midwife promotes antenatally and throughout labour a sense of the woman's ability to cope with the challenge of labour. Nicky Leap and colleagues' qualitative study of 10 women cared for by Albany group practice midwives in London, concluded that a relationship of continuity and trust with the midwife "enhanced women's ability to overcome fears and self-doubt about coping with pain and led to feelings of pride, elation, and empowerment after birth."[46]

It is down to midwives and birth activists to embrace these new understandings in order to support and protect physiological birth

A good place to start is to inform women of the Lamaze 'six healthy birth practices'.[47] These are:

- Let labour begin on its own.
- Encourage the woman to walk, move around and change positions throughout labour.
- Encourage the women to bring a loved one, friend or doula for continuous support.
- Avoid interventions that are not medically necessary.
- Encourage the woman to avoid giving birth on her back and encourage her to follow her body's urges to push.
- Keep mother and baby together.

The first five will reduce women's risk of having an unduly prolonged labour and are well supported by research evidence.

The midwife/birth attendant also needs a 'toolkit' of non-pharmacological techniques to support the woman. These techniques are discussed in depth in Penny Simkin and Ruth Ancheta's *Labour Progress Handbook*,[48] already in its second edition. The techniques they offer include maternal positions and movements such as asymmetrical lunging to help the occiput rotate, and comfort measures such as the use of water, support, massage and touch, acupuncture, hot and cold packs, food and drink, and others. Importantly, they also include psychological approaches. For example, a midwife can make an enormous difference in the early part of a woman's labour by providing information so that the woman doesn't become disheartened. She can explain the 'six ways to progress',[49] of which cervical dilation is only one element:

1 The cervix moves from posterior to anterior.
2 The cervix ripens or softens.
3 The cervix effaces.
4 The cervix dilates.
5 The fetal head rotates, flexes and moulds.
6 The fetus descends, rotates further and is born.

In addition, both the mother-midwife relationship and the environment for labour must be such that the woman feels 'safe enough to let go'[50] so that the woman can avoid 'emotional dystocia': the stalling of labour due to maternal fear and anxiety. By judicious use of language the midwife can also help a mother unblock emotions and free up labour so that it continues.[51] Another important point is that the midwife or birth attendant must be aware of her or his own stress levels and the deleterious effect the attendant's might have on a labouring woman.[52] As a wise obstetrician noted in 1969:[53] "A labour which is unduly prolonged is likely to give rise to one or more of three types of distress, namely maternal, fetal, or 'obstetrician's distress'. Of the three, the last may easily be the most dangerous!'"

Reasons to reject the 'old way' and find a better way forward

Adherence to rigid time limits is a simplistic, reductionist approach to the complexity of the finely balanced 'dance' of labour and, as I've shown, this approach is not supported by the available evidence. Indeed, I would argue that the straightjacket of the 'stages of labour' approach is oppressive to both midwives and women. To ascribe a spurious certainty where none exists is to strip midwives of their professional autonomy. Dealing with uncertainty, and using clinical skills and professional judgement is a hallmark of professionalism. Therefore, every midwife should have the skills to assess the progress of labour (which need not include routine vaginal examination), as well as her own 'non-pharmacological toolkit'. The 'ticking clock' of obstetric timekeeping is damaging to women as it undermines their bodily confidence, as well as their sense of agency and control.[54] It contributes to an overdiagnosis of delay in labour, which increases the risk of unnecessary medical intervention and operative delivery. Since the process of pregnancy and labour is unique for each woman now is the time for midwifery and obstetrics to rise to the challenge posed by 'unique normality.'[55]

Sarah Davies qualified as a midwife in 1982 and has worked in hospital and community settings and independently. She now teaches students and qualified midwives, as well as having an (extremely small) clinical caseload. Her students, the future guardians of normal birth, constantly challenge and inspire her. She has recently been involved with the Albany Action group, a group of mothers and midwives who came together to defend the caseload model of care after the untimely and deplorable closure of the Albany Midwifery Practice in London. She has written articles about this and other aspects of the maternity services in the UK in *AIMS Journal, British Journal of Midwifery, Practising Midwife* and in the *Healthcare Risk Report.*

References

1 Souza JP, Gulmezoglu AM, Lumbiganon P, et al , 2010. Caesarean section without medical indications is associated with an increased risk of adverse short-term maternal outcomes: the 2004-2008 WHO Global Survey on Maternal and Perinatal Health. *BMC Medicine* 8 (71).

2 van Dillen J, Zwart JJ, Schutte J, et al, 2010.Severe acute maternal morbidity and mode of delivery in the Netherlands. *Acta Obstetricia et Gynecologica Scandinavica* 89(11):1460-1465.

3 Pallasmaa N, Ekblad U, Aitokallio-Tallberg A, et al, 2010. Cesarean delivery in Finland: maternal complications and obstetric risk factors. *Acta Obstetricia et Gynecologica Scandinavica,* 89(7):896-902.

4 McCourt C (ed), 2010. *Childbirth, Midwifery and Concepts of Time.* Oxford: Berghahn Books.

5 Thompson EP, 1967. Time, work-discipline, and industrial capitalism. *Past and Present* 38(1): 56-97.

6 Thompson EP, 1967. Time, work-discipline, and industrial capitalism. *Past and Present* 38(1): 56-97.

7 Davis-Floyd R, 1987. The technological model of birth. *Journal of American Folklore* 100:479-95.

8 Martin M, 1987. *The Woman in the Body: a Cultural Analysis of Reproduction.* Milton Keynes: Oxford University Press: p66.

9 Murphy-Lawless, J, 2000. *Midwives, Power and Women's Time in Childbirth.* Presentation, European Congress for Out-of-Hospital Births, Aachen.

10 Shorter E, 1982. *Women's Bodies: A Social History of Women's Encounter with Health, Ill-Health, and Medicine.* Pelican Books. Cited in Murphy-Lawless J, 2000. *Midwives, Power and Women's Time in Childbirth.* Presentation, European Congress for Out-of-Hospital Births, Aachen.

11 Baird D, 1952. The cause and prevention of difficult labour. *American Journal of Obstetrics and Gynecology* 63:1200-1212.

12 Thompson EWL, 1963. Prolonged labour: Its management and prognosis. *Irish Journal of Medical Science,* 1926-1967; 38(7): 327-338, DOI: 10.1007/BF02953090.

13 O'Driscoll K, Stronge JM and Minogue M, 1973. Active management of labour. *British Medical Journal* 3:135-137.

14 Hodnett ED, Gates S, Hofmeyr GJ, Sakala C, Weston J, 2011. Continuous support for women during childbirth. *Cochrane Database of Systematic Reviews* 2011, Issue 2, Art. No: CD003766.

15 Walsh D, 2007. *Evidence-based Care for Normal Labour and Birth: a Guide for Midwives.* Routledge: London.

16 Friedman E, 1954. The graphic analysis of the progress of labour. *American Journal of Obstetrics and Gynecology.* 68:1568-75.

17 Walsh D, 2007. *Evidence-based Care for Normal Labour and Birth: a Guide for Midwives.* Routledge: London, p64.

18 Albers A, 2007. The evidence for physiologic management of the active phase of the first stage of labour. *Journal of Midwifery & Women's Health.* 52(3):207-215.

19 Philpott RH, Castle WM, 1972. Cervicographs in the management of labour in primigravidae: the alert line for detecting abnormal labour. *J Obstet Gynaecol Br Commonw,* 78: 592-8.

20 Studd J, 1973. Partograms and normograms of cervical dilation in management of primigravid labour. *British Medical Journal* 4: 451-5 Database of Systematic Reviews, Issue 4.

21 Lavender T, Hart A, Smyth RM, 2008. Effect of partogram use on outcomes for women in spontaneous labour at term. *Cochrane Database of Systematic Reviews* 8(4): CD005461.

22 Enkin M, Keirse MJNC, Neilson J, et al, 2000. *A Guide to Effective Care in Pregnancy and Childbirth.* 3rd ed. Oxford: Oxford University Press.

23 Albers L, 2001. Rethinking dystocia: patience please, *MIDIRS Midwifery Digest,* 11 (3):251-253.

24 Albers L, 2001. Rethinking dystocia: patience please. *MIDIRS Midwifery Digest,* 11 (3):251-253: p253.

25 Neal J, Lowe N, Ahijevych K, Patrick T, Cabbage L, Corwin E, 2010. Active labor duration and dilation rates among low-risk, nulliparous women with spontaneous labor onset: a systematic review. *Journal of Midwifery and Women's Health,* 55 (4): 308-318.

26 Neal J, Lowe N, Ahijevych K, Patrick T, Cabbage L, Corwin E, 2010. What is the slowest yet-normal cervical dilation rate among nulliparous women with spontaneous labor onset? *Journal of Gynecologic and Neonatal Nursing,* 39, 361-369.

27 Zhang J, Troendle J, Mikolajczyk R, 2010. The natural history of the normal first stage of labour. *Obstetrics & Gynaecology,* 115(4): 705–10.

28 National Institute for Health and Clinical Excellence (NICE), 2007. *Routine Intrapartum/ Care of Women and their Babies.* See http://www.nice.org.uk/nicemedia/live/11837/36280/36280.pdf [accessed 8 March 2011].

29 All Wales Clinical Pathway for Normal Labour available online at http://www.wales.nhs.uk/sites3/page.cfm?orgid=327&pid=5786 [accessed 12 April 2011].

30 Odent M, 2001. New reasons and new ways to study birth physiology. *International Journal of Gynaecology,* 72:S39-45.

31 Buckley S, 2004. Undisturbed birth—nature's hormonal blueprint for safety, ease and ecstasy. *MIDIRS Midwifery Digest,* 14 (2):203-209.

32 Duff M, 2005. *A study of labour.* Unpublished PhD dissertation, University of Technology, Sydney. Cited in: Winter C, Duff M, 2010. The progress of labour: Orderly Chaos? In McCourt C (Ed) 2010 *Childbirth, Midwifery and Concepts of Time.* Oxford: Berghahn Books, pp84-103.

33 Winter C and Duff M, 2010. The progress of labour: Orderly Chaos? In McCourt C (Ed) 2010 *Childbirth, Midwifery and Concepts of Time.* Oxford: Berghahn Books, pp84-103.

34 Simkin P, 1986. Stress, pain and catecholamines in labor: part 1. A review *Birth,* 13(4) 227-233,

35 Browne J, Chandra A, 2009. Slow midwifery. *Women and Birth* 22: 29-33.

36 Winter C, Cameron J, 2006. The 'stages' model of labour: deconstructing the myth. *British Journal of Midwifery;* 14:454-456.

37 Burvill S, 2002. Midwifery diagnosis of labour onset. *British Journal of Midwifery* 10(10):600-605.

38 Cheyne H, Dowding DW, Hundley V, 2006. Making the diagnosis of labour: midwives' diagnostic judgement and management decisions. *Journal of Advanced Nursing* 53:625-635.

39 McCourt C, 2010. Time in labour: themes from women's birth stories. Chapter 9, pp184-201 in McCourt C (ed), 2010. *Childbirth, Midwifery and Concepts of Time.* Oxford: Berghahn Books.

40 McCourt C, 2010. Time in labour: themes from women's birth stories. Chapter 9, pp184-201 in McCourt C (ed) 2010 *Childbirth, Midwifery and Concepts of Time.* Oxford: Berghahn Books p194.

41 Martin CJH, 2009. Effects of valsalva manoeuvre on maternal and fetal wellbeing. *British Journal of Midwifery,* 17(5):279-285.

42 Stevens M, 2010. *Time and Midwifery Practice,* Chapter 10, pp104-125 in McCourt C (ed), 2010. *Childbirth, Midwifery and Concepts of Time.* Oxford: Berghahn Books p194.

43 Kirkham M, 1999. The culture of midwifery in the National Health Service in England. *Journal of Advanced Nursing,* 30:732-739.

44 Davis-Floyd R, 1987. The technological model of birth. *Journal of American Folklore,* 100:479-95.

45 Jordan B, 1993. *Birth in Four Cultures*. 4th ed. Illinois: Waveland Press, p152

46 Leap N, Sandall J, Buckland S, Huber U, 2010. Journey to confidence: women's experiences of pain in labour and relational continuity of care. *Journal of Midwifery and Women's Health*, 55:234-242.

47 *Introduction to the Six Healthy Birth Practices*. Lamaze International. See http://www.lamaze.org/ExpectantParents/HealthyBirthPractices/tabid/251/Default.aspx [accessed 11 March 2011].

48 Simkin P, Ancheta R, 2005. *The Labor Progress Handbook*. 2nd ed. London: Blackwell.

49 Simkin P, Ancheta R, 2005. *The Labor Progress Handbook*. 2nd ed. London: Blackwell, p89.

50 Anderson T, 2010. Feeling safe enough to let go: the relationship between a woman and her midwife during the second stage of labour. Chapter 7 in Kirkham M (ed) *The Midwife-Mother Relationship* (2nd ed) Basingstoke, England: Palgrave Macmillan, pp116-143.

51 Simkin P, Ancheta R, 2005. *The Labor Progress Handbook*. 2nd ed. London: Blackwell, pp134-138

52 Odent M, 2004. Knitting midwives for drugless childbirth? *Midwifery Today*; 71: 21-22.

53 Donald I, 1969. *Practical Obstetric Problems.* 4th Ed. London: Lloyd- Duke Medical Books.

54 Murphy-Lawless J, 2000. *Midwives, Power and Women's Time in Childbirth.* Presentation, European Congress for Out-of-Hospital Births, Aachen.

55 Downe S, McCourt C, 2008. From being to becoming: reconstructing childbirth knowledges. In *Normal Childbirth: Evidence and Debate*. 2nd ed. Downe S (ed), pp3-27.

Which models of care most effectively promote normality?*

Robbie Davis-Floyd

The importance of ideology—what's in a name?

The 'medical model' shows us pregnancy and birth through the perspective of technological society, and from men's eyes. Birthing women are thus objects upon whom certain procedures must be done. The alternative model... which I will call 'the midwifery model... is a woman's perspective on birth, in which women are the subjects, the doers, the givers of birth.

Barbara Katz Rothman[1]

The co-edited volume *Birth Models That Work*[2] provides an educated tour of functional birth models whose practitioners are providing optimal maternity care and provides much of the basis for this chapter. All of the models presented in that book share a common ideology based on the fundamental notions that birth is normal and women are its protagonists. What should we call this shared ideology? It has received various names over time. It was first described in print by sociologist Barbara Katz Rothman in 1982 as the 'midwifery model of care'[1] and this label has since become internationally recognised as a useful signature by which to differentiate the philosophy and ideology of midwifery from that of obstetrics. Recognition of the difference between the two professions—midwives focus on normalcy, obstetricians on pathology—goes back centuries; serious discussions about the implications of those differences have been taking place since that time. Because midwives are the most numerous primary maternity care practitioners and have long engaged in discussion and reflection with each other and with social scientists about what it is that they do that works and doesn't work, they have continued to articulate and refine 'the midwifery model of care' (e.g. Rooks, 1999[3]). In many midwifery educational programmes around the world, this model is held out as an ideal for midwifery practice, while in others it is actively taught as the standard for midwifery care. Others have suggested other names for this model, in part to avoid identifying it with a particular profession and to acknowledge that many midwives over-medicalise their treatment of birth while some consultants and doctors (GPs) work very hard to practise 'the midwifery model'. To date there is no international consensus on the most appropriate name for the ideology and practice of supporting normal birth.

In *Birth as an American Rite of Passage*,[4] I expanded on Rothman's discussion of the differences between the 'medical' and 'midwifery' models of care, using the labels 'the technocratic model of birth' and 'the holistic model of birth' to name these contrasting paradigms. Some years later, I further expanded my understanding of the dominant paradigms operative in global maternity care to include a third paradigm, the humanistic model, which stretches across the divide between the technocratic and holistic models. As I noted in an earlier article,[5] humanists wish simply to humanise technomedicine–that is, to make it relational, partnership-oriented, individually responsive, and compassionate:

> *Humanism counterbalances technomedicine with a softer approach, which can be anything from a superficial overlay to profoundly alternative methods. It is superficially humanistic to decorate a technocratic labour room so the machines don't stand out so much; it is deeply humanistic to provide women with flexible spaces in which they have room to move around as much as they like, to be in water if they wish, to labour as they choose.*

Birth activists in all Spanish- and Portuguese-speaking countries appear to have reached consensus around the term 'humanisation'–they speak of *la humanizacion del parto y nacimiento* (the humanisation of birth), *parto humanizado* (humanised birth), etc. But to focus reform efforts on the humanisation of birth can only be a relevant strategy when birth is *dehumanised*, as indeed it is in many large Latin American hospitals, but not, generally speaking, in hospitals in the US and Canada, or in the UK, where the technocratic approach still prevails and yet women are humanistically treated–that is, with compassion and respect, and with support from companions they choose–which are the essential ingredients of a humanistic approach. And therein lies the rub: the humanistic paradigm is highly co-optable–I have witnessed some Latin American hospitals suddenly start calling their maternity care 'humanistic' simply because they decided to allow a partner to accompany the mother during labour or to allow mothers to stay with their babies in the freshly painted postnatal ward while many unnecessary interventions are still routinely performed.

If *humanistic* is to become as widely used in other countries as it is in the Hispanic world, we must be careful to distinguish the *superficial humanism* of the respectful and caring unnecessary caesarean from the *deep humanism* that acknowledges and facilitates the deep physiology and emotionality of birth, for example, through freedom of movement, upright positions for birth, and full emotional support and physical support.

The technocratic model of birth constitutes the hegemonic paradigm (i.e. one which involves dominance of one group over others) and it influences the attitudes and behaviours of biomedically-oriented birth practitioners.[5] This technocratic model views the mind as separate from the body and defines the body as a machine and the patient as an object (who may be referred to as 'The c/sec in Room 112'). Both definitions facilitate the distancing of practitioner from patient, the supervaluation of mechanical diagnoses via ultrasound and EFM, and the overuse of technological intervention designed to improve or correct the malfunctions of the maternal body-machine. In contrast, the humanistic model of birth places supreme importance on mind-body connection (the influence of mental and emotional states on the body, and vice versa), defines the body not as a machine but as an organism; most essentially, it stresses the importance of the caregiver-patient relationship.

The essence of a humanistic approach to birth is relationship, communication, and caring between patient and practitioner—a supervaluation of the needs of the individual instead of those of the institution.

The distinction between superficial and deep is key...

The distinction I mention above between superficial and deep humanism is key: *superficial humanism* involves beautifying the environment of birth, making the mother more comfortable, and treating her kindly and respectfully—but this approach can easily include the respectful and caring administration of multiple unnecessary technological interventions. Again, and in stark contrast, *deep humanism* goes much further, involving a profound understanding of the normal physiology of birth and how to facilitate it, and including an understanding of the power of the mother's emotions to affect the progress of labour. The *holistic model of birth* goes beyond the definition of the body as an organism to viewing it as an energy field in interaction with other energy fields. In the holistic view—one adopted by many midwives and some obstetricians—practitioners can preclude the need for technological interventions by intervening at the level of energy, changing or focusing the 'energy of birth' to facilitate optimal outcomes. (Jones, 2009 provides examples.[6])

Deep humanism involves a profound understanding...

Other descriptions of models exist. For example, In *Pursuing the Birth Machine*,[7] Marsden Wagner contrasted the medical model with the 'social model' of birth—a terminology followed by Lesley Barclay[8] in her discussions of midwives in Samoa. Of course, the social model is one that emphasises the sociality of birth. Dutch midwives speak of the 'physiological' model because their focus is on understanding and facilitating the deep physiology of birth.[9] Yet a focus on physiology can appear to minimise birth's social aspects, while a focus on sociality can seem to minimise the importance of physiology. Spreading out from France from the work of Bernard Bel and others is the term *naissance respectée* (respected childbirth)—a highly humanistic focus. US activists struggle with 'natural' vs 'normal' birth as their conceptual standard because both of these terms are problematic: nearly all human births are culturally shaped, and 'normal' is hard to define, especially when interventions are 'the norm' in hospitals. Anthropologist Brigitte Jordan utilised a 'biocultural' approach to her analysis of birth in four cultures[10]—and yet birth is more than a combination of biology and culture. It is therefore difficult to find terminology that communicates the full spectrum of essential values.

It is difficult to find terminology that communicates the full spectrum of essential values

Other nomenclature abounds in areas where individuals or organisations are aiming to improve care models. An international collaboration between WHO and UNICEF resulted in the creation of the *Baby-Friendly* Hospital Initiative, the focus of which is on facilitating successful breastfeeding. The Coalition for Improving Maternity Care (CIMS) in the US developed a national initiative based on a *mother-friendly* model of care (see www.mother-friendly.org).

The importance of ideology was definitively demonstrated by a systematic review of 137 reports on factors influencing women's evaluations of their childbirth experiences, carried out in 2002 by Ellen Hodnett.[11] Her objective was to summarise what is known about satisfaction with childbirth, with particular attention to the roles of pain and pain relief. The reports included in Hodnett's review included descriptive studies, randomised controlled trials, and reviews of intrapartum interventions. The results were as follows:

four factors—personal expectations, the amount of support from caregivers, the quality of the caregiver-patient relationship, and involvement in decision making—appear to be so important that they override the influences of age, socioeconomic status, ethnicity, childbirth preparation, the physical birth environment, pain, immobility, medical interventions, and continuity of care, when women evaluate their childbirth experiences.

The review's conclusion is that 'The influences of pain, pain relief, and intrapartum medical interventions on subsequent satisfaction are neither as obvious, as direct, nor as powerful as the influences of the attitudes and behaviors of the caregivers.' Attitudes and behaviours stem from particular philosophies, or paradigms, that form the template for the caregiver's beliefs about birth. In other words, *it's the model behind the model of practice that most determines the kind of care a practitioner will provide.*

The daughter organisation of the Coalition for Improving Maternity Care (CIMS), the International MotherBaby Childbirth Organization (IMBCO, has recently launched the *International MotherBaby Childbirth Initiative (IMBCI): 10 Steps to Optimal MotherBaby Maternity Services* (www.imbci.org). This Initiative organises itself around what its proponents have labelled the *MotherBaby Model of Care,* acknowledging its basis in the midwifery model. Its creators (including myself) chose the term MotherBaby to emphasise the integrity of this dyad. Two of its principles state:

The MotherBaby Model of Care promotes the health and wellbeing of all women and babies during pregnancy, birth, and breastfeeding, setting the gold standard for excellence and superior outcomes in maternity care. All maternity service providers should be educated in, provide, and support the MotherBaby Model of Care.

Midwives, who are the primary care providers for millions of birthing women in most countries, have developed a model of care based on the normal physiology, sociology, and psychology of pregnancy, labour, birth, and the postpartum period. The International MotherBaby Childbirth Initiative draws on the midwifery model of care and affirms that midwifery knowledge, skills, and behavior are essential for optimal MotherBaby care.[12]

As the International MotherBaby Childbirth Initiative (IMBCI) grows in influence and spreads over time, perhaps the term MotherBaby Model of Care will gain international dominance. Yet for now, wishing to name and describe the model that underlies optimal birth models, I note that *by definition midwives are or should be the primary guides and guardians of normal pregnancy and birth, while obstetricians, by definition, are or should be the backup providers dealing with conditions of actual danger or risk.*

The midwifery model as I define it here combines all elements of humanism with many elements of holism

Midwives are indeed primary practitioners in all of the models described in *Birth Models That Work*, and 'the midwifery model' seems to me at this point the most appropriate term to utilise. The midwifery model as I define it here combines all elements of humanism with many elements of holism. Although the midwives in the practices described in *Birth Models That Work* do practise according to this midwifery model, many thousands of midwives around the world are technocratically trained and do not. Nurses serve as primary birth attendants in some places, with varying results, and 'skilled birth attendants', with widely varying types of training, are now internationally promoted (e.g. by WHO). In almost every country one can find committed obstetricians who apply the 'midwifery model' daily in their practices. Thus I use the term 'MMOC practitioners' ('Midwifery-Model-of-Care Practitioners') to index those care providers who practise according to the ideology I describe in the following section.

The midwifery (humanistic/holistic) model of care

The midwifery model of care comes from a woman-centred perspective, defines women as active agents in pregnancy and birth, and sees the female body as normal in its own terms and pregnancy and birth as healthy, normal parts of women's lives. It takes a holistic, integrative approach, defining the body not as a machine but as an organism and an energy field in constant interaction with other energy fields.[5,13] It views mind and body as one and mother and baby as an inseparable unit... In fact, the use of the term 'motherbaby' in the International MotherBaby Childbirth Initiative indicates its authors' understanding of how profoundly the treatment of one affects the other. The safety and emotional needs of the mother and baby are the same; what is good for the mother is good for the child. As Rothman put it:

> *The medical model dichotomizes not only mind and body, but also mother and infant. Mother/fetus are seen in the medical model as a conflicting dyad rather than an integral unit. In the midwifery model, mother and fetus are genuinely one, and what meets the needs of the one meets the needs of the other. Emotional, physical, maternal and infant needs are not, in the midwifery model, at odds.*[14]

The family, not the institution, constitutes the most significant social unit, and the mother, not the practitioner, is the most significant birthing agent.

Birth as normal

Fundamentally, nature works well the vast majority of the time–birth outcomes are better when labour and birth are nurtured and supported but not interfered with. MMOC practitioners understand the deep physiology of birth. They know that labour, when allowed to flow, has its own rhythms–it can start and stop, speed up or slow down, take a few hours or a few days as the uterus tones and prepares and the mother works through her emotions. Facilitation is appropriate; intervention is usually inappropriate. MMOC practitioners use specific technologies (e.g. artifacts that facilitate upright positions like birthing balls, wall ladders, ropes, and chairs) and modalities (such as acupressure and visualisation) that work to support normal birth but generally minimise medical interventions, relying on a physiologically and emotionally supportive range of strategies and watchful vigilance. They read and understand the scientific evidence showing that labouring women should be encouraged to do as they please–to eat, drink, move about, rest. The first line of care for minor delays and complications is with low-tech interventions such as position changes, emotional support, massage, immersion in warm water, aromatherapy, herbs, homeopathy, hand maneuvres, and most fundamentally 'changing the energy' by working to create a more positive and trust-based atmosphere; higher-tech interventions are reserved for cases of true need. It is time that such modalities move into the mainstream.

... a woman's ability to bear labour pain can be greatly increased by nurturant care and a supportive ambience

MMOC practitioners see that labour pain is normal and that a woman's ability to bear it can be greatly increased by nurturant care and a supportive environmental ambience permeating what Ricardo Jones calls the 'psychosphere' of labour and birth.[6] Patience is the most essential attribute of the MMOC practitioner. In their chapter on Japanese maternity homes in *Birth Models That Work*, Matsuoka and Hinokuma explain midwives' emphasis on 'the importance of waiting': "Waiting does not mean so much time wasted or the time of just enduring pain for a birthing woman. It is a meaningful time, shared by the birthing woman, her family and the midwife together."[15] These midwives consider labour pain to be 'metamorphic': "a necessary process for a birthing woman as she grows into motherhood–to face her own self through the experience of pain." They believe that the comforting presence of the midwife and family members is enough to support the woman to experience this pain in a positive way; the pain is in fact positive because it is *productive* of the baby's birth and the woman's birth as a mother. They also see it as a way for the entire family and friends attending the birth to bond and thus they recognise the actual benefit of long hours of labour. MMOC practitioners are not afraid of labour pain or of watching women experience it; they know that their own calmness facilitates the woman's ability to move through the pain without the anxiety that increases it.

The importance of emotions and intuition

The uterus responds to the mother's emotional state; thus the best care is based not only on measurements and information but also on body knowledge and intuition.[16] In the midwifery model, experiential and emotional knowledge count as much as or more than technical knowledge. Essential attributes of maternity care include empathy, compassion, caring, and loving touch. MMOC practitioners know the importance of '*presence*: the ability to *be* fully with another person, completely attentive and focused, listening with an open heart'.[17]

Essential attributes of maternity care include empathy, compassion, caring, and loving touch

Reflective practice and preservation of knowledge

MMOC practitioners value and work hard to achieve cultural appropriateness and sensitivity, treating women as they wish to be treated and upholding their rights. They rely on introspection and case reviews with colleagues to reflect on what they are doing and they make efforts at improvement on an ongoing basis. They are aware of the de-skilling of obstetricians—who are increasingly taught simply to perform a caesarean for any complication—so they consciously work to learn and to preserve the myriad skills that some midwives and obstetricians have learned and recorded over time that can keep birth normal: massage; external cephalic version; positions and hand maneuvres for breech and twin delivery; variations on upright positions; stair-climbing or using a *rebozo* (shawl) to shake loose a stuck baby; non-medical means of stopping haemorrhage (since drugs are not always available). Such skills, and more, have long been part of the repertoire of traditional midwives in many regions and are consciously sought out by MMOC practitioners.[8,18-20] The midwifery model entails a two-way exchange—each group learns from and teaches the other, with mutual attitudes of respect.

Relationships of midwives and obstetricians: collaboration as key

As I noted above, the midwifery model positions the midwife as the guide and guardian of the normal birth process; her skills should be used to keep birth normal in the vast majority of cases and to identify and treat complications herself if she is qualified, or to seek appropriate medical help when she is not. (Globally, approximately 1% of midwives are male. I note with humour that my use of the word 'she' to apply to midwives in general is generally supported by male midwives themselves, who often tell me that they are very comfortable with developing 'their feminine side.') MMOC obstetricians work respectively and collaboratively with midwives and provide appropriate services for high risk and emergency births.

A midwifery model positions the midwife as the guide

If obstetricians who practise according to the midwifery model, such as those of the Netherlands, receive a client referred by a midwife for a risk or complication that later resolves, they will then re-classify her as normal and *refer her back* to midwifery care because they understand that normal birth is the midwife's specialty, while complicated conditions are theirs.

Community-based, caseload, and one-to-one midwifery: the importance of continuity of care

As illustrated in all of the chapters in *Birth Models That Work*, MMOC practitioners are more likely to be community-based, even if they use hospitals for birth. Their woman-centred ideology is reflected in the priority they place on continuity of care. When continuity of care is reflected in employment models, these may be described as 'team', 'caseload', or 'one-to-one' midwifery. The caseload model of care entails several midwives seeing the mother antenatally, getting to know her, and guaranteeing one of them will be present throughout her labour and birth.[21] The more common practice of hospital-based 'shift midwifery' interferes with full provision of the humanistic model—midwives leave after 8 or 10 hours no matter where the mother is in labour, a situation that can feel disruptive to the labouring mother. This situation can also produce anxiety for the midwife, especially when the midwife who is leaving was providing the midwifery model of care and knows that the midwife replacing her will not, and that the mother will find the sudden switch to technocratic care an unpleasant shock that may interfere with her ability to give birth successfully. But even shift midwifery can constitute a model that works when *all* staff midwives practise the MMOC, as is demonstrated at the Lichfield Maternity Unit described by Walsh,[22] where the departing midwife knows that her client will continue to receive the same kind of nurturant care that she was providing.

As at St George hospital in Sydney, Australia,[23] a number of midwives have found that caseload midwifery is not only better for the mother but also for the midwife—there is less burnout than is found in the 'team' model of care in which a group of midwives share the care of a large number of women. Women in the team system are less likely to build close continuous relationships with a particular midwife, and they are more likely to have midwives they do not know at their birth. The team model provides less continuity of carer and is associated with high levels of burnout for midwives.

'One-to-one' midwifery care means that the same midwife attends a pregnant woman throughout her antenatal, intrapartum, and postpartum care. This ideal, however, is very difficult to achieve—midwives have families and busy lives, and cannot always be present to one mother; caseload midwifery is the next best thing.

Caseload midwifery is the next best thing
to one-to-one care

The phrase 'the midwife follows the mother' means that the mother is free to choose her place of birth—home, freestanding birth centre, or hospital—and the midwife will attend her there. This principle represents an evidence-based ideal that has always been the norm in the Netherlands and was one of the founding principles of the midwifery renaissance in New Zealand[24] and Ontario, Canada.[25] Homes and freestanding birth centres are the places where the MMOC can be most fully applied, yet it is clear that the humanistic/midwifery approach can thrive in highly biomedical environments as well. Again, as Hodnett showed,[26,11] *it is the ideology of the practitioner, not of the society, that has the greatest effect on an individual birth.*

Practitioner education

Health care practitioners tend to practise as they were taught, so much so that when new information is presented, many long-time practitioners refuse to integrate or implement it because they are so habituated to doing things the way their teachers did.[13] A primary key to instilling the MMOC in nascent practitioners is the reform of professional education so that instead of being educated in the technology- and pathology-oriented biomedical approach to birth, student doctors, nurses, and midwives are educated in the humanistic- and normality-oriented midwifery model of birth. Such education is exemplified in medical, midwifery, and nursing training in the Netherlands;[9] in midwifery education in New Zealand[24] and Ontario, Canada,[25] the CASA School in Mexico,[18] in many US midwifery programmes;[27] and in Samoa,[8] where the best of both traditional and professional midwifery are incorporated into an integrated university-based degree that involves traditional midwives as teachers in the programme.

Effective leadership is essential in promoting and maintaining the Midwifery Model of Care

Leadership

In all of the models described in *Birth Models That Work*, effective leadership is essential in promoting and maintaining the MMOC—what Denis Walsh describes as 'a postmodern leadership style':[22]

Prior to [Helen's] coming, the staff structure was very hierarchical and relationships with both women and each other were formal and deferential. Helen ... addressed staff by their first names .... introduced informal visits for women considering booking at the centre .... she relaxed the institutional feel of the centre by deregulating visiting times, abandoning maternal postnatal observations, and morning routines like bed-making. She brought in midwifery-led care by negotiating the withdrawal of General Practitioners from intrapartum care and the setting up of an antenatal clinic at the unit, run by the midwives. She continued the refurbishment of the unit and deregulated staff work patterns. In all of these initiatives, she used a variety of methods in bringing about change. She worked with a supportive GP who mediated the changes in GP practice. With clinical changes, she used a combination of explaining her rationale and leading by example. Other staff were especially interested in upgrading the décor, and she gave them the freedom to lead this initiative. She built a team ethos by organising regular social outings and shared fund-raising activities. She eschewed role demarcations by encouraging all staff to be involved in the upkeep and cleanliness of the facility... "She would never say to us, could you make them a cup of tea? She would clean the kitchen out just like the rest of us" .... Over time, older members of staff who did not like the changes Anita was instituting left to be replaced with new ones who were inducted into the new philosophy.

Walsh notes that characteristics of this postmodern leadership style include flexibility, an integrated and team-based approach, a value on diversity, the aim to empower others, change as a constant, and a focus on people and relationships instead of places and things. His findings resonate with my own description of the 'postmodern midwife':[28]

With this term, I am trying to highlight the qualities that emerge from the practice, the discourse, and the political engagement of a certain kind of contemporary midwife—one who often constructs a radical critique of unexamined conventions and univariate assumptions. Postmodern midwives as I define them are relativistic, articulate, organized, political, and highly conscious of both their cultural uniqueness and their global importance... Postmodern midwives are scientifically informed: they know the limitations and strengths of the biomedical system and of their own, and they can move fluidly between them. These midwives play with the paradigms, working to ensure that the uniquely woman-centred dimensions of midwifery are not subsumed by biomedicine. They are shape-shifters, knowing how to subvert the medical system while appearing to comply with it, bridge-builders, making alliances with biomedicine where possible, and networkers ... [with a sense of mission around preserving and growing midwifery], and an understanding that for a midwife, the professional is always political: midwives and their colleagues must have an organized political voice if they are to survive. So postmodern midwives work to build organisations in their communities, join national and international midwifery organisations, and work within them for policies and legislation that support midwives and the mothers they attend.

Postmodern midwifery and postmodern leadership as I and Walsh describe them are profoundly characteristic of MMOC practitioners. This brand of postmodernism, eschewing hierarchy in favour of relationship and rigidity in favour of flexibility, encourages the levels of creativity, generativity, and out-of-box thinking that are essential to transcending the limits of the technocratic medical model in favour of what really works. In such efforts, the participation of consumers is extraordinarily important.[9,15,22,25,29]

Postmodern midwifery and postmodern leadership are profoundly characteristic of the midwifery model of care

Conclusion

The midwifery model of care, when fully implemented, improves the physiological, psychological, and social outcomes of pregnancy and birth and saves money for systems and families, exposing the need for the total reform of existing dysfunctional hegemonic models. The MMOC issues a clarion call to health organisations and individuals to replace technocratic models that don't work with midwifery models that do, at local, regional, and global levels, in order to reduce maternal and perinatal mortality and morbidity, empower women and their families, and facilitate healthy birth and breastfeeding. The end game of this much-needed ideological shift is healthy mothers and babies who can generate a more conscious and sustainable future for our human family.

**This chapter is revised and adapted from the "Conclusion" to Birth Models That Work (Davis-Floyd et al. 2009).*

Robbie Davis-Floyd is a medical anthropologist specialising in the anthropology of reproduction. An international speaker and researcher, she has given over 500 talks around the world in the past 10 years, and is author of over 80 articles and author, co-author, or co-editor of ten books, including *Cyborg Babies: From Techno-Sex to Techo-Tots* (1998), *Birth as an American Rite of Passage* (2nd edition 2004), *Mainstreaming Midwives: The Politics of Change* (2006), and *Birth Models That Work* (2009). She is Editorial Chair for the International MotherBaby-Friendly Initiative and a Board Member of the International MotherBaby Childbirth Organization (IMBCO).

References

1 Rothman BK, 1982. *In Labor: Women and Power in the Birthplace*. New York: W. W. Norton, p34.

2 Davis-Floyd R, Barclay L, Daviss B, Tritten J, 2009. *Birth Models That Work*. Berkeley and London: University of California Press.

3 Rooks J, 1999. 'The Midwifery Model of Care.' *Journal of Nurse-Midwifery* 44.4:370–74.

4 Davis-Floyd R, 2004 [1992]. *Birth as an American Rite of Passage*. Berkeley and London: University of California Press.

5 Davis-Floyd R, 2001. 'The Technocratic, Humanistic, and Holistic Models of Birth.' *International Journal of Gynecology and Obstetrics* 75, Suppl. no. 1:S5-S23, p15.

6 Jones R, 2009. Teamwork: An Obstetrician, a Midwife, and a Doula in Brazil. In *Birth Models That Work*, eds. R Davis-Floyd, L Barclay, BA Daviss, and J Tritten. Berkeley: University of California Press, pp. 271-304.

7 Wagner M, 1994. *Pursuing the Birth Machine*. Australia: Ace Graphics.

8 Barclay L, 2009. Samoan Midwives' Stories: Joining Social and Professional Midwives in New Models of Birth. In *Birth Models That Work*, eds. R Davis-Floyd, L Barclay, BA Daviss, and J Tritten. Berkeley: University of California Press, pp 119-140.

9 DeVries R, Weigers T, Smulders B, van Teiglingen E, 2009. The Dutch Obstetrical System: Vanguard of the Future in Maternity Care. In *Birth Models That Work*, eds. R Davis-Floyd, L Barclay, BA Daviss, and J Tritten. Berkeley: University of California Press, pp. 31-54.

10 Jordan B, 1993. *Birth in Four Cultures*. Prospect Heights, Ohio: Waveland Press.

11 Hodnett ED, 2002. 'Pain and Women's Satisfaction with the Experience of Childbirth: A Systematic Review.' *American Journal of Obstetrics and Gynecology* 186.5:S160–S172.

12 International MotherBaby Childbirth Initiative, 2008. Created by the International MotherBaby Childbirth Organization in collaboration with the Coalition for Improving Maternity Services and Childbirth Connection. www.imbci.org. p3.

13 Davis-Floyd R and St John G, 1998. *From Doctor to Healer: The Transformative Journey*. New Brunswick, NJ: Rutgers University Press.

14 Rothman BK, 1982. *In Labor: Women and Power in the Birthplace*. New York: W. W. Norton, p48.

15 Matsuoka E, Hinokuma F, 2009. Maternity Homes in Japan: Reservoirs of Normal Childbirth. In *Birth Models That Work*, eds. R Davis-Floyd, L Barclay, BA Daviss, and J Tritten. Berkeley: University of California Press, pp.223-226

16 Davis-Floyd R, and Davis E, 1997. 'Intuition as Authoritative Knowledge in Midwifery and Home Birth.' In *Childbirth and Authoritative Knowledge: Cross-Cultural Perspectives*, edited by R. Davis-Floyd and C. Sargent, 315–49. Berkeley and London: University of California Press.

17 Houston J, Foster J, Davenport A, Anderson A, Romano A, Lamprecht V, Frenkel G. No date. 'Weaving Traditional and Professional Midwifery: Midwives for Midwives in Guatemala.' Unpublished manuscript.

18 Mills L and Davis-Floyd R, 2009. The CASA Hospital and Professional Midwifery School: An Education and Practice Model That Works. In *Birth Models That Work*, eds. R Davis-Floyd, L Barclay, BA Daviss, and J Tritten. Berkeley: University of California Press, pp. 305-336.

19 Penwell V, 2009. Mercy in Action: Bringing Mother- and Baby-Friendly Birth Centers to the Philippines. In *Birth Models That Work*, eds. R Davis-Floyd, L Barclay, BA Daviss, and J Tritten. Berkeley: University of California Press, pp. 337-363.

20 Rattner D, Hamouche Abreu IP, Jose de Olivereira Araujo M, Franca Santos AR, 2009. Humanizing Childbirth To Reduce Maternal and Neonatal Mortality: A National Effort in Brazil. In *Birth Models That Work*, eds. R Davis-Floyd, L Barclay, BA Daviss, and J Tritten. Berkeley: University of California Press, pp. 385-414.

21 Reed B and Walton C, 2009. The Albany Midwifery Practice. In *Birth Models That Work*, eds. R Davis-Floyd, L Barclay, BA Daviss, and J Tritten. Berkeley: University of California Press, pp. 141-158.

22 Walsh D, 2009. Small Really Is Beautiful: Tales from a Freestanding Birth Center in England. In *Birth Models That Work*, eds. R Davis-Floyd, L Barclay, BA Daviss, and J Tritten. Berkeley: University of California Press, pp. 159-186.

23 Brodie P, Homer C, 2009. Transforming the Culture of a Maternity Service: St George Hospital, Sydney, Australia. In *Birth Models That Work*, eds. R Davis-Floyd, L Barclay, BA Daviss, and J Tritten. Berkeley: University of California Press, pp 187-212.

24 Hendry C, 2009. The New Zealand Maternity System: A Midwifery Renaissance. In *Birth Models That Work*, eds. R Davis-Floyd, L Barclay, BA Daviss, and J Tritten. Berkeley: University of California Press, pp 55-88.

25 MacDonald M, Bourgeault I, 2009. The Ontario Midwifery Model of Care. In *Birth Models That Work*, eds. R Davis-Floyd, L Barclay, BA Daviss, and J Tritten. Berkeley: University of California Press, pp 89-118.

26 Hodnett ED, 2001. 'Caregiver Support for Women During Childbirth.' *Cochrane Library,* Issue 4. Cochrane Database Syst Rev. 2002;(1):CD00199.

27 Kennedy H, 2009. 'Orchestrating Normal': The Conduct of Midwifery in the United States. In *Birth Models That Work*, eds. R Davis-Floyd, L Barclay, BA Daviss, and J Tritten. Berkeley: University of California Press, pp. 415-440.

28 Davis-Floyd R, 2005. 'Daughter of Time: The Postmodern Midwife.' *MIDIRS Midwifery Digest* 15.1. 32- 39 <AQ4>, pp.32-33

29 Gilmore E, 2009. The Northern New Mexico Midwifery Model, Taos, New Mexico. In *Birth Models That Work*, eds. R Davis-Floyd, L Barclay, BA Daviss, and J Tritten. Berkeley: University of California Press, pp. 239-269.

The birth centre as a place for normal birth

Susan Rutledge Stapleton

Definition

A birth centre is a freestanding (stand-alone) health care facility that is not a hospital, or it is a midwifery-led unit separate from the acute care obstetric unit of a hospital (alongside), where birth occurs following a normal pregnancy. The definition used by the National Perinatal Epidemiology group for a structured review of birth centre outcomes was:

> *"A birth centre is an institution that offers care to women with a straightforward pregnancy and where midwives take primary professional responsibility for care. During labour and birth medical services, including obstetric, neonatal and anaesthetic care are available should they be needed, but they may be on a separate site, or in a separate building, which may involve transfer by car or ambulance."*[1]

Birth centres are found in many countries, including the United Kingdom, Canada, Scandinavia, Europe, Canada, New Zealand, Australia, Mexico, and Japan. The American Association of Birth Centers (AABC) estimates that there are 200 birth centres in the United States.[2] A 2008 estimate by the National Childbirth Trust suggested that there were approximately 70 freestanding midwife-led units in England and Wales and 50 located alongside an obstetric unit.[3] The birth centre is not, however, merely a place. The definition of birth centre by the American Association of Birth Centers (AABC) includes the following:

Place A maxi-home rather than a mini-hospital

People Childbearing families and maternity care providers working together as a non-hierarchical team.

Programme of care Time- and education-intensive care that begins with the orientation visit and continues through postpartum and breastfeeding. Includes time to get to know mothers and families and understand their concerns and strengths.

Practice of midwifery 'With woman' care and an environment that supports autonomous midwifery.

Part of the system A collaborative model with systems in place for a seamless transition to acute and specialist care, should that be needed.[4]

Philosophy The birth centre philosophy maintains that pregnancy and birth are, until proven otherwise, normal physiological and psychosocial life events. Edwards and Byron describe the "social model of care" that is part of the birth centre philosophy as follows:

> *"Woman-centred care encapsulates terms such as trust, respect, empowerment, facilitation, and working in partnership with the woman and her family to maximise health outcomes. ... The social model acknowledges childbearing as part of the fabric of people's lives. Care is largely community based, linked with other agencies. Social support is recognised to be of equal importance to professional input in influencing outcomes for the woman, her baby and family."*[5]

Birth centre providers and staff

Care in birth centres is most often by midwives. In the United States, the National Center for Health Statistics reported that in 2006 , 0.25% of all births and 28% of all out-of-hospital births occurred in birth centres.[6] These figures under-report the number of women receiving care in birth centres since they do not reflect the women who laboured in birth centres and then gave birth in hospitals after intrapartum transfer. Certified nurse-midwives (CNMs) attended 59% of births that occurred in US birth centres in 2006, while other midwives attended 30%, and obstetricians (or doctors) attended 9%.[7] In other countries birth centres are almost universally midwifery-led units in which midwives take primary professional responsibility for care. Birth centre staff also generally include other professionals such as nurses, doulas, lactation consultants, and perinatal educators. Many birth centres use peer support, such as birth assistants, breastfeeding counsellors and teen mentoring by experienced mothers.

Criteria for birth centre elligibility

Screening begins when the woman enrols for antenatal care at the birth centre. Women who are candidates for birth centre care have no serious pre-existing medical problems such as pre-gestational diabetes, chronic hypertension, or serious psychiatric disorders. Women who have had a previous caesarean delivery are often considered too high risk to give birth in a birth centre; however, this issue is controversial.[8,9] More recently, both the Commission for the Accreditation of Birth Centers (CABC) and the American College of Obstetricians and Gynecologists (ACOG), based on more recent studies, have altered their positions to state that vaginal birth after caesarean (VBAC) may be appropriate and safe for certain women if occurring in freestanding birth centres that meet standards of relevant accrediting organisations, such as the CABC and the Accreditation Association for Ambulatory Health Care.[10] Women with a history of serious obstetric or medical conditions, with an antenatal experience which deviates from normal, or anticipating a birth which has a higher risk of complications than usual (e.g. malpresentation or post-dates pregnancy) are also not appropriate for birth centre care.

This careful screening continues at every antenatal appointment using risk criteria that have been mutually agreed upon by the birth centre providers and their collaborating obstetricians. Women who experience pregnancy complications, such as pre-eclampsia, preterm labour, malpresentation or significant anaemia, are required to give birth in the hospital, where their care may be managed collaboratively by the midwife/consultant team. This collaborative model assures a high level of continuity for those women who develop pregnancy complications.

A woman who is eligible for intrapartum care and birth in the birth centre is one who has a normal, uncomplicated antenatal experience as determined during regular antenatal care and screening, and for whom there is no reason to anticipate a serious complication during labour, as defined by generally accepted criteria of maternal and fetal health. For example, there should be no serious obstetric or medical conditions and a singleton fetus in a cephalic lie with a pregnancy that is neither preterm nor post-term.

Birth centre care

Childbearing families are guided in obtaining the knowledge they need to be active team members, make informed decisions about their care, and maximise their likelihood for a normal pregnancy and birth. Self-care is emphasised, including such activities as measuring one's own blood pressure and weight, and testing for proteinuria. Full access to the health record is provided, a practice that is the norm in some countries, but almost unheard of in the United States health care system. Clients are expected to know, for example, their blood type, baseline blood pressure, uterine growth pattern, gestational age and fetal heart rate range. Group antenatal care is common in birth centres in the United States.

The atmosphere of birth centres is relaxed with the goal of providing a home-like environment in which the mother is in charge and that supports physiological labour and birth. Women determine who will be with them during labour and birth; they take showers or baths; they eat, drink, and change positions as they desire. Interventions are used only as needed and only after discussion of the benefits and risks with the family. After birth, the mother, family and baby are not separated. The newborn examination is done on the mother's bed and used as an opportunity to educate parents and siblings about newborn appearance and behaviour, answer questions, and enhance the process of family bonding.

The birth centre model includes providing access to whatever level of care the mother and baby might need through collaborative relationships. As mentioned before, if complications arise that require medical or surgical intervention, the care of the woman or newborn is transferred to the consultant or neonatologist at the collaborating hospital. The birth centre midwives may continue to manage the mother's intrapartum and postnatal care in collaboration with the consultant. The midwives generally accompany the mother to the hospital, even if they are no longer managing her care, in order to provide support and continuity. Adherence to strict transfer criteria has resulted in good outcomes for these mothers and newborns, even when intrapartum complications occur.[11]

Information about the risks and benefits of childbirth in any setting is included in antenatal education to allow parents to make informed decisions about where they want to give birth. The midwives review unexpected events that can occur during childbirth, including emergencies, and how they would be managed in the birth centre. This discussion includes a list of complications that would require an antenatal referral to the collaborating consultant and/or a transfer of mother or baby during labour or postpartum to the collaborating hospital for care. Arrangements available for access to specialist and acute care for mother and newborn, if needed, are reviewed. Most birth centres conduct regular emergency drills, including drills with area emergency medical service personnel, and thus can tell families how an emergency transfer would proceed and how long the transport would take, depending on road or traffic conditions. Birth centre midwives, because of their constant attention during labour and their skill at anticipating problems, most often accomplish transfer to the hospital in a timely manner. Emergency transports are rare.

Care provided at birth centres is more time- and education-intensive than most consultant-based maternity care. In addition to the usual aspects of antenatal care, the providers in birth centres focus upon building the confidence of the childbearing couple in their ability to give birth and parent their infant. Standard antenatal tests are offered to women by their birth centre providers, as indicated, with information about the rationale, risks and benefits of each test. Such discussions are based upon a belief that the childbearing mother and her family are the leaders of the maternity care team.

Care during labour and birth in the birth centre continues this time-intensive, personalised approach with continuous support in labour by the midwife. Consistent with the evidence indicating that intermittent auscultation of the fetal heart tones is safe and effective for low-risk women,[12,13] birth centres use intermittent auscultation rather than continuous electronic fetal monitoring to monitor the fetus during labour. If the mother develops a condition for which continuous electronic monitoring is indicated, she is transferred to the hospital, as she is no longer considered low-risk.

Some birth centres have narcotic or non-narcotic analgesics available for pain relief during labour; however, pharmacological methods of pain relief are rarely needed and used only after non-pharmacological methods, such as hydrotherapy, position changes, massage, music, aromatherapy, and heat/cold have been tried. Current data from almost 5,500 births in over 60 birth centres in the United States indicate that 91% of mothers used no pharmacological methods of pain relief during labour, while 95% used one or more non-pharmacological methods. Most common among non-pharmacological methods was soaking in a tub of warm water, which was used by 33% of women.[14]

Neither induction or augmentation of labour with drugs nor epidural analgesia are offered in birth centres because of the risks involved with their use and the need for additional interventions, such as intravenous infusions, continuous electronic fetal monitoring, urinary bladder catheterisation, restricted activity, and operative delivery. Mothers needing these interventions are transferred non-urgently to the hospital. An indicated operative vaginal delivery is also considered a reason for transfer to the hospital since it is associated with an increased risk of maternal or neonatal conditions requiring acute care.

Throughout the intrapartum, and immediate postnatal and neonatal periods, risk criteria are continuously reviewed by the midwife to assure that mother and newborn remain appropriate for care in the birth centre. The length of stay in birth centres after birth ranges from 4-12 hours. Since the birth centre is designed as a short-stay facility, mothers or newborns requiring longer direct care and observation are admitted to the hospital for ongoing care.

Follow-up postnatal and newborn care in birth centres generally includes telephone calls, home visits, lactation support, and an office visit within the first two weeks after the birth. Current AABC data show that 72% of women giving birth in birth centres received one home visit, while 8.5% of women had two or more home visits. In addition, 27% of women who were transferred from the birth centre to the hospital in labour or postpartum also received one or more home visits. With a few exceptions, the home visits were made by birth centre staff.[14]

Standards, licensing and accreditation

The National Association of Childbearing Centers (NACC) was established in 1981 (initially as the Cooperative Birth Center Network) to support the development of birth centres in the United States. National standards for birth centres were written in 1983 and these included the criteria for low risk pregnancy and childbirth developed in 1974 by a committee of professionals representing obstetrics, neonatology, nursing, nurse-midwifery, and public health and were based on the best available evidence. In 2005, the organisation changed its name to the American Association of Birth Centers (AABC) (www.birthcenters.org). Blue Cross/ Blue Shield of Greater New York and New York State evaluated these risk criteria over a 16-month period, and validated their use.[15] Those initial criteria defining a low risk pregnancy and birth are currently used almost unchanged by birth centres in the United States.

In 1982, the American Public Health Association published 'Guidelines for the Regulation of Birth Centers' promoting state licensure of birth centres.[16] These guidelines continue to be used by US states to write regulations for licensing birth centres. 78% of US states currently license birth centres.[2]

After exploring mechanisms used by existing accrediting agencies, the newly formed NACC (now AABC) drafted preliminary procedures for national accreditation in 1983. In 1985 the independent Commission for the Accreditation of Birth Centers (CABC) was established. Accreditation is designed as an educational process for evaluating and maintaining quality and safety in birth centres and is comparable to that used by other agencies that accredit health care facilities or hospitals. As of late 2010, 45 US birth centres were accredited by the CABC. A number of US states either require accreditation based upon the *AABC Standards for Birth* Centers[17] or defer the state inspection for the years in which an accreditation site visit was carried out.

The NHS, as part of a comprehensive plan for promoting excellence in maternity services, made a commitment to guarantee childbearing families a choice of place of birth by 2009 that would include home birth, a local midwifery-led unit or birth centre and a hospital obstetric unit with care by a team of providers. This plan includes provisions for smooth transfer of care to an acute care setting if needed by the childbearing woman or her infant.[18]

Evidence supporting the birth centre model

There are no large randomised controlled trials comparing birth centre outcomes to hospital care. Most women are unwilling to be randomised to either an in- or out-of-hospital birth, thus randomised trials to compare the safety and effectiveness of various birth settings are not feasible. Other research designs, such as observational and practice-based research, have been used to provide good evidence on the safety of various birth settings, as described below. No study has reported worse outcomes for women or their infants cared for in birth centres in the United States than among those cared for in hospitals.

Systematic reviews have evaluated some interventions used in maternity care. Several of these interventions appear to be effective and are critical aspects of the birth centre model. They include:

- Antenatal pregnancy and childbirth education for the childbearing family[19,20]
- Continuous support during labour and birth[21]
- Non-pharmacological pain management during labour[22]
- Programmes supporting the initiation and continuation of breastfeeding[23]
- Midwifery-led care[24]

The National Birth Center Study and current data

The AABC maintains an online data registry for the prospective collection of perinatal data. The dataset currently holds data on over 40,000 pregnancies and nearly 25,000 births from 75 midwifery-led practices in the United States. The organisation also conducted the largest prospective study of birth centre care: the National Birth Center Study (NBCS).[25-28] This study reported on almost 18,000 women who had care at 84 birth centres in 35 states across the United States from 1985 to 1987. Data analysis was carried out on an intent-to-treat basis, thus women and infants transferred from the birth centres to the hospital were followed. Major findings of this study and from current registry data are as follows:

- **Transfer rates**

  In the NBCS, 14% of women who received antenatal care at a birth centre developed an antenatal complication that precluded out-of-hospital birth. Almost 90% of these complications occurred during the third trimester, the most common being post-term pregnancy. 12% of women admitted in labour to the birth centre were transferred to a hospital before giving birth. After birth, 4% of women and 4% of newborns were transferred to a hospital because of postnatal or newborn complications. Only 2.4% of all transfers were considered emergencies. The most common reasons for intrapartum transfer were failure to progress (43%), meconium stained amniotic fluid (11%), and non-reassuring fetal heart rate (8%).

- **Caesarean delivery rate**

  In the NBCS the caesarean delivery rate for women admitted to the birth centre in labour was 4.4% compared to a national average during the study period (1985 to 1987) of 24.4%. These deliveries occurred among the 12% of women transferred from a birth centre to a hospital during labour. Current AABC data indicate that among over 8,600 women admitted to a birth centre in labour, including those who were transferred to the hospital, from 2005-2010, 5.2% had a caesarean section.[9] The national caesarean delivery rate for the United States in 2007 was 31.8%.[29]

- **Infant mortality**

  Intrapartum and neonatal mortality in the NBCS was 1.3/1000 births (15/11,826 births); seven deaths were due to lethal congenital anomalies resulting in a corrected Intrapartum and neonatal mortality of 0.7/1000 births.[24] By comparison, low risk women delivering in three US hospitals had intrapartum and neonatal mortality rates of 1.0 to 4.3/1000 births.[27, 28]

- **Breastfeeding**

  In the NBCS, 78% of women who gave birth in a birth centre breastfed their infants, compared to a national rate at the time of 53% to 56%.[26] Current AABC data showed that 97% of women giving birth in a birth centre from 2005-2010 initiated exclusive breastfeeding, while another 1.2% combined breastfeeding with formula feeding. Only 1.3% did not breastfeed at all. In national US data, 75% of women initiated breastfeeding in 2007.[30] 85% of almost 5,000 women who gave birth in a birth centre from 2005-2010 and were seen for a 6-week postnatal visit were exclusively breastfeeding their infants. Another 1.3% were breastfeeding while sometimes giving formula. Only 5.8% of women were exclusively formula feeding at 6-weeks postpartum.[12]

Other studies

There have been a number of prospective and retrospective studies of care and outcomes in freestanding birth centres or alongside midwifery-led units in England,[31] Germany,[32] Norway,[33] Sweden,[35-37] Italy,[38] Brazil,[39] Australia,[40, 41] and the United States.[42-44] These studies have generally found that, with appropriately selected patients, these sites achieve perinatal outcomes comparable to, or better than, those for in-hospital care, with fewer intrapartum interventions and high rates of patient satisfaction. Systematic reviews have also affirmed the safety of birth centre care for low-risk pregnancies.[1,45,46]

One study compared the outcome of hospital-based midwifery care to the outcome of birth centre midwifery care in over 2,000 low-risk women. Women in both sites experienced similar rates of antepartum and intrapartum complications, but women whose care was by midwives *in hospitals* had more interventions during labour and birth. Major neonatal outcomes were similar for both groups, although the incidences of fetal distress, cord prolapse, and difficulty establishing respiration were significantly higher in the hospital group.[47] The authors noted that the hospital environment appears to promote an interventionist style of intrapartum management regardless of the provider.

Several studies, as well as cost data from the AABC member birth centres for the past 30-years, have shown that a normal birth in a birth centre is approximately 30-50% of the cost of a normal hospital birth in the same community.[48, 49, 50] Authors of a study of women giving birth at the National Health Service Edgware Birth Centre in England concluded that the mean cost to the health service of a woman giving birth there was £392.30, compared to £608.90 and £635.81 respectively at the two local acute obstetric units in the year 2000.[51]

Conclusions

The birth centre philosophy maintains that pregnancy and birth are normal physiological and psychosocial, events within a family. Midwives provide antenatal, intrapartum, and postnatal care at birth centres in a setting that is relaxed, more like a home than a hospital, and where the mother is in charge. Birth centre care is appropriate for women who are at low risk of developing maternal or fetal/neonatal complications antepartum, intrapartum, or postpartum. Observational studies have shown that midwives at birth centres can identify women who are at low risk for obstetric complications and provide care safely in the out-of-hospital setting. Birth centre care is less expensive than hospital maternity care, and achieves higher levels of patient satisfaction. Maternal and neonatal outcomes are comparable to those for low risk women cared for in traditional consultant- and hospital-based maternity care, but with fewer interventions and fewer caesarean deliveries, and higher rates of breastfeeding. As the authors of the NBCS concluded, "Few innovations in health service promote lower cost, greater availability, and a high degree of satisfaction with a comparable degree of safety. The results of this study suggest that modern birth centres can identify women who are at low risk for obstetric complications and care for them in a way that provides these benefits."[25]

Susan Rutledge Stapleton founded the Reading Birth & Women's Center in Reading, Pennsylvania, and was Director of that practice for 25 years, attending births in a freestanding birth centre, the hospital and mothers' homes. She is President of the Commission for the Accreditation of Birth Centers, the only national accrediting body for birth centres in the United States. She is also Chair of the Research Committee of the American Association of Birth Centers, and headed the task force to develop an AABC online perinatal data registry, the *Uniform Data Set*. She is currently primary investigator for the AABC multicentre, prospective *National Study of Optimal Birth.*

References

1 Stewart, M., McCandlish, R., Henderson, J. Brockhurst, P. *Review of evidence about clinical, psychosocial and economic outcomes for women with straightforward pregnancies who plan to give birth in a midwife-led birth center, and outcomes for their babies. Report of a structured review of birth center outcomes.* Oxford: National Perinatal Epidemiology Unit; 2005. http://www.npeu.ox.ac.uk/files/downloads/reports/Birth-Center-Review.pdf [Accessed September 12, 2010].

2 Personal Communication with Kate Bauer, Executive Director, American Association of Birth Centers. Perkiomenville, PA, November, 2010.

3 National Childbirth Trust. NCT Briefing: Midwife-led units, community maternity units and birth centers. August, 2008. http://www.nctpregnancyandbabycare.com/_.../MS2Midwife-ledunits.pdf [Accessed October 1, 2010].

4 American Association of Birth Centers. *How to Start a Birth Center Workshop Manual: Exploring Innovation in Maternity Care.* Perkiomenville, PA. March 2010.

5 Edwards G., Byron, S. editors. *Essential Midwifery Practice: Public Health.* Oxford: Blackwell Publishing; 2007, page 209.

6 MacDorman, M., Menacker, F., Declercq, E. Trends and characteristics of home and other out-of-hospital births in the United States, 1990–2006. National vital statistics reports: 58(11). Hyattsville, MD: National Center for Health Statistics. 2010.

7 Births: Final Data (annual reports). National vital statistics reports. Hyattsville, MD: National Center for Health Statistics. http://www.cdc.gov/nchs/births.htm [Accessed November 2, 2010].

8 Lieberman E., Ernst, E., Rooks, J., Stapleton, S., Flamm, B. Results of the national study of vaginal birth after cesarean in birth centers. *Obstetrics and Gynecology.* 2004; 104(5, Part 1):933-42. http://journals.lww.com/greenjournal/Fulltext/2004/11000/Emergency_Peripartum_HysterectomyExperience_at_a.9.aspx# [Accessed September, 2010].

9 Albers, L. Safety of VBAC's in birth centers: choices and risks. *Birth* 32 (3): September 2005. http://www.birthgirlz.com/.../Birth_Leah_Albers_review_of_VBAC_study.pdf

10 News, Birth 2007; 34:352.

11 DeJong, R.,Shy,K.,Carr,K., An out-of-hospital birth center using university referral. *Obstetrics and Gynecology*, 1981;58(6):703-7.

12 American College of Nurse Midwives. Clinical Practice Bulletin No. 9. March 2007. http://www.midwife.org/memberFiles/education/jmwh_clinical_practice_bulletin.pdf [Accessed December 2010].

13 Alfirevic Z, Devane D, Gyte GML. Continuous cardiotocography (CTG) as a form of electronic fetal monitoring (EFM) for fetal assessment during labour. Cochrane Database of Systematic Reviews 2006, Issue 3. Art. No.: CD006066. DOI: 10.1002/14651858.CD006066. http://www2.cochrane.org/reviews/en/ab006066.html [Accessed December 2010].

14 Stapleton, S. Presentation at the American Association of Birth Centers' Birth Institute, *35,000 and Rising - Report of Preliminary UDS Data and Validation Study.* Newport Beach, CA. September, 2010.

15 Blue Cross and Blue Shield of Greater New York. Maternity Center Association's Childbearing Center: 1976-1977 Cost Analysis. Health Affairs Research, New York 1978.

16 American Public Health Association. Guidelines for Licensing and Regulating Birth Centers. American Journal of Public Health 1983; 73. http://www.birthcenters.org/pdf/apha_guidelines.pdf [Accessed September, 2010].

17 American Association of Birth Centers. *Standards for Birth Centers.* Perkiomenville, PA. 2003.

18 Department of Health, National Health Service. *Maternity Matters: choice, access and continuity of care in a safe service.* London. 2007. http://www.dh.gov.uk/prod_consum_dh/groups/dh_digitalassets/@dh/@en/documents/digitalasset/dh_074199.pdf. [Accessed November, 2010].

19 National Institutes of Health. US Preventative Health Service. Caring for Our Future: the Content of Prenatal Care. A Report of the Public Health Service Expert Panel on the Content of Prenatal Care. Bethesda, MD. 1989.

20 Gregory K, Johnson C., Johnson T., Entman S. The content of prenatal care: update 2005. *Women's Health Issues.* 16(4), July 2006: 198-215.

21 Hodnett E., Gates S., Hofmeyer G., Saklaa C. Continuous support for women during childbirth. *Cochrane Database of Systematic Reviews.* 2007, Issue 3. Art. No.: CD003766. DOI: 10.1002/14651858.CD003766.pub2. http://www.childbirthconnection.org/pdfs/continuous_support.pdf [Accessed September 12, 2010].

22 Simkin P., O'Hara M. Nonpharmacologic relief of pain during labor: systematic reviews of five methods. *American Journal of Obstetrics and Gynecology.* May 2002; 186(5 Supplement): S131-59.

23 Sikorski J., Renfrew M., Pindoria S., Wade A. Support for breastfeeding mothers: a systematic review. *Paedriatric and Perinatal Epidemiology* 17(4) October 2003: 407-17.

24 Hatem, M., Sandall, J., Devane. D., Soltani, H., Gates, S. (2008) Midwife-led versus other models of care for childbearing women. *Cochrane Database of Systematic Reviews*, Issue 4. Art. No.: CD004667. DOI:10.1002/14651858.CD004667.pub2.

25 Rooks J., Weatherby N., Ernst E., Stapleton S; Rosen D; Rosenfield A. Outcomes of care in birth centers: The National Birth Center Study. New England Journal of Medicine; 321(26):1804-11. http://www.nejm.org/doi/pdf/10.1056/NEJM198912283212606 [Accessed June, 2010].

26 Rooks, JP, Weatherby, NL, Ernst, EK. The National Birth Center Study. Part I–Methodology and prenatal care and referrals. *Journal of Nurse Midwifery* 1992; 37:222.

27 Rooks, JP, Weatherby, NL, Ernst, EK. The National Birth Center Study. Part II–Intrapartum and immediate postpartum and neonatal care. *Journal of Nurse Midwifery* 1992; 37:301.

28 Rooks, JP, Weatherby, NL, Ernst, EK. The National Birth Center Study. Part III–Intrapartum and immediate postpartum and neonatal complications and transfers, postpartum and neonatal care, outcomes, and client satisfaction. *Journal of Nurse Midwifery* 1992; 37:361.

29 Hamilton B., Martin J., and Ventura S. (2009). Births: Preliminary data for 2007. National vital statistics reports, Web release; 57(12). Hyattsville, MD: National Center for Health Statistics. Released March 18, 2009. http://www.cdc.gov/nchs/data/nvsr/nvsr57/nvsr57_12.pdf [Accessed December 13, 2009].

30 United States Centers for Disease Control and Prevention (CDC). *Breastfeeding Report Card -- United States, 2010.* http://www.cdc.gov/breastfeeding/pdf/BreastfeedingReportCard2010.pdf [Accessed November 11, 2010].

31 Reddy K., Reginald P., Spring J., Nunn L., Mishra N. A freestanding low-risk maternity unit in the United Kingdom: does it have a role? *Journal of Obstetrics and Gynaecology.* June 2004;24(4):360-6.

32 David M., von Schwarzenfeld H., Dimer J., Kentenich H. Perinatal outcome in hospital and birth center obstetric care. *International Journal of Gynaecology and Obstetrics.* May 1999;65(2):149-56.

33 Schmidt N., Abelson B., Oian P. Deliveries in maternity homes in Norway: results from a 2-year prospective study. *Acta Obstetrics and Gynecology of Scandinavia.* August 2002; 81(8):731-7.

34 Waldenstrom, U, Nilsson, CA, Winbladh, B. The Stockholm birth center trial: maternal and infant outcome. *British Journal of Obstetrics and Gynaecology* 1997; 104:410.

35 Waldenstrom, U, Nilsson, CA. A randomized controlled study of birth center care versus standard maternity care: effects on women's health. *Birth* 1997; 24:17.

36 Waldenstrom, U, Nilsson, CA. Experience of childbirth in birth center care. A randomized controlled study. *Acta Obstetrics and Gynecology of Scandinavia* 1994; 73:547.

37 Gottvall, K, Grunewald, C, Waldenstrom, U. Safety of birth center care: perinatal mortality over a 10-year period. *British Journal of Obstetrics and Gynaecology* 2004; 111:71.

38 Morano, S, Cerutti, F, Mistrangelo, E, Pastorino, D., Benussi M., Costantini S., Ragni N. Outcomes of the first midwife-led birth center in Italy: 5 years' experience. *Archives in Gynecology and Obstetrics* 2007; 276:333.

39 Campos, S, Lana, F. Results of childbirth care at a birthing center in Belo Horizonte, Minas Gerais, Brazil]. *Cadernos de Saude Publica (Reports in Public Health)* 2007; 23:1349.

40 Byrne, JP, Crowther, CA, Moss, JR. A randomised controlled trial comparing birthing center care with delivery suite care in Adelaide, Australia. *Australian and New Zealand Journal of Obstetrics and Gynaecology* 2000; 40:268.

41 Tracy, SK, Dahlen, H, Caplice, S, et al. Birth centers in Australia: a national population-based study of perinatal mortality associated with giving birth in a birth center. *Birth* 2007; 34:194.

42 Jackson, DJ, Lang, JM, Swartz, WH, Ganiats TG, Fullerton J, Ecker J, Nguyen U. Outcomes, safety, and resource utilization in a collaborative care birth center program compared with traditional physician-based perinatal care. *American Journal of Public Health* 2003; 93:999.

43 Eakins, PS. Free-standing birth centers in California. Program and medical outcome. Journal of Reproductive Medicine 1989; 34:960.

44 Garite TJ, Snell BJ, Walker DL, Darrow VC. Development and experience of a university-based, freestanding birth center. *Obstetrics and Gynecology* 1995; 86:411.

45 Hodnett, ED, Downe, S, Edwards, N, Walsh, D. Home-like versus conventional institutional settings for birth. Cochrane Database Syst Rev 2005; :CD000012.

46 Stewart, M, McCandlish, R, Henderson, J, and Brocklehurst, P. Report of a Structured Review of Birth Center Outcomes. National Perinatal Epidemiology Unit, Oxford University, December, 2004. (Revised July, 2005).

47 Fullerton, JT, Severino, R. In-hospital care for low-risk childbirth. Comparison with results from the National Birth Center Study. *Journal of Nurse Midwifery* 1992; 37:331.

48 Swartz, W, Jackson, D, Lang, J, Ecker J.,Ganiats T., Dickinson, C.,Nguyen U. The BirthPlace collaborative practice model: results from the San Diego Birth Center Study. Primary Care Update for Obstetricians and *Gynecologists* 1998; 5:207.

49 Health Insurance Association of America. Research Bulletin: The Cost of Maternity care in the United States, Washington DC, 1989.

50 American Association of Birth Centers. Biannual Surveys of Birth Center Operations. Perkiomenville, PA 2006.

51 Saunders D, Boulton M, Chapple J et al. *Evaluation of the Edgware Birth Center.* Edgware: Barnet Health Authority; 2000.

pause to think and talk...

...about birth centres and MLUs (midwifery-led units)

1 Do you think it makes a difference whether a birth centre is stand-alone or attached to a large maternity unit? If you think there are any differences, what are these in terms of atmosphere, facilities, staff and equipment?

2 Where should a free-standing birth centre ideally be situated in a town or village? How should it be presented and marketed to residents of that area? What should the outside look like? Should there be soundproofing?

3 How is it possible to make a birth centre of any kind 'home-like'?

4 Consider the kind of décor you think most appropriate for a birth centre:

- ♥ in the reception area
- ♥ in the main labouring rooms
- ♥ in rooms where family and friends wait
- ♥ in rooms which are only reserved for birth centre staff

Think in terms of colour, light/lighting and materials/textures, as well as in terms of features (e.g. curtains vs blinds, flowers, equipment).

5 What kind of food and drink should be provided for pregnant and labouring women (and their companions), in your view, and how freely should they be given access to meals, snacks and refreshments?

6 How should pregnant women be prepared for labour and birth in a birth centre? To what extent do they need to feel 'at home' in the environment and how could this potentially be achieved? What do you think of Michel Odent's practice (when he was manager of the maternity unit in Pithiviers, near Paris) of holding weekly singing sessions for pregnant women and new mothers in the unit where labour and birth also took place?

7 Do you think murals, paintings and wall hangings are helpful in a birth centre? If so, what kind of imagery is most appropriate and facilitative of normal birth? Should clients be able to bring in their own artwork?

8 Could or should testimonials from past clients be part of the display which pregnant women see when they visit a birth centre? What role could photos also play? Do TVs and books help or hinder birthing processes?

9 Taking into account the fact that people can potentially come and go freely when women labour and birth at home, what kinds of policies should there be in a birth centre towards birth companions? Should any limit be placed on numbers? If free access is given, how can an atmosphere of privacy also be sustained around labouring women?

10 How freely do you think midwives working within a birth centre should welcome other professionals—e.g. obstetricians, GPs and doulas? Should appointments be encouraged or stipulated, or free access allowed? What would the advantages and disadvantages be of each policy?

Promoting home birth in accordance with the best scientific evidence

Ole Olsen

Birth can be a joyous and miraculous event. It creates and extends a family and can bring pride and happiness. And it can also be a highly emotional experience. At its best it is an undisturbed, relaxed, intense, private, friendly, and perhaps even sexual experience. All good reason to choose a home birth. So does anyone care about science and statistics in that context? The media does not. Too many obstetricians do not. But quite a few pregnant women and their partners do care about science. They wonder if the dream birth is safe and secure.

When my wife got pregnant with our first child 20 years ago, she had already discussed the possibilities of a home birth with a close friend who had planned a home birth. I thought it might be a good idea—but I also wondered how much more dangerous it might be compared to a planned hospital birth. I had heard about all the advantages that you can read about later on in this book. But I had also heard many people say that it could very well turn out to be dangerous and that it was an irresponsible and selfish choice which disregarded the importance of that baby's health. I needed to find out about the statistical evidence.

As a statistician working in a medical environment, I imagined that it would be fairly easy to find some reliable statistics. Not so. On the contrary, I discovered it had been a field of heavy controversy for a century[1] or more. So I decided (after our son's birth) to apply for some funding and do a systematic review of the safety of planned home birth compared to planned hospital birth for pregnant women without serious complications living in the Western world in settings with experienced homebirth attendants available. In other words, I wanted to do a comparison that reflected our own situation as closely as possible.

As a statistician I imagined it would be fairly easy to find some reliable statistics. No so! It was a field of controversy.

Midwives and doulas who want to promote home birth also need to know a bit about the statistics. Not because they should expect to be able to convince any obstetricians, journalists or policy makers about the safety and the benefits of a planned home birth by means of the existing scientific facts—but in order to be prepared for discussion. History has shown that most obstetricians in most countries and most journalists are immune to even the best scientific studies. They often prefer pre-scientific thinking and stories with a scary, dramatic twist. But if you want to be prepared for a discussion about the safety of home birth, please read on here.

Statistics, safety and science

Back in the 1990s I identified six comparative studies of sufficient scientific quality from Australia, the United States, England, The Netherlands and Switzerland.[2] The perinatal mortality rate was very low for these selected uncomplicated pregnancies and the rate of interventions was generally lower in the homebirth group. My conclusion was that there was 'no significant difference in perinatal mortality' when I compared women who had planned a home birth with similar women who had planned a hospital birth; the confidence interval was not compatible with extreme excess risks in any of the groups (odds ratio 0.87, 95% confidence interval 0.54 to 1.41). Overall, the best available evidence in the 1990s did not provide any strong reason to promote either home or hospital birth at the cost of the other.[2]

Since then several much larger studies have been published, which more or less studied the same question. First of all, the Dutch finally published data to show the comparative safety for approximately half a million Dutch births preselected to be low risk according to the Dutch system.[3] Nobody else can provide such extensive, comparable and well registered data because no other country has home birth as such an integral part of the health care system and no other country has a homebirth rate of around 30%; in most other developed countries it is around or below 1%. The Dutch study shows that various measures of perinatal mortality are comparable and that no significant differences are found between planned home and planned hospital birth. When the comparisons are adjusted for parity, gestational age, maternal age, socioeconomic status and ethnic background the observed difference in mortality is very, very small and the direction of the difference depends on the exact choice of measure (relative risks in the range 0.97-1.02). It is difficult to imagine a closer race between planned home and planned hospital birth. Thus, we can be fairly sure that there are no good reasons, as far as perinatal mortality is concerned, to promote either hospital or home birth.

What about other potential harms to mother or baby, such as lacerations or birth trauma? The Dutch did not report them. But as most morbidity outcomes are much more common than perinatal death, we do not need such large studies to reach statistical certainty. Several good comparative studies have been carried out recently. The largest one[4] comprises more planned home births than the aggregate of all studies included in my old meta-analysis. It shows that all measures of serious maternal morbidity were lower in the planned homebirth group, typically 10-30% lower and that rates for all interventions were lower, typically 20-60%. The study did not report on birth trauma to the newborn, but another large study[5] showed that birth trauma was three times as frequent in the hospital birth group (involving, for example, cerebral haemorrhage; fractures of the clavicle, long bones or skull; fascial nerve injury or nerve injury affecting movement of a child's shoulder, arm, and hand). One might well hypothesise that the higher amount of birth trauma occurring in hospital environments is caused by the high number of interventions during birth in the planned hospital birth group.

Other potential harms to mother or baby were not reported

Maybe the results of the statistical studies should not come as a surprise, at least not to a biologist. Natural selection should be expected to have selected those individuals who are able to reproduce, and this should be particularly true for a species, like ours, which has a low number of offspring. Many animals will seek a quiet and undisturbed environment for birth. Any danger or disturbance will (for good reasons) halt the birth process; equally so for a planned transportation to hospital followed by an ongoing 'meet-new-people' ceremony. Finally, bacteria in the natural environment will usually be non-threatening whereas a move to a new environment will challenge the immune system with new infectious threats. In relation to birth this is more of a challenge because the immune system of the baby is mainly supplied from the mother during the last part of pregnancy and later through breastfeeding.

But is a planned home birth with an experienced homebirth caregiver backed up by a well equipped hospital department always a better solution than a planned hospital birth? The first part of the answer lies with the condition that there should be an experienced homebirth caregiver in attendance. The comparative studies that I have quoted all demand some sort of experienced homebirth caregiver. Caregivers, of whatever kind (whether midwife, nurse-midwife, family doctor or obstetrician), will usually not agree to attend what they would consider to be high risk births at home. However, their selection criteria vary and are based on a range of factors, including their experience, national legislation, proximity and collaboration with hospitals. Of course, this means that for cases where all experienced homebirth caregivers consider it too risky to plan for a home birth, we will never get the statistics to prove or disprove the validity of their judgement. Thus, at the moment we only have evidence available to promote planned home birth as the better solution for fairly uncomplicated pregnancies.

Science as a battlefield?

As I wrote in the introduction, most obstetricians, politicians and media are not willingly convinced by science and statistics. They seem to prefer narratives, tales and stories filled with fear, danger, blood, high costs and death—and on top of that: distorted science.

A recent example to substantiate this claim is a press release with the heading 'Planned home births associated with tripling of neonatal mortality rate vs planned hospital births', based on the article 'Maternal and newborn outcomes in planned home birth vs planned hospital births: a metaanalysis'.[6] It immediately influenced newspaper headlines in many countries. When I first read the press release I was baffled. The press release and the conclusion immediately evoked a feeling that something was not right. How could these results in any way be compatible with the results from the extremely large Dutch study[3] published just one year earlier? People who knew the existing research about homebirth safety could only be surprised. If the extremely large Dutch study had been included in the metaanalysis its relative size compared to all other studies would have meant that the overall result in the metaanalysis would have been determined almost solely by the Dutch results. So either the Dutch study was not included in the metaanalysis or the metaanalysis was somehow flawed. In either case the outcome of the metaanalysis and the press release would be misleading—and this was indeed the case, as we shall soon see. Nevertheless, the lay press, *The Lancet*[7] and the *BMJ*[8] presented the conclusions of the metaanalysis without asking any critical questions.

A quick inspection of the metaanalysis showed that many basic errors had been made

A quick inspection of the metaanalysis showed that many basic errors had been made when the study was conducted, that the presentation of the analysis was far from transparent, and that the large Dutch study seemed to have been left out in the comparisons of neonatal mortality rates, without reason. This led to a flood of letters to the editors, some of which were published.[9,10] However, the journal in which the paper was originally published seemed reluctant to publish any critique of the original paper and seemed even more reluctant to correct the errors or retract the paper, as was suggested.[11]

This willingness to distort science is not something new among obstetricians, nor is the reluctance to get the errors corrected. And, unfortunately, these attitudes are not restricted to home birth. In relation to ultrasound screening of all pregnancies the most promising study turned out to be based on a distortion of the scientific findings.[12] It took more than 16 years, and the efforts of many activist scientists, to get the full manuscript published. For years the first author resisted strong pressure to publish while at the same time the misleading data was included in non-Cochrane meta-analyses and misled public health policy all over the world. Nevertheless, the first author was elected world president for the International Society of Ultrasound in Obstetrics and Gynecology even though, during his entire career, he had acted against good scientific practice. In 1984 he stated in several places that he would actively work against any regulations on the use of the new technique. In 1987 he was brought to the Norwegian Council on Medical Ethics, and in 1989 he was found guilty of having campaigned for the introduction of a new service by claiming, contrary to his best knowledge, that all fetal developmental deviations could be discovered by ultrasound and subsequently treated and thus that it would be unethical not to make this service publicly accessible. In 1990 he was accused of underreporting scientific results, then in 2000 the Norwegian Council on Scientific Dishonesty described his work as 'poor workmanship' and 'contrary to good research practice'. All reported outcome data were changed in the full publication, which—as I said—had been delayed for 16 years, and all changes were in the direction of reducing the claimed benefit of screening, Several of the changes to the final paper were significant.

This man's work was described as 'poor workmanship'

In the case of another high-tech intervention (Doppler ultrasound in high risk pregnancies) the most promising study was excluded from the relevant Cochrane review soon after the senior author of the study was accused of several cases of fraud and after he had been unable to verify the published data included in the Cochrane review.[13] Nonetheless, the outdated Cochrane review was used as an argument for the introduction of the technology in Denmark with the words: "It is a very long time ago that a diagnostic test procedure with such a dramatic effect has been ready for implementation" (my translation). This claim was made despite the fact that the significant effect in the first Cochrane review had completely disappeared in the updated version.[13] As in the routine ultrasound screening example above, the senior author was not just any ordinary doctor: he had prominently acted as an associate editor at the *British Journal of Obstetrics and Gynaecology* while his non-verifiable research had been published. In the leading Danish medical journal the outdated review was promoted in an editorial despite the fact that the misleading review had already been excluded from the Cochrane review and a less promising update had been published.[13]

Thus, it seems that even the most prominent obstetricians have a strong will to promote high-tech interventions, while at the same time opposing the safety of home birth. And they seem willing to do so irrespective of the means needed to achieve their aims. What's more, the media often willingly promote their 'facts' and the associated view on the world. Why is this the case?

A UK sociologist, Furedi,[14] points out that Western societies seem to have become dominated by a 'culture of fear'. We have never been so safe, yet never have we been so fearful. The need to 'be careful' dominates our cultural imagination. According to Furedi, we belong to "a culture that continually inflates the danger and risks facing people". He goes on to say that "Activities that were hitherto seen as healthy and fun ... are now declared to be major health risks". He even says that "to ignore safety advice is to transgress the new moral consensus". A US sociologist, Glassner,[15] adds that "The scope of our health fears seems limitless ... we continue to fret over already refuted dangers". He explains that the main reason for these attitudes is "that producers of TV news magazines routinely let emotional accounts trump objective information". But he also adds that "a wide array of groups, including business, advocacy organisations ... and political parties, promote and profit from scares." Glassner concludes that immense power and money await those who tap into people's fears.

However, Glassner adds that despite the fact that "of the several institutions most culpable for creating and sustaining scares the news media are arguably first among equals". He also says they are also the most promising candidates for positive change. "News organisations are distinguished from other fear-mongering groups because they sometimes bite the scare that feeds them".[15] Maybe we will have to accept that the best choice of birthplace can only be communicated in subgroups via the Internet and only maintained by strong and self-confident caregivers who are able to stay out of mainstream healthcare while still maintaining friendly, professional relationships with independent mainstream obstetricians for cases where a transfer might be needed.

Or maybe it is time to reclaim science?—to liberate science from those who seem to see science mainly as a means to promote their own personal career and their own subspecialty at the cost of patients, women, colleagues and other medical subspecialties. Maybe it is time instead to use science to solve real problems and to promote good solutions?—and thereby maybe also motivate the news media to 'bite the scare that feeds them'?

Science as a way forward?

The evidence based on observational studies in favour of home birth is now so strong that it could hardly get any better. Given all these benefits of home birth, with no inherent dangers for mothers or babies, it is probably time to promote home birth more actively. However, any sceptical obstetrician may (and will), of course, claim that self selection into the planned home birth group is so strong that it explains all the observed benefits. On the other hand, the same sceptics must also admit that selection may only explain part of the difference, or none at all. The usual way of reaching agreement in contemporary medicine is to set up a randomised trial. In this case that would mean offering healthy women with a normal pregnancy information about the results from the best observational studies, the potential benefits and harms from a planned home birth and the potential benefits and harms from a planned hospital birth and finally to invite any woman who could not make up her mind as to where to give birth to participate in the trial.

Would that be possible? It has been a common assumption that the obvious place to set up such a trial would be in the Netherlands.[16] I disagree. It is the least obvious place. Women in the Netherlands are already well-informed and they have the freedom to choose a planned home birth or a planned hospital birth as they please. They live in a culture where they have already considered both options and know about them from family and friends prior to their own first pregnancy. So why should Dutch women be in doubt? They very rarely are. Nevertheless, it seems to come as something of a surprise to the authors of the Dutch trial (many obstetricians and no midwives) that women "highly value their autonomy", "want to decide themselves" and thus did not join the trial.[16] In a critical commentary following the paper, emeritus professor in medical ethics, Raanan Gillon, states that "the interest of the individual patient [here: the pregnant woman] should always be put ahead of the interest of science".[16]

On the other hand, outside the Netherlands, in countries where few home births take place, a trial would make sense. It would provide many women with useful information; it would give them options they had never thought of before; and it would give them a chance to think and discuss these options, their benefits and drawbacks. And if the women—after discussion with partner, family and friends, and maybe after additional talks with professionals—still could not make up their minds, they would be offered entry into a randomised trial. Under these circumstances participation in a trial would not overrule autonomy or personal decisions.

Actually, when the pros and the cons are on such incomparable scales and in such different dimensions, it is very human to leave decision-making to the dice, to allow oneself to be relieved from the heavy burden of decision-making. Caesar did so when he pondered whether to cross Rubicon or not (*ālea iacta est*—"the die has been cast"), and the same aleatoric principle has for long been known as an instrument for decision making in one of the oldest classical Chinese texts, the *I Ching*, though it involved flipping coins or throwing yarrow stalks rather than throwing a dice.

Ethical committee approvals of RCTs have previously been obtained in the Netherlands[16] and in the UK.[17] Professional caregivers have been involved in setting up these trials. All that we need is to find a setting that will fully respect pregnant women and their preferred type of decision-making.

In this trial it would be essential to present the most useful information and the best evidence about planned home and planned hospital birth, to offer both standard hospital care and homebirth care in an atmosphere of professional collaboration and, throughout the process, to respect the pregnant women's autonomy and integrity. In this way, as well as contributing to the evidence on the effects and side-effects of the two places of birth, it would be possible to study the role of information and collaboration in the decision-making process.

Implications for the organisation of healthcare

As yet, there is no strong evidence in favour of hospital birth for selected, low-risk pregnant women. Observational studies suggest that planned home birth may lead to fewer complications, fewer interventions and fewer neonatal problems. Whether further research is needed is a matter of judgement. If policy planners wish to make recommendations or restrict individual women's choice, further trials must be carried out prior to such steps.

As yet, there is no strong evidence in favour of hospital birth for selected, low-risk pregnant women

In countries and areas where it is possible to establish a homebirth service backed up by a modern hospital system, low-risk pregnant women should be offered the possibility of considering a planned home birth and they should be informed about the quality of the available evidence to guide their choice.

Ole Olsen is a mathematical statistician by education and has a research career mainly with issues related to public health, e.g. screening, occupational health or childbirth. He has noticed that every entry into a new field is also an entry into a new professional context with dogmas, hierarchies and fights. One question repeatedly crops up: which 'established truths' are based on science and which are based on traditions or power? He has also taught evidence-based medicine (and scepticism in general) to midwives, doctors, physiotherapists and nurses for many years. He has two children, both of whom were born at home.

References

1 Tew M. Safer Childbirth?: A Critical History of Maternity Care. Chapman and Hall 1990.

2 Olsen O. Meta-analysis of the safety of home birth. Birth. 1997;24:4-13; discussion 14-6.

3 de Jonge A, van der Goes BY, Ravelli AC, Amelink-Verburg MP, Mol BW, Nijhuis JG, Bennebroek Gravenhorst J, Buitendijk SE. Perinatal mortality and morbidity in a nationwide cohort of 529,688 low-risk planned home and hospital births. BJOG. 2009;116:1177-84.

4 Hutton EK, Reitsma AH, Kaufman K. Outcomes associated with planned home and planned hospital births in low-risk women attended by midwives in Ontario, Canada, 2003-2006: a retrospective cohort study. Birth. 2009 Sep;36:180-9.

5 Janssen PA, Saxell L, Page LA, Klein MC, Liston RM, Lee SK. Outcomes of planned home birth with registered midwife versus planned hospital birth with midwife or physician. CMAJ. 2009;181):377-83. Epub 2009 Aug 31.

6 Wax JR, Lucas FL, Lamont M, Pinette MG, Cartin A, Blackstone J. Maternal and newborn outcomes in planned home birth vs planned hospital births: a metaanalysis. Am J Obstet Gynecol. 2010;203(3):243.e1-8.

7 Mayor S. Study shows higher rates of neonatal mortality with planned home births. BMJ2010;341:c3551. (2 July.)

8 Anonymous. Home birth--proceed with caution. Lancet. 2010 Jul 31;376 (9738):303.

9 Gyte G, Dodwell M, Newburn M, Sandall J, Macfarlane A, Bewley S.Safety of planned home births. Findings of meta-analysis cannot be relied on. BMJ. 2010 Jul 27;341:c4033. doi: 10.1136/bmj.c4033.

10 Gyte G, Dodwell M, Macfarlane A. Editorials about home birth--proceed with caution. Lancet. 2010 Oct 16;376(9749):1297

11 Horton R. Offline: Urgency and concern about home birth. Lancet. 2010 Nov 27;376(9755):1812.

12 Olsen O. Correction of data delayed for 16 years. Lancet. 2001 Apr 28;357 (9265):1360-1.

13 Olsen O, Gøtzsche PC. [The necessity of electronically updated meta-analyses: Doppler ultrasound in obstetrics as an example] Ugeskr Laeger. 1996 Dec 30;159 (1):27-8. Danish

14 Furedi F. Culture of fear revisited: risk-taking and the morality of low expectation. Cassell. 1997.

15 Glassner B. The Culture of Fear: Why Americans are Afraid of the Wrong Things. Basic Books. 1999.

16 Hendrix M, Van Horck M, Moreta D, Nieman F, Nieuwenhuijze M, Severens J, Nijhuis J. Why women do not accept randomisation for place of birth: feasibility of a RCT in The Netherlands. BJOG. 2009 Mar;116:537-42; discussion 542-4.

17 Dowswell T, Thornton JG, Hewison J, Lilford RJ, Raisler J, Macfarlane A, Young G, Newburn M, Dodds R, Settatree RS. Should there be a trial of home versus hospital delivery in the United Kingdom? BMJ. 1996;312(7033):753-7.

Maternal mental health: an overlooked need of mothers and its impact on positive childbirth

Shannon Senefeld

Mental health problems around the world

The World Health Organization estimates that more than 150 million people suffer from depression globally, while another 26 million suffer from schizophrenia and 125 million from alcohol use disorders.[1] Depression and anxiety disorders are most prevalent amongst women when they are in their childbearing years.[2] The World Health Organization estimates that 1 in 3 to 1 in 5 women in developing countries and 1 in 10 in developed countries experience a significant mental health problem during pregnancy or after childbirth.[3]

Mental health problems in pregnancy

The etiology of mental health problems is as diverse as the mental health problems themselves. Much research has been conducted on the physiological changes that occur during pregnancy that may be linked with a change in mood.[4] Other risk factors for perinatal mental health problems include being single, being in an unsupportive relationship, a previous history of stillbirth or repeated miscarriages, poverty and economic hardship, and a lack of practical support.[5] Research has begun to explore the role that sleep disruption during the perinatal period may play in affecting mood.[25] One significant predictor of mental health problems during the perinatal period is a history of abuse. Studies estimate that women who have been exposed to intimate partner violence are 3 to 5 times more likely to experience a mental health problem than those who have not experienced such violence.[6]

One of the most commonly documented mental health concerns during the antenatal period is depression.[7] Many pregnant women also have specific anxiety related to childbirth. One study in Sweden interviewed pregnant women with psychosomatic complaints believed to be related to their fear of childbirth and found that 73% of the women expressed anxiety over delivery related to a lack of trust in maternity staff, while 65% feared their own incompetence; 55% feared the death of mother, baby or both; 44% feared intolerable pain; and 43% feared a loss of control during childbirth.[18] A small intervention trial examined the efficaciousness of targeted support for women who had elevated anxiety related to childbirth. In this trial, 68% of women initially requested a caesarean section, but after individualised psychological and maternity support, 38% agreed to vaginal delivery, while 30% underwent elective caesarean section. The study found that psychological therapy was cost-effective over elective caesarean section.[19]

Less common mental health concerns include eating disorders and psychosis. Although anorexia is less common during pregnancy due likely in fact to the reduced fertility rates associated with anorexia, bulimia may still pose a threat to some women during the perinatal period. Research suggests that many eating disorder symptoms may actually improve during pregnancy. However, women with eating disorders during pregnancy are more likely to have obstetric problems including miscarriage and premature or low-birth weight infants.[10] Women with schizophrenia have been demonstrated to be more likely to experience preterm labour, low birth weight, and stillbirth.

While the exact etiology of maternal mental health issues remains unknown, the impact of these issues is becoming startlingly clear. Research demonstrates that pregnant women who are diagnosed with depression or anxiety during their pregnancies have higher rates of fatigue, nausea, headache, back pain, bowel problems, dizziness, insomnia, palpitations and chest pain, and fainting.[8] Bloom, Curry, and Durham found that psychosocial distress was positively associated with accessing healthcare services more frequently, which the researchers hypothesise may be a way for women with psychosocial distress to ask for help from healthcare providers.[9]

Mental health in the intrapartum period

Research is steadily emerging that demonstrates that women with mental health problems suffer greater obstetric complications[11] and/or preterm labour.[12] An estimated 40% of births in the United States are complicated by some form of mood disorder.[13] Depression has been demonstrated to affect obstetric outcomes in a variety of ways.[14] Studies of women with depression have shown an increased need for pain relief during labour[16] and increased negative experiences related to childbirth.[17] These outcomes are then linked to increased fear of childbirth in future pregnancies, thus creating a vicious cycle of reinforced fear. Women with anxiety and women with eating disorders during pregnancy have both demonstrated greater obstetric interventions including delivery by caesarean section. [10, 19]

In addition to premorbid mental health disorders affecting the intrapartum period, additional psychosocial factors can directly affect intrapartum outcomes. Certain variables, including adequate support during childbirth, are associated with more positive feelings toward childbirth in the months and years after the event and these could be significant in terms of the normality or otherwise of birth outcome. For example, one Cochrane review found that women who were continuously supported during labour experienced higher rates of spontaneous vaginal births, used fewer pain medications, experienced shorter labours, and were more likely to be satisfied with the overall childbirth experience. Another study also found that healthcare provider support can increase the perceived levels of control of women in the intrapartum period and lead to reduced anxiety. Research also suggests that the continuous presence of trained support staff can reduce the likelihood of medication for pain relief, operative vaginal delivery, caesarean delivery, and that this ongoing support can reduce the length of labour. The importance of maternal mental health in the intrapartum period therefore cannot be underestimated when considering its impact on obstetric outcomes.

Maternal mental health problems postpartum

The negative impacts of untreated mental health problems extend beyond the antenatal period into the postnatal period, affecting not only the women, but also their infants. While nearly 80% of women experience the 'baby blues', 10% to 20% actually go on to meet the criteria for a major depressive episode as outlined in the Diagnostic and Statistical Manual of Mental Disorders, 4th Edition (DSM-IV).[22] Postnatal depression has increasingly become recognised as a serious complication of childbirth.[23] While postnatal depression is gaining recognition, it is also important to note that the onset of many of these symptoms actually begins during pregnancy with many women. Recent research demonstrated that while 9% of women had probable depression scores at 8 weeks after delivery, 14% had probable depression scores at 32 weeks of pregnancy.[24] These results suggest that depressive symptoms may frequently begin during the antenatal period with long-lasting effects.

Depression among mothers in low-resource environments has been linked to lower infant birth weight, increased rates of malnutrition and stunting, increased diarrhaeal disease, infectious disease and hospital admission, along with a decrease in completion of immunisation schedules among children.[26] In addition, maternal depression has been shown to negatively affect the overall development of children in their infancy and early years.[27] For example, women with depression are less likely to look their infants in the face, and these infants show long-term effects, including showing fewer facial expressions, smiling less, and crying more.[28]

Infants of depressed mothers show long-term effects

While depression has typically been reviewed as one of the most common mental health concerns in the antenatal period, anxiety has also emerged more recently in the literature as a parallel concern of mounting proportions. Select research has found the same rates for postnatal depression and anxiety disorders (18%) using a structured interview technique.[29] Additional research found that 28% of women endorsed sub-clinical difficulties with generalised anxiety in the postnatal period with an additional 4% meeting DSM-IV criteria for generalised anxiety disorder.[30] Less than 3% of the women in the study met criteria for major depressive disorder, demonstrating that postnatal generalised anxiety disorder may have a higher prevalence than postnatal depression. This research strongly supports the need to screen for both perinatal depression and anxiety simultaneously.

Postnatal generalised anxiety disorder may have a higher prevalence than postnatal depression

Psychosis is relatively rare, and although the incidence is often difficult to determine due in large part to pre-existing serious mental health diagnoses such as schizophrenia, the overall incidence rate is estimated to be 1 to 2 per 1000 deliveries.[20] Screening for psychosis in the postnatal period is also important, especially for women with postnatal depression. While postnatal psychosis is rare, occurring in only 0.1% of all deliveries, it most often resembles a manic or mixed episode.[21] If a manic or mixed episode is present during the perinatal period, clinicians should also screen for psychosis.

How the normality or otherwise of birthing mode affects postnatal feelings needs further research. Some research has suggested that women experiencing a caesarean have decreased mood and self-esteem in the postnatal period. However, a meta-analysis in 2006 found no significant association between caesarean births and postnatal depression. Research has also found that women who undergo emergency caesarean sections have higher rates of post-traumatic intrusive stress reactions in the postnatal period. Instrumental and surgical interventions during delivery have also been associated with a negative impact on first postnatal contact between mothers and babies. Thus, research remains mixed in terms of how birthing choices and modes affect postnatal mental health. Additional research on the interaction between birthing choices and mental health outcomes in the short- and long-term postpartum is warranted.

Addressing mental health in perinatal care

While the prevalence and existence of mental health issues and disorders is well established, less research has been conducted on how to address these issues to promote positive birth experiences and ultimately, sustained positive child outcomes. To what extent 'positive' means 'normal'—and how that is defined—are areas which require additional exploration. What we can do now, before these questions are answered, is draw on the emerging evidence base. The National Institute of Health and Clinical Excellence (NICE) published guidelines on the clinical management of antenatal and postnatal mental health that offer several concrete recommendations on responding to the needs of expectant mothers.[31] For example, NICE recommends establishing a firm continuity of care, so that women with pre-existing mental disorders can continue to receive treatment for these disorders while also receiving antenatal care, which means coordinating care across providers. NICE also recommends that healthcare providers screen closely for mental health issues during antenatal appointments. NICE recommends that two main questions are asked of women during antenatal appointments to identify possible perinatal depression.[32]

- During the last month, have you often been bothered by feeling down, depressed or hopeless?
- During the last month have you often been bothered by having little interest or pleasure in doing things?

If a woman responds that she has been bothered by such feelings, NICE recommends that she is then asked a third question:

- Is this something you feel you need or want help with?

The World Health Organization offers additional screening questions for anxiety ("How much of the time during the last month have you been a very nervous person?") and psychosis ("Have you been receiving any special messages from people or from the way things are arranged around you?").[33]

Midwives, in particular, may play a great role in screening for any emerging issues and could closely monitor women during the perinatal period.[34] However, while many midwives are interested in providing additional mental health services, few midwives are adequately trained to do so.[35] While midwives could play a particularly helpful role throughout the pregnancy period and most certainly during the labour and delivery phase, many may not have had the advanced training to enable them to be as successful as possible.

Antidepressants have been shown to be effective in treating perinatal depression, which is not especially surprising given that selective serotonin reuptake inhibitors (SSRIs) have been found to be effective in the treatment of depression in general.[36,37] However, no one SSRI has shown superiority in the treatment of perinatal depression, and antidepressants must be carefully prescribed for this population, as many antidepressants are contraindicated in pregnant women and among breastfeeding mothers.[38]

Cognitive and behavioural interventions for anxiety and depressive disorders are considered well established, empirically validated treatments.[39] Support groups also show promise among some pregnant women.[40] General social support is also important including an open relationship with the relational partner and regular socialisation with friends.[41] Thus, a variety of non-pharmacological options are available for responding to depression and anxiety during pregnancy, and the benefit of such options likely increases positive outcomes related to the acute labour and delivery phase.

As previously mentioned, research also suggests that the continuous presence of trained support staff can reduce the likelihood of medication for pain relief, operative vaginal delivery, caesarean delivery, and reduce the length of labour.[42] Additionally, the Confidential Enquiry into Maternal And Child Health (CEMACH) reported in several triennial reports that suicide and psychiatric issues were the leading causes of indirect maternal death in the UK.[43]

The World Health Organization (WHO) offers hopeful statistics related to maternal mental health, estimating that 70% to 80% of women with maternal mental disorders can be treated successfully and recover.[44] WHO offers guidance that the woman and her partner (as appropriate) be involved in the full continuum of care, including education and treatment options. Further, WHO estimates that most mental health disorders can be screened and managed at primary healthcare facilities and integrated into ongoing, standardised care.[45]

Conclusions

Maternal mental health is an often overlooked gap in perinatal care. Yet, the research clearly demonstrates the need to address this component of women's healthcare. Data demonstrates that depression and anxiety alone can have serious effects on women's healthcare and the outcomes of their pregnancy, including the childbirth process. There are clearly options for responding to the needs of women during pregnancy that hold much promise. Yet, frontline healthcare providers are often not trained specifically to respond to the present need. Additional staffing to address the mental health needs of pregnant women, along with dedicated training for midwives and other frontline healthcare professionals would fill a much needed gap, improving overall perinatal outcomes for both the woman and her child in a cost-effective manner. Undoubtedly, mental health and birthing are related in a symbiotic relationship, with mental health being a determinant of birthing choices and birthing outcomes. Less well known is how birthing choices affect mental health in both the short- and long-term. The question as to whether or not a normal birth (however that is defined) can promote improved mental health also needs to be addressed.

Shannon Senefeld is a Senior Technical Advisor for international health and HIV programmes at Catholic Relief Services in Baltimore, MD, where she specialises in mental health and psychosocial support aspects of health programming. Additionally, she has worked as a therapist in a variety of US-based healthcare settings and is currently completing her pre-doctoral residency in clinical psychology at Mt. Washington Pediatric Hospital in Baltimore, MD. Shannon holds an MA in International Development from George Washington University in Washington, DC, and an MA in Clinical Psychology from Argosy University in Washington, DC. She anticipates being awarded a doctorate of clinical psychology in summer 2011. She has two children.

References

1 World Health Organization. (2010). Mental Health and Development: Targeting people with mental health conditions as a vulnerable group. Geneva. Downloaded October 25, 2010 from http://www.who.int/mental_health/policy/mhtargeting/en/index.html.

2 Blehar, M. C. (2003). Public health context of women's mental health research. *Psychiatry Clinics of North America, 26*(3), 781–799.

3 World Health Organization. (2008). Improving Maternal Mental Health. Available at: http://www.who.int/mental_health/prevention/suicide/Perinatal_depression_mmh_final.pdf.

4 Russell, J.A., Douglas, A.J., & Ingram, C.D. (2001). Brain preparations for maternity — adaptive changes in behavioral and neuroendocrine systems during pregnancy and lactation. An overview. *Prog Brain Res, 133*, 1-38.

5 *Maternal mental health and child health and development in low and middle income countries*. Report of the WHO meeting. Geneva, World Health Organization,

2008. Available at: http://www.who.int/mental_health/prevention/suicide/mmh_jan08_meeting_report.pdf.

6 Golding, J.M. (1999). Intimate partner violence as a risk factor for mental disorders: a meta-analysis. *J Fam Viol,14*, 99–132.

7 van Bussel, J., Spitz, B., & Demyttenaere, K. (2006). Women's Mental Health Before, During, and After Pregnancy: A Population-Based Controlled Cohort Study. *Birth, 33*, 4, 297-302.

8 Evans, J., Heron, J., Francomb, H., Oke, S., & Golding, J. (2001). Cohort study of depressed mood during pregnancy and after childbirth. *British Medical Journal, 323*(7307), 257–260.

9 Bloom, T., Curry, M.A., & Durham, L. (2007). Abuse and psychosocial stress as factors in high utilization of medical services during pregnancy. *Issues in Mental Health Nursing*, 28:849–866.

10 Buck, A. (2009). Perinatal mental health. *Practice Nurse, 27*, 27-8, 30-1.

11 Andersson, L. et al. (2004). Implications of Antenatal Depression and Anxiety for Obstetric Outcome. *Obstetrics and Gynecology*, 104, 467-476.

12 Alder, J. et al. (2007). Depression and anxiety during pregnancy: a risk factor for obstetric, fetal and neonatal outcome? A critical review of the literature. *J Matern Fetal Neonatal Med, 20*, 189-209.

13 O'Hara MW. Postpartum Depression. In: Alloy LB (Ed.) Series in Psychopathology; (pp 1–27). New York: Springer-Verlag 1995.

14 Field, T. et al. (2004). Prenatal depression effects on the fetus and the newborn. *Infant Behavior and Development*, 27, 216-229.

15 Andersson, L. et al. (2004). Implications of Antenatal Depression and Anxiety for Obstetric Outcome. *Obstetrics and Gynecology*, 104, 467-476.

16 Andersson, L. et al. (2004). Implications of Antenatal Depression and Anxiety for Obstetric Outcome. *Obstetrics and Gynecology*, 104, 467-476.

17 Field, T. et al. (2004). Prenatal depression effects on the fetus and the newborn. *Infant Behavior and Development*, 27, 216-229.

18 *Sjögren , B.* (1997). Reasons for anxiety about childbirth in 100 pregnant women. *Journal of Psychosomatic Obstetrics and Gynecology, 18*, 266 - 272.

19 Sjögren B, Thomassen P. (1997). Obstetric outcome in 100 women with severe anxiety over childbirth. *Acta Obstet Gynecol Scand, 76(10)*, 948-52.

20 Buck, A. (2009). Perinatal mental health. *Practice Nurse, 27*, 27-8, 30-1.

21 Payne, J. L. (2007). Antidepressant Use in the Postpartum Period: Practical Considerations. *The American Journal of Psychiatry, 164*, 1329-33.

22 Payne, J. L. (2007). Antidepressant Use in the Postpartum Period: Practical Considerations. *The American Journal of Psychiatry, 164*, 1329-33.

23 Gold, L.H. (2002). Postpartum disorders in primary care: diagnosis and treatment. *Prim Care, 29(1)*, 27–41.

24 Evans, J., Heron, J., Francomb, H., et al. (2001). Cohort study of depressed mood during pregnancy and after childbirth. *Brit Med Journal, 323*, 257–60.

25 Ross, L.E., Murray, B.J., & Steiner, M. (2005). Sleep and perinatal mood disorders: A critical review. *J Psychiatry Neurosci, 30*, 247-256.

26 World Health Organization. (2008). Improving Maternal Mental Health. Available at: http://www.who.int/mental_health/prevention/suicide/Perinatal_depression_mmh_final.pdf.

27 *Maternal mental health and child health and development in low and middle income countries.* Report of the WHO meeting. Geneva, World Health Organization, 2008. Available at: http://www.who.int/mental_health/prevention/suicide/mmh_jan08_meeting_report.pdf.

28 World Health Organization. Maternal mental health and child health and development. Available at: http://www.who.int/mental_health/prevention/suicide/MaternalMH/en/index.html.

29 Muzik, M., Klier, C.M., Rosenblum, K.L., et al. (2000). Are commonly used self-report inventories suitable for screening postpartum depression and anxiety disorders? *Acta Psychiatr Scand, 102(1)*:71–3.

30 Wenzel, A., Haugen, E.N., Jackson, L.C., et al. (2006). Prevalence of generalized anxiety at eight weeks postpartum. *Arch Women Mental Health 6(1)*, 43–49.

31 National Institute of Health and Clinical Excellence (NICE). (2007). *Antenatal and postnatal mental health: clinical management and service guidance.* http://guidance.nice.org.uk/CG45.

32 National Institute of Health and Clinical Excellence (NICE). (2007). *Antenatal and postnatal mental health: clinical management and service guidance.* http://guidance.nice.org.uk/CG45.

33 World Health Organization. Maternal mental health and child health and development. Available at: http://www.who.int/mental_health/prevention/suicide/MaternalMH/en/index.html.

34 Taylor, C., Richens, Y., & Burbeck, R. (2007). Mental health and childbirth. *Midwives, 10:4*, 176-177.

35 Ross-Davie, M., Elliott, S., Sarkar, A., & Green, L. (2006). A public health role in perinatal mental health: Are midwives ready? *British Journal of Midwifery, 14*, 330-334.

36 Andersson L, Sundstr¨om-Poromaa I, Bixo M, et al. (2003). Point prevalence of psychiatric disorders during the second trimester of pregnancy: A population-based study. *Am J Obstet Gynecol, 89*(1), 148–154.

37 Maurer-Spurej, E., Pittendreigh, C., Misri, S. (2007). Platelet serotonin levels support depression scores for women with postpartum depression. *Journal of Psychiatry and Neuroscience, 32*, 23-9.

38 Payne, J. L. (2007). Antidepressant Use in the Postpartum Period: Practical Considerations. *The American Journal of Psychiatry, 164*, 1329-33.

39 Weisberg, R.B., & Paquette, J.A. (2002). Screening and treatment of anxiety disorders in pregnant and lactating women. *Women's Health Issues, 12(1)*, 32–36.

40 Misri, S., & Kostaras, X. (2002). Benefits and risks to mother and infant of drug treatment for postnatal depression. *Drug Saf, 25(13)*, 903–911.

41 Goebert, D., Morland, L., Frattarelli, L., Onoye, J., & Matsu, C. (2007). Mental Health During Pregnancy: A Study Comparing Asian, Caucasian and Native Hawaiian Women. *Matern Child Health Journal*, 11:249–255.

42 Hodnett E.D. (1999) Caregiver support for postpartum depression, (date of most recent substantive amendment; 15 October 1998). The Cochrane Library, Oxford.

43 *Confidential Enquiry in Maternal and Child Health (CEMACH). Why Mothers Die (1997-1999). London: RCOG, 2001; CEMACH. Why Mothers Die (2000-2002). London: RCOG, 2005; CEMACH. Why Mothers Die (2003-2005). London: RCOG, 2007.*

44 World Health Organization. Maternal mental health and child health and development. Available at: http://www.who.int/mental_health/prevention/suicide/MaternalMH/en/index.html.

45 World Health Organization. Maternal mental health and child health and development. Available at: http://www.who.int/mental_health/prevention/suicide/MaternalMH/en/index.html.

The value of lay support in protecting normal birth: the doula's role

Adela Stockton

For the purposes of this chapter, I use the term 'normal' to mean 'completely physiological' birth. That is, without induction, augmentation, continuous fetal monitoring or episiotomy, without the use of pharmacological pain management, and without any restriction on the mother's positioning or movement.

If, as some caregivers suggest, preserving the physical birth environment is key to protecting the normal physiology of labour, it would make sense that birth attendants or supporters are included as an integral part of this picture too. According to obstetrician and natural birth pioneer Michel Odent, the mother needs to feel safe and therefore able to access her primal brain in order to connect effectively with the powers of the birth process.[1,2] Midwife and author Ina May Gaskin talks about the 'sphincter law', explaining that the cervix is a sphincter which—like the rectum—will not function on demand; a birthplace where the mother feels private and unobserved therefore, Gaskin reiterates, is essential to support the progress of labour.[3,4] GP, homebirther and author of *Gentle Birth, Gentle Mothering,* Sarah Buckley, proposes that maintaining an 'undisturbed' environment will support the labouring woman to keep producing the 'cocktail of hormones' that are essential to her ongoing birth journey.[5] A mother who wishes to fulfil her ability to birth gently, may or may not be well-informed of the value of protecting her birth environment to this end. Yet no matter how well she has prepared, much can still be affected by the integrity of the people who are present around her at the time. Mostly, the labouring woman will be accompanied by her partner and the midwife in attendance, but increasingly, and in view of encouraging research findings in favour of normality at doula-supported births[6], expectant parents are turning to lay companions for additional support during childbirth.

Originating from ancient times, when female family members or neighbours would gather to support the birthing family, one direct precursor to the modern doula's role in Europe was the Medieval 'godsibb'. This 'Sister of God' literally 'accompanied' mothers during birth and stayed on afterwards to help out with other children and household chores.[7] The idea of the 'childbirth companion' was resurrected by US medical anthropologist, Dana Raphael, in the 1970s, when she coined the term 'doula' from the Greek, meaning 'serving woman', and reinterpreted it to mean *"the person who supports the mother so that she can breastfeed"*.[8,9] US paediatrician John Kennell and neonatologist Phyllis Klaus, whose research findings had shown that sustained support from another woman during labour increased the mother's chances of experiencing a normal birth,[10] took the concept a step further. In partnership with colleagues Marshall Klaus, Penny Simkin and Annie Kennedy, and with the aim that every expectant woman should have access to someone to 'mother the mother', in 1992 they set up

DONA International (Doulas of North America), establishing the definition of the contemporary doula as "a woman who serves other women" during the time around childbirth.[11] Interestingly, in the South African Sesotho language, the word *dula* means 'to sit',[12] a sense which may alternatively resonate more soundly with women who doula, for indeed, the doula's work can frequently involve long hours of simply sitting quietly alongside the labouring woman or new mother.

The doula's work can involve long hours of simply sitting

The doula role first appeared in the UK in the 1990s through the work of the women of the Hansy Josovic Maternity Trust, who provided support to birthing families within the Orthodox Jewish community in London.[13] It was perpetuated by childbirth activist and social anthropologist Sheila Kitzinger's pioneering work—with National Childbirth Trust teacher Diana Parkinson—in establishing a network of lay companions or 'birth sisters' to support expectant women in Holloway prison.[14,15] In 2001, inspired by Kitzinger and Odent's philosophies on natural birth, a group of like-minded women, some of whom were already supporting birthing families, set up the non-profit network Doula UK as a peer group support organisation for doulas run by doulas.[16] A variety of doula courses, both independent as well as state-provided, duly evolved across the country.[17,18] Over the past decade, the popularity of the lay childbirth companion has spread throughout much of the rest of Europe, frequently fuelled by the teachings of Odent in liaison with experienced doula Liliana Lammers (Paramana Doula course), and Debra Pascali Bonaro of DONA International. Growing doula communities can now also be found in Australia, the Middle East and South Africa, as well as in many other countries around the globe.[19,20]

Growing doula communities can now be found around the globe, e.g. in Australia, the Middle East and South Africa

So what exactly does a doula do and what is it that makes her role so significant within the realm of protecting normal birth? As a *lay* person, there is no statutory requirement for a doula to be 'trained', 'qualified' or 'certified'; while she may work in a 'professional way', she is not a 'trained professional'. Usually, she will have undertaken a short course of study, however, and may be affiliated to a doula network for the purposes of peer support and ongoing learning. However, as Odent points out: *"If the focus is on the training of the doula rather than on her way of being and her personality, the doula phenomenon will be a missed opportunity."*[21] The key to her skill-building lies in developing self-awareness, honing reflective and listening skills, adopting an attitude of humility and integrity, and practising mindfulness of ego, little of which can be formally taught. In Kitzinger's view, doula-ing is *"an opportunity to use skills which have not previously been recognised as marketable—understanding and insight, sympathy, warm friendship, a capacity to communicate effectively and at an intimate level."*[22] Much therefore depends on the integrity of the individual doula. Nevertheless, organisations DONA International and Doula UK, have set standards for basic learning and essential skills; membership requires that novice doulas not only complete an approved course but also commit to an initial period of mentorship with an experienced doula as they start out supporting clients.[23,24]

Usually a mother herself, experienced in birth and parenting, the doula's role is to provide sustained psychosocial support—mother to mother, sister to sister—to the birthing woman and her family.[25] Importantly, she is selected and chosen by the mother or couple-to-be, and works to support fathers too. When enlisted for a birth, the doula takes plenty of time to meet with the parents during pregnancy to prepare for the birth of their baby, listening to their hopes and fears, helping with their birth plan, and building up a relationship of trust and understanding. She may additionally teach some form of breath and bodywork sessions, such as pregnancy yoga or aquanatal classes, to which her clients will be invited. Not qualified to give advice, the doula supports the mother's informed choice however, and works at promoting normality by explaining the health and well-being benefits of physiological birth. She can point parents towards further relevant resources, facilitating their ability to prepare well for birth and make decisions for their maternity care in the way that feels right for them. Doulas are frequently taken on during a second pregnancy when the mother has experienced a traumatic birth with her firstborn, one which may have left her feeling disempowered and distressed. Revisiting the circumstances under which their previous birth required medical intervention can encourage parents to explore how they might prefer to plan things differently next time around. While, despite everyone's best efforts, obstetric emergencies can occur unexpectedly or for no apparent reason, conversely, there are times when the need for further intervention may have arisen as a result of a medical procedure in the first place, such as when the artificial rupture of membranes for augmentation of labour causes a cord prolapse.[26] It is possible, however, that the mother's birth space may have been 'disturbed' initially in a much more subtle way, by strangers entering the room or as a result of fearful attendants or through the administration of pain medication. Any neocortical stimulation can cause interruption to the flow of oxytocin or endorphins, which in turn may slow labour down and/or reduce the woman's pain threshold, inviting the first step to a potential ensuing 'cascade of intervention'.[27,28] Having her previous birth story heard by someone who she trusts not to judge her—especially if things did not go as anticipated—can be the start of a healing journey for some mothers.[29] Knowing that she has a confidante to help her (and her partner) to protect her birth space may instil the beginnings of a renewed sense of confidence and a more positive attitude towards the birth to come.

During labour, the doula provides sustained emotional and practical support for both mother and father according to their individual needs; her role is to hold a safe space for their birth story to unfold. While working to support mother-led care, she also aims to respectfully complement the midwife's clinical role, striving to maintain a calm, harmonious ambience in the birthing room. The doula may, at her client's request, advocate through supporting or directly reiterating the mother's wishes, even, for example, if asked by parents to protect their privacy by sitting outside their birthing room to 'guard' the door.

Some doulas are trained in complementary therapies such as aromatherapy, homeopathy, reflexology or hypnobirthing, which the mother or father may choose to use as additional intrapartum comfort or support measures. Yet these skills do not necessarily make her a better doula. Doula-ing is so often much less about 'doing' than about 'being',[30] and her mindful presence beside the parents can simply be enough to facilitate their confidence as they pass through the rite of passage of birth and into their roles as new mother or father, whether for the first or subsequent time. The doula is careful to help preserve an 'undisturbed' birth environment until after the placenta is safely delivered, and stays with the mother or couple to support skin-to-skin contact with the new baby and the initiation of breastfeeding, as the parents wish. She will return to visit the new family at least once during the first postnatal week, unless they have enlisted her to provide support throughout the postpartum period, when she may continue work with them until the baby is around 6-8 weeks old.

So how has the demand for the lay birth companion, in *addition* to the midwife, arisen? Despite the fact that the benefits of continuous one-to-one *midwifery* care in protecting normality have long been established, it could be argued that the midwife's traditional role in providing emotional and spiritual care has largely been usurped by the doula, with midwifery attendance at births focused more around clinical need only.[31] A recent study undertaken in Sweden claims that midwives are simply no longer able to provide psychosocial support due to lack of time and resources, suggesting why this role therefore now lies with the doula.[32] Furthermore, as research midwife Professor Rosemary Mander proposes, the doula may be 'the answer to the obstetrician's prayer'.[33] Not only does physiological birth with physically, as well as emotionally healthy mothers and babies come at considerably less cost to the state,[34] but also the doula is funded by the service-user rather than the provider. Even in the case of the state-provided doula, her salary will be considerably less than that of a midwife. Fundamentally, however, the rise in popularity of the doula has been drive by mothers and fathers, who increasingly realise the value of emotional support around childbirth. Indeed, research shows that with the support of an additional person who is not part of the hospital system, labouring women are less likely to need augmentation, are less likely to request an epidural or other pain medication and their births are up to 50% less likely to end in caesarean section.[35,36,37] Both mothers and fathers are more likely to feel a greater sense of satisfaction from a doula supported birth experience,[38,39,40,41] breastfeeding is more likely to go well,[42,43,44] and the new mother is less at risk of suffering from postnatal illness.[45,46]

If it is recognised that there is value in promoting normal, natural birth, then responding to the evidence that additional support from a known lay companion during labour is effective to this end, surely makes sense. Whether hired independently, enlisted through a funded or charitable initiative or provided by the state, with her trusted, nurturing presence and gentle touch, a doula upholds the heart and soul of birth in a way that can be largely neglected through the medicalised approach; through 'mothering the mother', she brings a little of the traditional sense of community back to childbirth. The labouring woman, protected in her wishes for birth and in the knowledge that her partner is well supported too, is better able to focus on birthing her baby instinctively and gently, when most times, birth will go well. In view of the increasing inaccessibility of emotional and practical support through midwifery care—regardless of the current global humanitarian push towards protecting normal birth—it would seem appropriate therefore that the doula's role is perpetuated. DONA International's mission statement proposes "a doula for every woman who wants one"[47] and if this means less risk of birth trauma with improved health and well-being for mothers, babies and fathers, then why not?

Adela Stockton's passion lies in encouraging expectant mothers and fathers towards protecting the gentle birth of their babies and to secure the support and care that feels right for them during the childbirth year. Former midwife, now doula/doula educator, she also prepares women as lay companions for birthing families through her Mindful Doulas course. Author of popular book *Birth Space, Safe Place: emotional wellbeing through pregnancy and birth* (Findhorn Press), Stockton's articles on doulas and gentle birth appear, amongst others, in *MIDIRS Midwifery Digest*, *AIMS Journal*, *Practising Midwife* and *Juno* magazine. Her new book about the UK/European doula movement *Gentle Birth Companions: doulas serving humanity* was published this year (2010). Website: www.adelastockton.co.uk

References

1 Odent, M. *Primal Health* Clairview Books: East Sussex, 2007

2 Odent, M. *The Scientification of Love.* London: Oxford University Press, 1999

3 Gaskin, IM. *Ina May's Guide to Childbirth* Bantam Books: New York, 2003

4 The Farm Midwifery Center (Ina May Gaskin), 2010 [Online] Available from: http://www.thefarmmidwives.org/ [Accessed 5 November 2010]

5 Buckley, S. *Gentle Birth, Gentle Mothering* Celestial Arts: Berkeley, California, 2009

6 Hodnett, ED., Gates, S., Hofmeyr, GJ. & Sakala, C. Continuous support for women during childbirth. *Cochrane Database of Systematic Reviews,* 2007, Issue 3

7 Dictionary.com [Online] Available from: http://dictionary.reference.com/browse/gossip [Accessed 4 October 2010]

8 Raphael D. *The Tender Gift: Breastfeeding.* Englewood Cliffs, New Jersey: Prentice-Hall, 1973

9 Raphael, D. Interview with Reiko Kishi, *Breastfeeding and Doula Support.* Child Research Net, 2005 [Online] Available from: http://www.childresearch.net/SCIENCE/DIALOGS/2007/index.html [Accessed 4 October 2010]

10 Klaus, MH., Kennell, JH., Robertson, SS. & Sosa, R. Effects of social support during parturition on maternal and infant morbidity. *British Medical Journal,* 1986, 293, pp.585-587

11 Klaus, M., Kennell, J., Klaus, P., Simkin, P. & Kennedy, A. *DONA International Founders: Mothering the Mother.* [Online] Available from: www.dona.org/aboutus/founders.php [Accessed 5 November 2010]

12 Olivier, J. *Sesotho Online* [Online] Available from: www.sesotho.web.za/dipolelo.htm [Accessed 5 November 2010]

13 Ne'eman Staff, Y. Hansy Josovic Activists from Stamford Hill Go to Venice, *Dei'ah veDibur Information & Insight*, 9th August 2006 [Online] Available from: http://chareidi.shemayisrael.com/archives5766/eikev/ahjmcekv66.htm [Accessed 4 October 2010]

14 Kitzinger, S. *Mothers and babies in prison*, 2010 [Online] Available from: http://www.sheilakitzinger.com/Prisons.htm [Accessed 5 November 2010]

15 Birth Companions. *How we started*, 2009. [Online] Available from: http://www.birthcompanions.org.uk/howstarted.html [Accessed 4 October 2010]

16 Doula UK. *Minutes of the First Meeting of The Independent Doula Association* 10th February, 2001 [Online] Available to Doula UK members from: http://www.doula.org.uk/content/duk/members/Previous_Meetings_Minutes.asp [Accessed 4 October 2010]

17 Doula UK. *How to become a doula*, 2010 [Online] Available from: http://www.doula.org.uk/content/duk/become/How_to_become_a_Doula.asp [Accessed 5 November 2010]

18 Goodwin Volunteer Doula Project [Online] Available from: http://www.goodwindoulas.org/ [Accessed 7 December 2010]

19 L'association de Doulas de France. *The European Doula Guide*, 2007 [Online] Available from: http://www.doulas.info/cahier2.php [Accessed 5 November 2010]

20 Stockton, A. *Gentle Birth Companions: doulas serving humanity*. Dumfries: McCubbington Press, 2010

21 Odent, M. Ch 15 The Future of the Midwifery-Obstetrics Relationship, *The Farmer and the Obstetrician* London: Free Association Books, 2002, p.123

22 Kitzinger, S. *UK 'doula movement'*. IN: Stockton, A. *Gentle Birth Companions: doulas serving humanity*. Dumfries: McCubbington Press p. 21 Personal email to: Adela Stockton, 30th April, 2009

23 DONA International. *Birth Doula Certification: become a birth doula*, 2005 [Online] Available from: http://www.dona.org/develop/birth_cert.php [Accessed 5 November 2010]

24 Doula UK. *Journey to being a doula*, 2005 [Online] Available from: http://www.doula.org.uk/content/duk/become/Journey_to_Being_a_Doula.asp [Accessed 5 November 2010]

25 Klaus, MH., Kennell, JH. & Klaus, P. *The Doula Book*. Cambridge, MA: Perseus Publishing, 2002.

26 Levy, H., Meier, PR & Makowski, EL. Umbilical cord prolapse. *Obstetrics & Gynecology* 1984; 64(4):499-502

27 Buckley, S. Undisturbed Birth—nature's hormonal blueprint for safety, ease and ecstasy. *MIDIRS Midwifery Digest*, June 2004, 14(2), pp.203-209

28 Buckley, S. What disturbs birth? *MIDIRS Midwifery Digest*, Sept 2004, 14(3), pp.353-359

29 Wilkie, T. 2005. Tina's Story. In: D. Vernon, ed. 2005. *Having a Great Birth in Australia*. Canberra City: Australian College of Midwives

30 Doula UK. *Journey to being a doula*, 2005 [Online] Available from: http://www.doula.org.uk/content.duk/become/Journey_to_Being_a_Doula.asp [Accessed 5 November 2010]

31 Beake, S., McCourt, C. & Page, L. (eds) *Evaluation of One-to-One Midwifery* Second Cohort Study July 2001 NHS Hammersmith Hospitals Trust/TVU London [Online] PDF available from: http://www.wolfson.tvu.ac.uk/mid/.../Evaluation%20report%20dec2001.pdf [Accessed 5 November 2010]

32 Lundgren, I. Swedish women's experiences of doula support during childbirth. *Midwifery*, April 2010, Vol 26(2), pp.173-180

33 Mander, R. Is the doula merely the answer to an obstetrician's prayer? *MIDIRS Midwifery Digest* 2002, 12(1), pp.8-12

34 NHS Institute for Improvement and Innovation. Promoting normal birth: benefits for patients and benefits for NHS. [Online] Available from: http://www.institute.nhs.uk/building_capability/general/promoting_normal_birth.html [Accessed 5 November 2010]

35 Klaus MH, Kennell JH, Robertson SS, Sosa R. Effects of social support during parturition on maternal and infant morbidity. *British Medical Journal* 1986, 293:585–587

36 Khreisheh, R. Support in the first stage of labour from a female relative: the first step in improving the quality of maternity services. *Midwifery* 2009 (article in Press)

37 Trueba, G., Contreras, C., Velazco, MT., Lara, EG. & Martínez, HB. Alternative Strategy to Decrease Cesarean Section: Support by Doulas During Labor. *Journal of Perinatal Education* Spring 2000, 9(2), pp.8-13

38 Berg, M. & Terstad, A. Swedish women's experiences of doula support during childbirth *Midwifery*, 2006, Vol 22, pp.330-338

39 Lundgren, I. Swedish women's experiences of doula support during childbirth. *Midwifery*, April 2010, Vol 26(2), pp.173-180

40 McGrath, SK. & Kennel, JH. A Randomized Controlled Trial of Continuous Labor Support for Middle-Class Couples: Effect on Cesarean Delivery Rates. *Birth* 2008, 35(2), pp.92-97

41 Koumouitzes-Douvia, J. & Carr, CA. Women's Perceptions of their Doula Support. *Journal of Perinatal Education* 2006, 15(4), pp.34-40 [Online] Available (PDF) from: http://www.ncbi.nlm.nih.gov/pmc/articles/PMC1804309/#citeref12 [Accessed 4 October 2010]

42 Campbell, D., Scott, KD., Klaus, MH. & Falk, M. Female Relatives or Friends Trained as Labor Doulas: Outcomes at 6 to 8 Weeks Postpartum. *Birth* Sept 2007, Vol 34(3), pp.220–227

43 Mottl-Santiago, J., Walker, C., Ewan, J., Vragovic, O., Winder, S. & Stubblefield, P. A hospital based doula program and childbirth outcomes in an urban, multicultural setting. *Maternal and Child Health Journal* May 2008, Vol 12(3), pp.372-377

44 Langer, A., Campero, L., Garcia, C. & Reynoso, S. Effects of psychosocial support during labour and childbirth on breastfeeding, medical interventions, and mothers' wellbeing in a Mexican public hospital: a randomised clinical trial. *British Journal of Obstetrics & Gynaecology* Oct 1998, 105(10), pp.1056-63

45 McComish, JF. & Visger, JM. Domains of Postpartum Doula Care and Maternal Responsiveness and Competence. *Journal of Obstetric, Gynaecologic & Neonatal Nursing* Mar/Apr 2009, Vol 38(2), pp.148-156

46 Goldbort, J. Postpartum depression: Bridging the gap between medicalized birth and social support International. *Journal of Childbirth Education* Dec 2002

47 DONA International *History & Mission*, 2005 [Online] PDF available from: http://www.dona.org/aboutus/mission.php [Accessed 5 November 2010]

Useful contacts

- AIMS (Association for Improvement of Maternity Services) www.aims.org.uk —campaigning group for parents, midwives and childbirth, UK
- Australian Doulas http://www.freewebs.com/australiandoulas/—doula network, Australia
- Birth Companions http://www.birthcompanions.org.uk—doulas supporting women in prison, UK
- Da-a-luz http://www.da-a-luz.co.uk —lay midwifery/holistic pregnancy centre, Spain
- Developing Doulas http://developingdoulas.co.uk/—doula preparation course, Cambridge, UK
- Doulas de France http://www.doulas.info—national doula organisation, France
- DONA International http://www.dona.org—leading doula organisation, North America and beyond
- Doula UK http://www.doula.org.uk—leading national doula organisation, UK
- Mindful Doulas http://www.adelastockton.co.uk—doula preparation course, Scotland, UK
- Sarah Buckley's website http://www.sarahbuckley.com/—articles, books
- Sheila Kitzinger's website http://www.sheilakitzinger.com/—articles, books
- The Farm Midwives http://www.midwiferyworkshops.org/midwifery_services.html —traditional midwifery centre founded by Ina May Gaskin, US
- Womb Ecology http://wombecology.com/—articles & books by Michel Odent

KEY QUOTES: RESEARCH

1 "Research clearly shows that interfering with the normal physiological processes of labour and birth increases risk factors and complications for both mother and baby. ... it is important to understand that these routine interventions can have consequences not only for a woman's labour and birth, but also for the mother and baby immediately after birth and/or some time later, even up to adulthood." (Els Hendrix)

2 "...when used routinely as a first line agent, epidural analgesia can create problems that could have been avoided. ... It is time we told the truth about epidural analgesia—to colleagues and women—and engaged in a truly informed decision-making discussion with women about its optimal use." (Michael Klein)

3 "What is essential [for physiological third stage care] is that a holistic, psychophysiological approach means that the woman and baby are both healthy at the end of the second stage, there is immediate and sustained skin-to-skin contact after the birth, the cord remains intact at least until it stops pulsing, if not through the fourth stage too, the environment remains peaceful, the focus is on the woman and baby and the woman's condition is unobtrusively observed for an hour after the birth of the placenta." (Kathleen Fahy and Carolyn Hastie)

4 "The midwifery model of care, when fully implemented, improves the physiological, psychological, and social outcomes of pregnancy and birth and saves money for systems and families, exposing the need for the total reform of existing dysfunctional hegemonic models." (Robbie Davis-Floyd)

5 "Birth centre care is less expensive than hospital maternity care, and achieves higher levels of patient satisfaction. Maternal and neonatal outcomes are comparable to those for low risk women cared for in traditional physician and hospital-based maternity care, but with fewer interventions and fewer caesarean deliveries, and higher rates of breastfeeding." (Susan Routledge Stapleton)

6 "As yet, there is no strong evidence in favour of hospital birth for selected, low-risk pregnant women. Observational studies suggest that planned home birth may lead to fewer complications, fewer interventions and fewer neonatal problems." (Ole Olsen)

7 "Undoubtedly, mental health and birthing are related in a symbiotic relationship, with mental health being a determinant of birthing choices and birthing outcomes. Less well known is how birthing choices affect mental health in both the short- and long-term." (Shannon Senefeld)

8 "Whether hired independently, enlisted through a funded or charitable initiative or provided by the state, with her trusted, nurturing presence and gentle touch, a doula upholds the heart and soul of birth in a way that can be largely neglected through the medicalised approach; through 'mothering the mother', she brings a little of the traditional sense of community back to childbirth." (Adela Stockton)

pause to think and talk...

...about research

1 Has any of the research surprised you so far?

2 Do you now use, or frequently witness, interventions which you know are not evidence-based?

3 Do you now use, or frequently witness any interventions which prevent women from having normal births?

4 Do you feel any need to change your current practice?

5 If you observe colleagues engaging in practices which seem non-facilitative of normal outcomes what do you do? What *could* you do?

6 To what extent do you feel the women you care for enjoy true informed consent, particularly as regards pharmacological pain relief such as epidurals? Are there any risks you are currently not telling women about?

7 Which approach do you and your colleagues currently take for the third stage of labour? How many women do you inform of the possibilities?

8 How would you feel about working in a birth centre?

9 Would you like to work in the community, supporting home births?

10 Having reconsidered the research relating to home births, if you were previously against or hesitant about home birth, would you consider a rethink? What would change if large numbers of women suddenly started opting for home birth? Consider staffing, transport, equipment and drugs.

11 To what extent is a hospital you know like a birth centre?

12 Why are birth centres set up, who sets them up and what are the day-to-day logistics, do you think? Are there major differences between stand-alone units and ones which are attached to maternity hospitals?

13 What do you do when you suspect or discover that anyone in your care has issues with mental health? What *could* you do in small and big ways?

14 How do you feel about doulas? If you are a midwife or obstetrician, are you happy to work with one? If you're a doula, what is your experience of working with caregivers of various types? How can the situation be optimised for the sake of the women you are caring for?

15 If you are interested in exploring an area of practice further yourself, how would you go about setting up a research project?

16 What do you feel is the value (or otherwise) of publishing data from any research you do, or audit data you collect?

17 Which areas of practice have been influenced by research or audits during your own career?

18 Who could you collaborate with to carry out research in your local area or beyond?

reflect and share further...

The material here and overleaf is intended to help you reflect on research relevant to the topics covered here and perhaps do some research yourself too.

Change

1. How could you effectively research different caregivers' attitudes towards the historical development of professional structures over the centuries, particularly over the last few decades?
2. How could you accurately research and map out influential events in the history of childbirth? What types of events would you need to track?
3. How would you rank types of influence within various professions and agencies? To what extent do the following play a part in influencing attitudes and action?
   - experts' opinions
   - pronouncements from associations (e.g. RCOG or the RCM)
   - research data published in journals which are readable and popular, but not peer-reviewed
   - research data published in peer-reviewed journals
   - pressure from the media, either intentional or accidental
   - litigation, or the fear of litigation
   - individuals campaigning for change
   - groups campaigning for change
   - publishing companies and their publications
   - social networking via Facebook, Twitter, etc
   - conferences
   - government campaigns

   How could you research the power any or all of the above have exerted over the last few decades in influencing change in maternity care?
4. How could you set up research projects which effectively investigated people's attitudes towards time (i.e. the use of partograms, induction, etc)?
5. How could you research outcomes of different attitudes towards time?
6. What kind of data would you need to gather in order to accurately quantify the costs of various treatments, equipment and/or approaches to care?
7. How could you explore caregivers' motivation to adopt various models of care, considering cost factors, convenience and power?
8. How could you find creative solutions to current systems by conducting research into a) caregivers' and consumers' attitudes, and b) different systems operating in different countries? What challenges would be involved?

Pain

1. What research do you know of on pain experienced by women in labour?
2. What research do you know of on pain experienced by women postnatally?
3. Do you agree that pain is 'better' when birth is 'physiological' than when it is experienced in the lead-up to having an epidural and afterwards (before the second stage)?
4. In your view, to what extent is the pain a woman experiences linked with a) her preparation for labour, b) her expectations, c) her choices regarding pain relief (both pharmacological and non-drug-based), d) the support she has in labour, e) her personal resources for coping?
5. Do you see pain in childbirth as being positive or negative?
6. Why do some women report pain relief as being inadequate? How could you research women's perceptions of the 'adequacy' or otherwise of pain relief?
7. Why do some women reportedly continue to request epidurals or caesareans for subsequent births, even after they have had a bad experience with either of these for an earlier labour/birth?
8. Considering the hormonal landscape of birth, to what extent do you think a woman's emotions (e.g. fear) are associated with pain experienced? How could you research this further?
9. Why, according to some research, are women sometimes satisfied with pain relief, but *not* satisfied with their overall experience of birth? How could you research this further?
10. How could you set up a research project to further explore how and why different women experience pain or other sensations during labour and birth?
11. What kind of research project could you set up in order to research women's memories of childbirth, particularly in terms of pain and pain relief?
12. How could you research positive (non-painful) physical sensations associated with birth—e.g. intrapartum orgasm or postnatal euphoria—and what kinds of conclusions would you expect to come to?
13. What kind of research would effectively explore caregivers experience of and attitudes towards pain during pregnancy, labour and the puerperium?
14. How could you find out more about interactions which occur between pregnant and labouring women and caregivers on the subject of pain?
15. How could you research how pain relief is promoted or discouraged generally within cultures around the world?

Birth experience

13 What research do you know of which has investigated women's experience of birth? Do you know of any research which has investigated men's experience of birth? How would you set up a research project?

14 What research evidence can you find on rates of tearing after different types of birth—a) entirely physiological, b) vaginal but with opioids, c) vaginal with an epidural in place, d) vaginal with other forms of pain relief?

15 What research evidence can you find on maternal outcomes—in terms of mortality and morbidity for different types of birth in different contexts?

16 What research evidence can you find on neonatal outcomes—in terms of mortality and morbidity for different types of birth in different contexts?

17 How could you go about research attitudes towards stillbirth in different places and subcultures, a) amongst families who have experienced miscarriage, b) amongst families who have experienced stillbirth and c) amongst families who have had a live baby?

Postnatal scenarios

18 How could you further research possible causal links between pain relief of any kind and later problems?

19 What kind(s) of pain relief would you personally choose to research and why? How would you set up an effective research project?

20 How could you investigate underreporting of postnatal problems which are possibly associated with the use of pain relief during labour?

21 What kinds of material would you need to explore in order to research the historical development of pain relief and use of the caesarean section as a 'solution' to the 'problem' of vaginal birth?

22 How could you research how women's attitudes towards pain relief compare before and after they have experienced childbirth themselves?

23 What kind of research project would you set up in order to find out whether or not pharmacological pain relief affects maternal and neonatal alertness?

24 What kind of research project would you set up in order to find out whether or not pharmacological pain relief affects mother-baby bonding?

25 How could you research longer term effects of birth approaches of various kinds, fairly representing all types of birth, including entirely physiological?

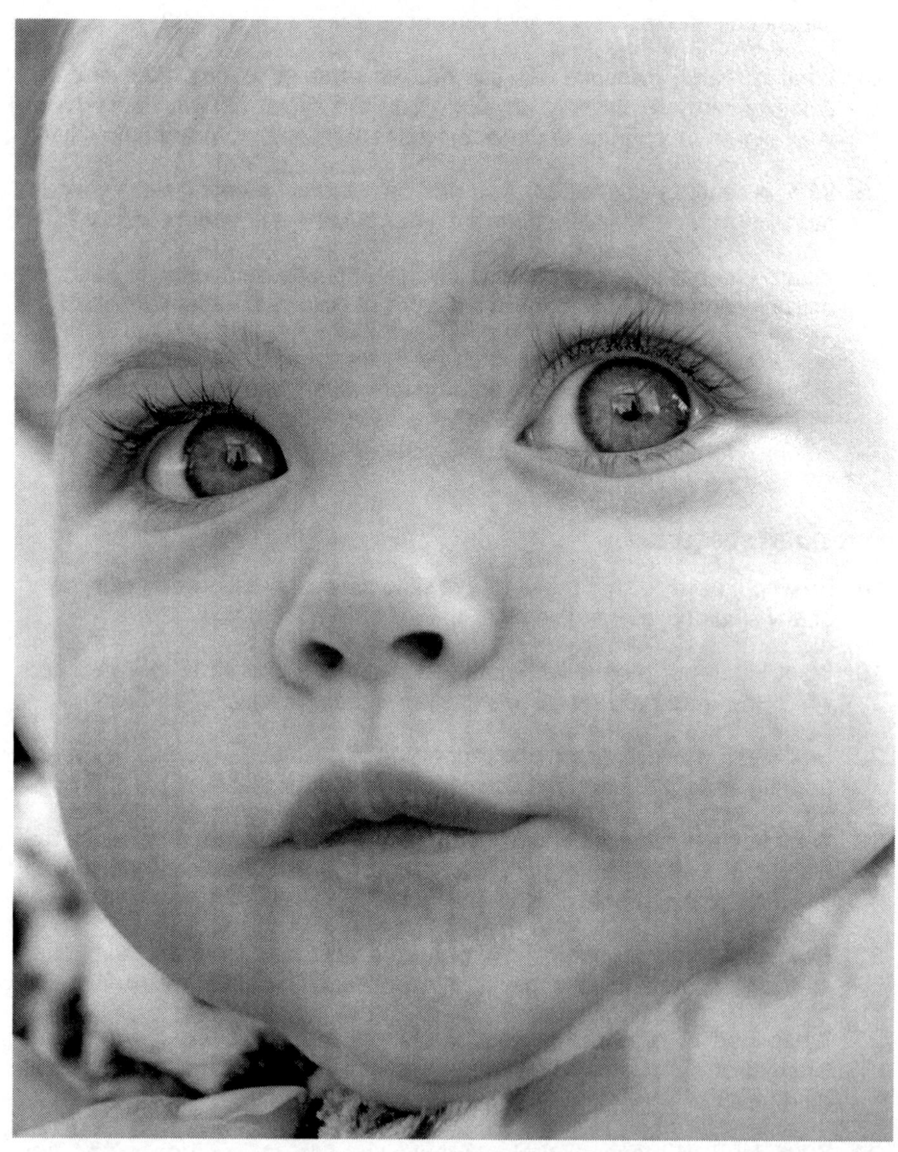

part two: reflections

- reasons for intervention
- RCTs and everyday practices
- harmonising technology and biology
- power and professionalism
- embedding normality in the curriculum
- reclaiming meanings from home births
- learning from traditional cultures
- normality and midwifery in China
- principles for change in developing countries
- inspiration from 'natural' caesareans
- ways and reasons to promote home birth
- founding midwifery today

Why a section on reflections? And where does it all lead?

As you probably know, reflection has become a key part of many courses. However, although we may be forced to reflect when we're on a course or participating in some kind of in-service training, how much do we continue on our own? How much do we allow our pre-conceived ideas to be challenged? Most importantly, perhaps, if we do change our views, how prepared are we to help facilitate real change?

Since this book is about *promoting* normal birth, I'm hoping you will use it to help you do just that. Perhaps, in order to be effective we need to a) have some ideas about what needs to be changed and how this can be done, b) have a vision, and c) have a good idea how we can fit into the change process personally.

This reflections section of the book should help with ideas generation. In the book *Stoking Your Innovation Bonfire,* author Kelly Braden talks about 'idea fatigue'.[1] There is plenty of wonderful material here to help you avoid that!

Considering the vision we need to develop next, Jack Welch, former CEO of General Electric, apparently once said, "Good business leaders create a vision, articulate the vision, passionately own the vision, and relentlessly drive it to completion."[2] Do you know what a better world of birth would be like? What do we want to promote precisely? How are we going to go about doing that? This brings us to the third key to effective change... How are we each personally going to take part?

Braden identifies nine roles in the innovation process:[3]

- **The Revolutionary:** Are you the kind of person who has lots of ideas and plenty of interest in shaking up systems and people?! Can you inspire others?
- **The Conscript:** Do you prefer to keep your head down and just take action? Can you help someone who is more of a 'revolutionary'?
- **The Connector:** Are you good at bringing people together so as to create synergy and effective change? Who could you usefully introduce or encourage?
- **The Artist:** Is your talent to do with refining ideas and making them even better?
- **The Customer Champion:** Are you tuned in to pregnant women's needs and so in touch with your clients that you can communicate their needs to others?
- **The Troubleshooter:** Do you have knowledge or expertise to help solve problems?
- **The Judge:** Are you good at realistically assessing what will work in practice?
- **The Magic-Maker:** Is your role to harness resources to make ideas reality?
- **The Evangelist:** Are you good at making people—both clients and caregivers—believe in ideas and can you help to gather the support necessary for real change?

As you read, consider where you can fit in. Will your thoughts lead to useful action?

References

1 Braden K, 2010. *Stoking Your Innovation Bonfire: A Roadmap to a Sustainable Culture of Ingenuity and Purpose.* New Jersey: John Wiley, p9.

2 Braden K, 2010, p63.

3 Braden K, 2010, p64-.66

Reasons for intervention... but no justification

Ricardo Herbert Jones

The broken bridge

According to various writers and experts, contemporary science occupies the space vacated by religion in social imagination, offering the same promises of redemption and elevation that were historically created by religious organisations. In the West, images of progress permeate the media, relating technology to health, creating an ethos of medical jingoism towards combating diseases, often drowning out the critical thinking of alternative voices. An ideology of transcendence and salvation through technological sophistication that will ultimately redeem us from human limitations has come to predominate in our thinking—Robbie Davis-Floyd (1992, 2004) calls this ideology 'the technocratic model of birth and health care'.[1,2] Yet nowadays, in the light of rising costs in healthcare, it appears that this technocratic model is a bubble about to burst, and it becomes clear that there is a need to build a space for dialogue between scientific evidence and everyday medical practice.

Noting the lack of scientific support for the many routine obstetric practices applied to pregnancy and childbirth, in 1979 the World Health Organization (WHO) established the European Perinatal Study Group, inviting multiple social actors for a debate about these routine practices. Among the representatives were obstetricians, neonatologists, midwives, nurses, perinatal epidemiologists, health administrators, economists, psychologists, sociologists and consumers. The fundamental idea and main objective of these meetings, financed and promoted by WHO, was not to deal with high risk pregnancies, but rather to work with the majority of healthy women facing the challenges of pregnancy and birth. At the beginning of their discussions, in the early 1980s, the term 'evidence-based medicine' was not yet in common use and had not achieved the importance it has today as the primary clinical guide for medical practice. The European Perinatal Study Group was groundbreaking in its challenge to current practice standards in many areas of childbirth care, using scientific evidence as the main criterion for determining which procedures should be part of routine practice, and which ones should be abandoned for lack of scientific consistency. This pioneering group conducted a study of literature from around the world on perinatal and obstetric practices; only 10% of medical interventions were truly based on satisfactory scientific evidence.[3]

More recently, in 2005, studies conducted by Bergsjo confirmed there were still great variations in obstetric practices, with little or no difference in perinatal out-comes.[4] These variations occurred between countries, within countries, between districts, even between hospitals, proving that perinatal practice is not based on the best scientific evidence, but rather on the opinions and beliefs of the local doctors, especially the ones with the most prominence and prestige.

These studies, which critically appraised obstetric practice and the recommendations of major institutions and illuminated the gap between medical practice and scientific evidence, can be considered the first global effort to transform obstetrics into a specialty tightly linked to science.

In the United States, two large 'Listening to Mothers'[5] surveys conducted by Childbirth Connection reinforced the conclusion that typical obstetric practices —high rates of caesareans, episiotomies, lithotomy position for birth, syntocinon induction and augmentation, electronic fetal monitoring and other invasive procedures—are far from evidence-based.

The routine use of these non-evidence-based procedures has spread in recent decades from the Western world to many countries in the developing world. The repercussions are varied and complex. If scientific evidence is not the main guide to professional conduct in maternity care in the West, what are the real triggers for action? Why the distance between the recommendations of WHO, national health authorities, the Pan American Health Organization (PAHO), the Cochrane Library and other renowned institutions—and everyday practice in maternity wards? Why is there a gap between evidence-based medicine and current obstetric practice? Why is there currently such a shaky bridge between science and obstetric care?

I suggest that there are hidden forces determining these practices and that they are not rationally but *pre-rationally* guided. What so many studies reveal is the magnitude and power of biomedical mythologies, which are still standing after decades of scientific proof of their inadequacy. Hierarchical and totemic mythological constructions determine standard obstetric practice. People in positions of authority hold the power to establish routines and protocols and they are under little or no pressure to link these routines and protocols to sound science; the 'eminence' of a caregiver has become more important than the 'evidence' of research. Despite its scientific pretence, contemporary obstetrics follows the same authority models found over ten millennia of cultural evolution.

Mind the gap

Professionals who attend human birth are normally guided by 'standards of care', or protocols established by authority figures in the institutions in which they work. The origin of these protocols is multifactorial. Some of them are truly based on scientific evidence but, as we shall see, that is far from being the rule. According to epidemiologist Marsden Wagner:

> *"... if the evidence shows that a certain practice is extremely risky (such as thalidomide, diethylstilbestrol, X-rays, etc) it is likely that this conduct will be discarded from protocols. But if the evidence offers support for a practice that favours doctors (e.g. fetal monitoring should be used when there is hormonal induction and epidural), it will be standardised. If a practice is uncontroversial and beneficial, but not favourable to the doctor (e.g. vertical position for delivery) the likelihood of it being standardised in any particular obstetric service is very weak, and this is the reason why we have such a big gap between scientific evidence and everyday practice in obstetric centres."*[6]

The painful truth about contemporary maternity care is that its criteria are not focused on the patient; they were displaced to the doctor, the current owner of authoritative knowledge about birth, mostly over the course of the 20th century. Part of this domination occurred through the near extermination of midwives and the 'feminine obstetrics' they provided. (This was certainly the case in Brazil, as well as in the US and Canada.) Today, in Brazil, almost all deliveries take place in hospitals, taking women away from their normal environment and their families. Birth went from being a social experience to a medical one, and this dislocated the birthing mother from her previous role as protagonist. Doctors and their instruments became the main actors in the drama of labour. Women were left the task of carrying the child during pregnancy so that at the end the child could be received by doctors—the keepers of health and well-being, on behalf of society and its institutions. This profound cultural shift inevitably had repercussions which had an equal impact on society, culture and healthcare practices.

The painful truth about contemporary maternity care is that its criteria are not focused on the patient

In Brazil, by the 1970s, following the American model, intervention had become the norm and it was untrammeled in its development. In that same decade in the US, a huge childbirth activist movement arose which was dedicated to challenging the routine use of obstetric procedures and to returning birth to women. The power of this movement is the reason why caesarean rates today in the United States, while way too high at 32%, have not reached the 43% caesarean rate of contemporary Brazil. Note, too, that this rate encompasses the huge Amazon region, where caesareans are few, so is in fact far higher in urban areas. In fact, in Brazilian cities, particularly in the case of upper- and middle-class women, caesarean rates have reached 85%.[7] Even during normal births, which are an increasingly rare occurrence, most women are given medication that is potentially dangerous for the baby, and a 'cascade of interventions' is triggered that easily leads to the surgical interruption of labour.[8] Epidurals have almost become mandatory in maternity wards.

Today, there is a large and growing childbirth movement in Brazil dedicated to 'the humanisation of birth'. Following the lead of a number of pioneering obstetricians and midwives, this movement crystalised in the year 2000 at a conference in Fortaleza, the site of the former WHO conference. This conference was attended by around 2,000 people, many of whom have gone on to become passionate advocates of normal birth. Sadly, though, in spite of 10 years of effort, these people have not yet succeeded in achieving any reduction in the overall caesarean rate in Brazil; nevertheless, they have accomplished significant change in particular hospitals and have inspired many out-of-hospital birth facilities to open.

Brazilian obstetric intolerance of practices which depart from the current norm (at any one time) has much in common with religious discrimination. Similar attitudes prevail in other countries and perhaps explains the persecution of midwives in Hungary[9] and the Czech Republic,[10] as well as the ostracism and vilification of midwives and holistic obstetricians in the United States and Brazil. Corporate medicine in many countries remains inured against any attempt to challenge or even discuss childbirth protocols. To regulate the protection of basic human rights, such as a couple's right to choose the place of birth, the European Court of Human Rights recently found it necessary to speak, concluding that it is a basic human right to choose where a birth should take place.[11]

It is a basic human right to choose where a birth takes place

Among the reasons for the observed asymmetry between scientific evidence and what we really witness in obstetric care, the following can be suggested...

Rituals

As we've seen, obstetric protocols and standards of care are based not on scientific evidence but on 'hidden' cultural factors. According to Davis-Floyd, when obstetricians rely on their 'personal experiences' as justification for their wholesale adoption of routine procedures, they are simply exhibiting the habituation they have internalised to doing things *the way they have always been done.*[11] Davis-Floyd analyses the routine procedures of obstetrics as rituals to which obstetricians have become, over their years of training, habituated and thus subservient.[1] They do it the same way, over and over again, and then they can't imagine any other way of doing it.

But why should we believe that the protocols and routines of hospitals are in fact 'rituals', controlled by powerful, irrational (or pre-rational) forces and connected to the deep values of our culture? To better understand this proposal it is necessary to understand the concept of ritual that Robbie Davis-Floyd developed[1,2]

> *"A 'ritual' can be defined as a repetitive, patterned and symbolic enactment of a cultural belief or value."*

Thus, the patterned repetition of behaviours within the context of obstetric practice could fit perfectly in the concept of ritual, as long as these behaviours are *symbolic representatives of beliefs and social values.* Davis-Floyd also notes that that:

> *"The belief system of a culture is enacted through rituals, and an analysis of these rituals may lead us directly to the understanding of this belief system."*[13]

In *Birth as an American Rite of Passage*,[1] Davis-Floyd analyses enemas (washing/cleansing), the use of indiscreet hospital gowns, the separation from family that many women are forced to endure, the shaving of pubic hair, the IV, artificial induction and augmentation of labour, electronic fetal monitoring, episiotomy and caesarean section as modern rituals that express and display deep cultural values and beliefs regarding the 'dirtiness' of feminine biological processes, the ongoing patriarchal devaluation of women, and the deep cultural valuation of high technology. The moment of birth is one of profound sensory opening, and it constitutes the best possible cultural moment to reinforce women's inferior place in society and enact and display a profound cultural belief in high technology as superior to natural processes. Davis-Floyd notes that:

> *"Sometimes, existing values and beliefs are clarified as they are represented, but often the deeper values that a ritual expresses are from the order of the unconscious, rather than being consciously determined."*[13]

She goes on to explain that medical habituation to standard obstetric procedures develops in the body, over time, usually outside of consciousness. Reason and rationality give way to the power of ritual habituation. In other words, even if a procedure is shown to be risky or non-evidence-based, this will usually not be sufficient to threaten its use on a large scale in the short term. For example, rationally showing the inadequacy of the lithotomy position, enemas, shaving and the unrestrained use of episiotomies, has not proven to be an effective way to eradicate routines that are obviously inadequate and risky for both mother and baby. The reasons for this failure lie in the fact that reasons for the use of these interventions are rooted deeply in the unconscious mind of caregivers. Even though, as Davis-Floyd demonstrates, rituals are not static and permanent—we don't sacrifice virgins or burn witches at the stake any more, for example—the modification of rituals only occurs when the constitutive bases of these rituals are altered, i.e. when the very roots of a practice are pulled out. When they are not, we can only mask the ritual and transform it superficially (using goats instead of virgins, birthing women instead of witches). Only through a revolution in cultural values will we be able to change these entrenched procedures.

Culture and advertising

Brazil has a culture that clearly associates access to high technology with social status. People from the middle and upper classes have more access to 'cargo' (things, objects, possessions), in the words of Jared Diamond.[14] The more they have, the more distance they keep from nature and the closer they get to technology. Media plays an unquestionable role in 'mediating' relationships between individuals and establishing society's codes of values and behaviour. The *British Medical Journal* recently published a research article about Brazilian women's magazines and the issue of birth.[15] 20 years of publications about normal delivery and caesarean section were analysed. The result was not surprising: the majority of the publications didn't use good sources of information. The representations of caesarean were incomplete and tended to de-emphasise risks. These magazines are targeted at the middle class, the sector of population with the highest caesarean rates. The study showed that when women reproduce they tend to embrace values that glorify technology applied to birth and belittle their own intrinsic ability to give birth safely.

A myth recently challenged was the idea that the high caesarean rates in Brazil (and in other countries) were due to women's demand for surgical births. However, a recent study published in the *British Medical Journal of Obstetrics and Gynecology* in 2011 shows that only a small percentage of women express the desire to have a scheduled caesarean.[16] This study reflects the same conclusions reached by Joe Potter and Kristine Hopkins in their study of caesareans in Brazil: women don't demand caesareans... obstetricians do.[17] Another factor is one that comes from the world of celebrities. 9 out of 10 female Brazilian 'pop stars' have their babies by caesarean section, most of them with renowned obstetricians. (As the British say, they are simply 'too posh to push'. These young women, the 'opinion makers' and an example for adolescents to follow, associate caesareans with luxury, power and fame. The result must surely be fans who think: "If she can have a caesarean and stay beautiful sexy and charming, so can I". It's worth noting, though, that Gisele Bündchen, the famous Brazilian model, had a home birth in water in the United States, which initiated an interesting debate regarding the humanisation of birth in the Brazilian media.

Convenience

It is obvious that in a world controlled by time, deliveries can present a challenge to the contemporary preference for practicality and expediency. A birth can take 10, 12, 24 hours or more, demanding the presence of a professional that can offer safety and support for the patient in labour throughout the process. In contemporary models of care, an obstetrician has difficulties juggling tasks, jobs, vacations, leisure, and paperwork with the eventuality of a birth. The attempt to control the beginning and end of labour can be seen in the alarmingly high rates of labour induction (the use of hormones to induce contractions) and scheduled caesareans. For example, in the city of Porto Alegre, the capital of a state in the extreme south of Brazil, in 2006 the caesarean rate fell dramatically from around 1,400 on weekdays to just over 1,000 on Saturdays and under 800 on Sundays. Clearly, convenience for the obstetricians must have been a factor in determining the rate on any particular day, not just medical indications.[18] Convenience must clearly also explain why in the city of Rio de Janeiro a 2011 study from the organisation FIOCRUZ revealed that 92% of all caesareans were being conducted prior to the onset of labour.[19]

In reporting on these statistics, I am not attempting to blame any groups of people or corporations... I am simply trying to suggest that motivations unrelated to the well-being of both mother and baby are unquestionable realities and it seems clear that these realities (based on motivations) produce consequences. These consequences can be clearly measured and they are responsible for many problems in maternity care. Some of these results can be seen in the caesarean rate, which is 43% in Brazil,[20] and over 30% in the United States.[21] WHO concludes that, when adequate care is provided for a woman in labour "there is no justification for a caesarean incidence above 15% anywhere in the world".[22] The exaggeratedly high rates of intervention are a clear indication that some kind of conflict of interests exists that is strong enough to modify medical behaviours and procedures.

As Marsden Wagner says "the social layer [the well-fed, well-to-do] that least needs this operation is the one that makes more use of it."[23] ANS (the Brazilian National Agency of Supplementary Health) states that 84.5% of middle-class patients have their babies by caesarean section,[24] which means that 4 out of 5 women in this social class undergo major surgery in order to give birth to their babies, without worrying about any of the associated risks.

A major issue here is the very low payments given to professionals who attend childbirth, who are paid by insurance companies. In many Brazilian cities, payment barely exceeds R$ 200,00 (£75.00 or US$121.50).[25] In 2010 the obstetric association of São Paulo (SOGESP) launched a campaign criticising the fact that attendance at a birth was paid the amount usually paid to a hairdresser for a perm. Even the filming crew that records the birth usually gets up to five times more money than the obstetrician.

Another fact related to convenience is the inadequacy of obstetrics training in medical schools and during medical residencies. Training is increasingly focused on pathology and on the resolution of problems and diseases so trainee obstetricians end up devoting little attention to the complex process of learning how to attend a normal delivery. The more professionals (ultra) specialise, the more they lose touch with the normal physiology of birth and push themselves away from the multiple skills they will need in order to safeguard and facilitate a normal birth. Birth assistance is a complex and integrative ability developed over millennia. The 'reduction' of birth to a predictable series of mechanical events removed from the professionals that attend it obscures and obviates the obstetrician's abilities to achieve full understanding of the psychological, emotional and spiritual elements of the birth process. More and more, obstetricians know less about how to deal with the emotional demands of birth, meaning that they unconsciously direct patients towards behaviours which mean they can be treated in the way they were trained. Since caesareans cut down the time care is needed they don't interfere with a professional's leisure time, they don't clash with appointments in their private practice, they don't involve the anguish which comes with dealing with the unknown... and since caesareans represent a medical procedure for which the obstetrician is better trained, they must seem to be a natural solution to the dilemmas of birth. Unfortunately, mothers and babies are the ones who keep paying the bill, monetary and otherwise.

Mothers and babies are the ones who keep paying the bill

Fear

In the early 1990s there was a strong wave of medical lawsuits in countries like England, where at that time 85% of doctors had already been sued once, and 65% twice.[26] In Brazil the medical culture of litigation has not yet reached this critical point, but the fear of the courtroom is already making Brazilian doctors practise defensive medicine. São Paulo's Medical Council admitted this in a letter to the Public Ministry in 2007, when it explained that out of the 31 lawsuits against obstetricians in that state between 2001 and 2006, 29 (over 93%) were brought against obstetricians who had assisted a normal delivery and only two (less than 7%) were against obstetricians who had performed caesareans.[27] In the state of Rio Grande do Sul, the same reality appears: obstetricians are the medical specialists that get sued the most.[28]

In spite of the fact that ACOG (the American Congress of Obstetrics and Gynecology) itself presented a pronouncement criticising the unrestricted use of continuous fetal monitoring in 1995,[29] the use of fetal monitoring did not decrease at that point, even in deliveries that were expected to be normal. The indiscriminate use of this technology, which continues today, is based on obstetricians' fear that the absence of clear documentation of fetal well-being might be used against them in court. The overuse of this technology stems in part from the insecurity and fear that obstetricians have of the legal system and results in an attitude of self-protection, but can also result in wrong interpretations of fetal distress. These faulty interpretations of monitor readings lead to interventions and caesareans in profusion. On many occasions an obstetrician's fear is the first trigger of a 'cascade of interventions' in maternity care.

In contrast to the US, the legal system in Brazil does not emphasise monetary compensation for bad medical outcomes. Therefore, there is no culture of million-dollar lawsuits against professionals due to unfortunate medical sequelae or even patient death. The penalties issued by the Medical Councils are of a moral order and in legal courts (civil and criminal) the penalties are never large, unlike in American courts. In Brazil, perhaps because of the devoutly Catholic Christian culture, where money is considered 'dirty' and both life and pain are considered unquantifiable, putting a monetary value on human life as compensation for a bad medical result seems strange and even immoral. (Thus, while lawsuits might destroy a doctor's reputation, they don't usually affect his finances to the point of destroying them.) This is why Brazil has never created a widespread and consistent system of medical insurance, much less a mandatory one. The existing insurance systems are very 'shy' and of very low coverage. Having said all this, in Brazil we are indeed currently witnessing an extraordinary growth in the number of lawsuits against medical professionals in the medical councils. Obstetricians in Brazil (but also in many other Western countries) are among the most sued of professionals, and almost all lawsuits in obstetrics are related to care provided during a normal delivery. We almost never see accusations against doctors who overuse interventions, especially caesareans, even when outcomes are bad.

According to Davis-Floyd, medical professionals who overuse technology, even in non-evidence-based and dangerous ways, are covered by a protective cultural cloak, which she codes as 'the technological imperative': "If the technology exists, it must be used."[30] She goes on to say that this imperative is based on 'the myth of technological transcendence'—one of the most powerful myths of modern civilisation. Since we collectively believe in the redemptive and curative powers of technology, this belief—which is pre-rational in character—is the main guide for our behaviour.

Even obstetricians who aim to practise evidence-based medicine are not protected because their inevitable fear of lawsuits is bound to make them behave defensively. This is likely to lead them to constantly increase their use of interventions and, consequently, there will be an ongoing increase in rates of birth-related morbidity.[31] We therefore need to build a system to protect professionals who assist birth in a humanistic way, and this should be based on evidence, not on the authority of local medical authorities. The discussion of this new approach should come from a group made up of five parties: consumers, midwives, obstetricians, prosecutors and judges. These five parties need to develop a new understanding of birth risks and then inform and educate the population about the increasing risk of the liberal use of interventions. In other words, they need to disclose the reality of the 'technological mythology'. If we, as a society, don't manage to do this, caregivers will inevitably become increasingly fearful of litigation and will continue to work in a defensive way. This will lead to more interventions being carried out, simply because these protect the obstetrician inasmuch as he or she is acting out the fallacious contemporary myth—that technology must be the best way forward... i.e. he or she is following the 'technocratic imperative'. Since, ultimately, this inappropriate use of interventions causes more harm than good the only way forward is to change the mythology underlying maternity care. This should just be the starting point to completely transforming current systems of maternity care.

Money

The power of local and national economic interests in birth is far from subtle. Universities, hospitals, and doctors work closely with the birth industry, which has access to doctors, patients, and highly-trained medical researchers. As a result, they can profit from sponsoring studies on the use of technology that are published in medical journals and presented at conferences. Doctors and other professionals can promote their careers through studies financed by the drug and technology industry and thereby achieve recognition and status. Undeniably, since medicine was transformed into a multi-billion business, pressure from large pharmaceutical companies has grown stronger every day. Hospitals make more profit from surgery and the longer hospitalisation it requires, and this makes it necessary to maintain hospitals above a critical level, and use the same logistics as hotels. Hospital costs are kept extremely high due to the use of qualified professionals who are called to work there and the purchase and maintenance of the latest generation of high-tech equipment.

Hospitals seem to need management by profit-based capitalism

Hospitals have therefore become expensive companies that appear to need to be managed according to the laws and logistics of profit-based capitalism, which means safeguarding security and investment made, and managing risk. The 'raw material' of hospitals is the patient—an entity which must be transformed into money. In other words, a hospital works with the same mandate as any ordinary commercial enterprise: it needs to cut costs and increase profits. Considering birth in this light, it is clear that a caesarean patient consumes less time in the delivery room and that consumer rotation is consequently faster. Even if this were not a factor, an obstetrician can organise his life more easily by scheduling caesareans, because this means that less time will be spent with each client and more time will be left for money-making private appointments. In fact, many Brazilian obstetricians attend caesareans in industrial assembly-line fashion: five or six patients are lined up for treatment and all procedures are carried out on the same morning so that the normal randomness of birth cannot interfere with the obstetrician's lifestyle—his or her office time, holidays, fun and family time.

If birth really were simply a mechanical process that benefited from technological intervention, there would be no problem here. Unfortunately, this mechanistic and profit-based treatment of birth has many negative repercussions for the well-being of the mother, the baby, and the family as a whole.

Fixing the bridge

The basic founding principle of medicine, 'First, do no harm,' implies that all medical practice should primarily be beneficial to the patient and not to the professionals or the system. This Hippocratic Oath, if fully implemented, would ensure that the non-medical factors of *ritual, convenience, culture, fear and money*—which, as I've outlined above, are clearly related to the interests of professionals—should never interfere with the protocols and routines of maternity care or of health care in general. Unfortunately, reality shows us that standard obstetric protocols and routines reflect only the ideological bias of influential doctors, who are uniformly subject to the hegemonic technocratic model of birth.

Renowned birth anthropologist Brigitte Jordan states that:

> *"To legitimate a form of knowledge as authoritative it is necessary to devalue all other forms of knowledge".*[32]

Perhaps this explains why normal birth (and particularly home birth) is undermined in places where caesarean rates are high... The authoritative knowledge held, in this case, by obstetricians, only works to reinforce the technocratic model through direct transmission from one generation of obstetricians to the next, with very little consideration of the scientific evidence.

According to Marsden Wagner, health professionals who work with a humanistic approach focused on women's needs and preferences and based on sound scientific evidence are frequently treated as 'heretics' or threats to the system.[33] In the words of Brigitte Jordan:

> *"Those who link themselves to alternative knowledge systems tend to be considered backward, ignorant, naïve or 'trouble makers'. Whatever they say about the negotiation of the routine obstetric practices, for example, is considered irrelevant, ungrounded or unrelated to the subject".*[34]

As we have seen, the list of contemporary interventions where there is a discrepancy between practice and scientific evidence is a long one. Most contemporary obstetricians in most countries who routinely apply interventions are influenced by the 'hidden forces' I have discussed, i.e. non-medical factors that benefit professionals, their institutions and corporations. Thus, humanistic change comes slowly, if at all.[35]

To give a very clear example, the definitive work on the negative effects of routine episiotomy and the lack of any evidence supporting the routine use of this procedure date from 1987, which is over 20 years ago.[36] Nevertheless, episiotomy is still performed in the vast majority of vaginal deliveries in Brazil. The reason for this is that its introduction, in the mid-20th century, harmonised strongly with a consistent social belief in the superiority of technology ('technological transcendence' in Davis-Floyd's analysis), in addition to supporting and sustaining the cultural view rooted in patriarchy of 'women's essential defectiveness'.

As I wrote in my book, "Humanising birth is the restitution of agency to women".[37] This concept incorporates autonomy and freedom as superior values to be developed and stimulated. It is in line with the words of many great thinkers, from Christ to Erich Fromm, who see freedom as the ultimate goal, the one where all our efforts should lead. To reframe birthing women as protagonists in birth rather than passive patients means putting women back at the centre of everyone's attention and decision-making processes and relegating medical staff as helpers and consultants. In order to do this, it is not enough just to keep the focus on the woman; she needs to be empowered so that she can really regain her freedom. In other words, we need to offer each pregnant woman a hope, encouragement and inspiration so that she can light her own path through the birthing experience and successfully move through the challenges of the birth event towards a new dawn, with a baby in her arms.

Human birth is a process which has involved millennia of improvement and it is a constitutive part of who and what we are as individuals and as a species. Our essential connection to our mother's love created the psychological substrate that ultimately produced rationality and language. The personal 'imprints' produced by the way each individual puts him- or herself into the world is a fundamental part of each person's constitution. For this reason, every human birth is a patchwork of countless meanings, from hormonal to cultural, including psychological, emotional, and spiritual aspects. Therefore, the birth of our babies should never be managed and controlled by the cultural factors of time, money or power, as outlined above.

Only by understanding these intangible and powerful forces will we be able to overcome beliefs that are not supported by scientific evidence. Once achieved, this understanding will empower us to provide mothers and babies with the best, evidence-based practice we can manage so as to facilitate mothers' transition to motherhood and babies' entry into the world. Only by gaining this understanding can we be guides and guardians through the most amazing, transformative 'rite of passage' that exists in the world: the birth of a child.

Ricardo Herbert Jones is an obstetrician-gynecologist and homeopath, the representative of CIMS for Brazil and a spokesperson and advocate for humanisation in childbirth. He is the author of *Memorias do Homem de Vidro* (Memoirs of the Man Made of Glass) (Porto Alegre, Brazil) in which he describes his paradigm shift towards an interdisciplinary and humanised approach to childbirth. In Brazil he is a professor of national and international courses for doulas and perinatal educators and internationally, he frequently speaks at conferences on the humanisation of childbirth. He is also the father of two hospital-born children.

References

1 Davis-Floyd, Robbie. 2004 (orig published 1992), Birth as an American Rite of Passage. Berkeley and London: University of California Press.

2 Davis-Floyd, Robbie. 1987 Obstetric Training as a Rite of Passage, in Obstetrics in the United States: Woman, Physician, and Society, Robert Hahn, ed. Special Issue of the *Medical Anthropology Quarterly*, 1(3): 288-318.

3 Fraser C, Selected perinatal procedures, *Acta Obstetrica et Gynecologica Scandinavia*, supplement 117,1983.

4 http://onlinelibrary.wiley.com/doi/10.1111/j.1471-0528.1983.tb09279. x/abstract [accessed 13 February 2011].

5 Declerc E, Sakala C., Corry M., and Appelbaum S. Listening to Mothers II: Report of the Second National US Survey of Women's Childbearing Experiences, Executive Summary. New York. Childbirth Connection, 2006.

6 Wagner, M., *Bad Habits*. 1999/2000. *AIMS Journal* 11(4).

7 http://www1.folha.uol.com.br/folha/equilibrio/noticias/ult263u597422.shtml [accessed 13 February 2011].

8 http://www.childbirthconnection.org/article.asp?ck-10182 [accessed 13 February

2011].

9 http://www.guardian.co.uk/world/2010/oct/22/hungary-midwife-agnes-gereb-home-birth [accessed 13 February 2011].

10 http://tasz/hu/en/news/victory-strasbourg-cause-home-birth [accessed 13 February 2011].

11 http://ipsnews.net/newTVE.asp?idnews=54171 [accessed 13 February 2011].

12 Davis-Floyd, R. *Birth as an American Rite of Passage*, 2nd ed. Berkeley and London: University of California Press, 2004.

13 Davis-Floyd, R. *Birth as an American Rite of Passage*, 2nd ed. Berkeley and London: University of California Press, 2004.

14 Diamond J, 1999. *Guns, Germs and Steel: The Fates of Human Societies*. New York, W,W. Norton.

15 http://www.ncbi.nlm.nih.gov/pubmed/21266421 [accessed 13 February 2011]

16 Mazzoni A, Althabe F, Liu N, Bonotti A, Gibbons L, Sánchez A, Belizán J. Women's preference for caesarean section: a systematic review and meta-analysis of observational studies. *BJOG* 2011;118:391–399.

17 Joseph E. Potter PhD, Kristine Hopkins PhD, Anibal Faúndes MD, Ignez Perpétuo MD, PhD. Women's Autonomy and Scheduled Cesarean Sections in Brazil: A Cautionary Tale. *Birth*, Volume 35, Issue 1, pages 33–40, March 2008.

18 http://lproweb.procempa.com.br/pmpa/prefpoa/cgvs/usu_doc/ev_sinasc_2006.pdf [accessed 13 February 2011].

19 http://www.fiocruz.br/ccs/cgi/cgilua.exe/sys/start.htm?infoid=1539&sid=9 [accessed 13 February 2011].

20 http://tabnet.datasus.gov.br/cgi/deftohtm.exe?sinasc/cnv/pnvbr.def [accessed 13 February 2011].

21 http://www.cdc.gov/nchs/fastats/delivery.htm [accessed 13 February 2011]

22 Ana P. Betrán, Mario Merialdi, Jeremy A. Lauer, Wang Bing-Shun, Jane Thomas, Paul Van Look, Marsden Wagner. Rates of caesarean section: analysis of global, regional and national estimates. *Paediatric and Perinatal Epidemiology*, Volume 21, Issue 2, pages 98–113, March 2007.

23 Wagner M., *Pursuing the Birth Machine: The search for appropriate birth technology*. Sidney: Ace Graphics,1994.

24 http://www1.folha.uol.com.br/folha/equilibrio/noticias/ult263u597422.shtml [accessed 13 February 2011].

25 http://www.febrasgo.org.br/?op=300&id_srv=2&id_tpc=5&nid_tpc=&id_grp=1&add=&lk=1&nti=511&l_nti=S&itg=S&st=&dst=3 [accessed 13 February 2011].

26 Capstick J & Edwards P Trends in obstetric malpractice claims, *Lancet*, vol 336, pp 931, 1990.

27 Ofício 022/07 CRM-SP.

28 Costa, S.M. A questão das cesarianas. Revista Brasileira de Ginecologia e Obstetrícia vol.27 nº.10 Rio de Janeiro Oct. 2005.

29 American College of Obstetricians and Gynecologists. Fetal Heart Rate Patterns: Monitoring, Interpreta-tion, and Management. *ACOG Technical Bulletin* 207.

Washington, DC: ACOG, 1995.

30 Davis-Floyd, R Culture and Birth: The Technocratic Imperative. *International Journal of Childbirth Education*, 9(2):6-7, 1994.

31 Jones RH. 2009. Teamwork: An Obstetrician, a Midwife, and a Doula in Brazil. In *Birth Models That Work*, eds Robbie Davis-Floyd, Lesley Barclay, Betty-Anne Daviss, and Jan Tritten. University of Cal-ifornia Press, pp. 271-304.

32 Jordan, B. Birth in Four Cultures, Waveland Press, Prospect Heights, Illinois, US,1993.

33 Wagner M A Global Witchhunt, *Lancet,* Vol 346, pp 1020-22,1995.

34 Jordan B, 1993. *Birth in Four Cultures*. Prospect Heights, Illinois: Waveland Press.

35 Wagner M. Bad Habits. *AIMS Journal* 11(4). 1999/2000.

36 Thacker SB, Banta HD. Benefits and risks of episiotomy: an interpretive review of the English language literature, 1860-1980. *Obst Gynecol Surv*, 38(6):322-338, 1983.

37 Jones RH, 2004. Memórias do Homem de Vidro—Reminiscências de Um Obstetra Humanista. Porto Alegre: Editora Idéias à Granel.

RCTs and everyday practices... a troubled relationship

Jette Aaroe Clausen

Translating problems into research questions—not an innocent task

The randomised controlled trial (RCT) has been much celebrated in midwifery and obstetrics in recent decades and plays an important role in constituting midwifery and obstetrics as scientific practices. RCTs became attractive to midwifery in the late 1980s and were even more widely referred to throughout the 1990s. This call for evidence from randomised trials came with a call for less interventionist maternity care.[1] At first RCTs seemed to get the job done; the trials documented that many interventions in pregnancy and childbirth were unjustified and as midwives and obstetricians increasingly referred to RCTs this made the RCTs themselves acquire more status and authority.

It is now taken for granted that evidence always improves maternity care. Evidence has gained a hegemonic status in midwifery and obstetrics (i.e. it carries great weight). However, there is no such thing as a free lunch and Murray Enkin, co-author of *Effective Care in Pregnancy and Childbirth*,[1] a supporter of midwifery and a firm believer in evidence-based medicine, has now called for humility:

> *"Above all, we need humility. The power of randomised trials, particularly as they feed into official health care guidelines, is enormous. They are a form of advice unlike ordinary advice; because of pressure to conform, there may be no option to refusal. The 'scientific evidence' has achieved a mythical status. It is excessively powerful rhetoric, a tool that so easily has become a weapon."*[2]

Nowadays, it seems that nothing is too small, too big, too simple or too complex to be tested in a randomised trial. RCTs are used to test interventions as diverse as the Pinard and the electronic fetal monitor, epidurals and birthing pools; they are also used to determine the best way for a midwife to place her hands at birth and to evaluate different birth settings. However, turning everyday choices and interventions into research questions is not an innocent task. The Belgian philosopher Isabelle Stengers urges us to slow down our reasoning and consider if we have asked the right question when setting up a trial.[3] The way a research question is phrased defines the boundaries of the world that we can explore.

I take Stengers' suggestion seriously and in the following sections I shall take you on an exploratory journey into evidence and antenatal care practices. You, the traveller, should be prepared to encounter acting artefacts and emergent bodies. Unlike, obstetric texts that subscribe to an essentialist approach to technology and the body, I will present a post-constructivist and non-essentialist take on technology. Such a move has consequences; it means that we cannot take for granted that we know what a technology or a body is—we have to remain open, and explore what they are in a particular practice.

What prompted my question about the relationship between the randomised trial and everyday midwifery practices was a short piece of text in the Danish National Guidelines for Maternity Care[4] that states that listening to the fetus has no effect on perinatal mortality and morbidity. The author(s) nevertheless suggested that the midwife could use a Sonicaid because this would provide women with a good experience. Being a midwife and having done research in the field of Science and Technology Studies (STS)[5] this little text seemed 'noisy'. I say 'noisy' here in the sense of something which triggers a protest or a complaint. 'Noisy stories' are stories which do not conform to a common-sense understanding of technology as a mere tool, which is used because it provides an effective *means* to an *end*. In other words, when a story is 'noisy' it suggests that more is going on in clinical practice than that which is explained in traditional textbooks and in evidence-based discourse. However, this 'noise' is not heard by everyone because the noisiness of a story will vary depending on how the reader is positioned. Personally, I hear the 'noise' as a result of working in the fields of midwifery and STS. I therefore found myself asking various questions... Why did the Danish National Board of Health suggest that midwives use a Sonicaid? Why did they expel the Pinard? And why did they frame it as a good experience? To develop my analysis I draw on theoretical resources from the field of Science, Technology and Society Studies (STS) as well as on interviews with midwives and on my own experience as a midwife.

Different monitoring practices in antenatal care

'Listening to the stomach' is an integrated part of antenatal care in a range of countries. Either a Pinard or a Sonicaid is used. There are many different Pinards: they come in wood, plastic, metal and they can be long or short. In some places midwives also use other kinds of stethoscopes such as the DeLee. (This is a stethoscope that is placed between a woman's abdomen and the midwife's forehead. The midwife places the two 'listening-in' tubes in her ears.) A Sonicaid is a handheld ultrasound device. There are also several versions of the Sonicaid; some display the heart sound on a small screen while others do not; some have loudspeakers whereas others are used with earplugs meaning that the only person who hears the sound is the person who has the earplugs in. In this analysis I restrict myself to the wooden Pinard and the Sonicaid with a display, without earplugs, because they are the artefacts that midwives use in Denmark (as well as in many other places around the world) in antenatal care.

'Listening to the stomach' and 'listening to the fetal heart', are often understood as synonymous acts. To an outside observer who does not have an intimate knowledge of these practices it can seem quite plausible that what goes on in these practices is what obstetric textbooks describe as 'listening to the fetal heart'. Historically, the stethoscope and the heart became closely linked together. The stethoscope, introduced by the French doctor René Laënnec in 1816, was an important tool for constituting modern medicine. Laënnec developed stethoscopes made of glass, metal and wood, and finally he settled on the shape of a thin, approximately 30cm long, hollow cylinder, that has much in common with the type of stethoscope that midwives use today. Laënnec used the stethoscope to diagnose lung and heart diseases but his experiment with stethoscopes was by no means innocent. Stanley Reiser, a doctor and historian, describes the introduction of the stethoscope in medicine as equivalent to that of the letterpress to Western culture[6]—it changed practice. Olesen points out that the introduction of the stethoscope marked a shift away from situated conversation towards universal, reproducible diagnosis.[7] Prior to the stethoscope it had not been possible to establish unequivocal connections between a patient's narrative and outer physical signs on the one hand, and the anatomical features hidden inside the body on the other.[7]

The etymological roots for the word 'stethoscope' refer back to the Greek work for 'chest' and 'I view'. Laënneck belonged to what has been called the French school, a group of doctors who stressed that symptoms were to have diagnostic relevance, a thought that today seems self-evident, but which was not so at the beginning of the early 1800s. Laënneck assumed that the sounds that he could hear in the stethoscope could provide him with information about diseases that resided *within* the body—diseases that could be verified by a post-mortem examination, i.e. confirmed visually.[7]

Instruments often travel from one practice to another and that was also what the Pinard did. When the Pinard first entered maternity care, it was still a tool that provided knowledge about the inside of the body. Jacques-Alexandre Lejumeau de Kergaradec (1787-1877), a student of Laënnec's, brought the stethoscope to maternity care when he applied a stethoscope to the abdomen of a woman at term in 1819. Lejumeau de Kergaradec described how he had expected to hear the fetus splashing in water, but was surprised to hear a 'double sound', and realised that this must be the fetal heart. Listening to the fetal heart was not the only thing that Lejumeau de Kergaradec hoped the Pinard could help him do. He writes, among other things, about the use of the stethoscope to confirm pregnancy, twin gestation, fetal position, and the location of the placenta. He described his ideas in a book[8] and thus provided a vehicle for the Pinard to travel and gain followers. As time has passed, some of Lejumeau de Kergaradec's ideas have vanished, whereas the idea of listening to the fetal heart is still accepted. I haven't been able to ascertain when the Pinard came to be used routinely in antenatal care practices, but it was certainly much later.

What purpose do Pinards and Sonicaids serve in contemporary antenatal care? And in what respect are these pieces of equipment similar or different? The theoretical resources that I need in order to move beyond mute and passive technology (i.e. the understanding of technologies as neutral means to an end) are found in Science, Technology and Society Studies (STS). STS is a diverse and interdisciplinary field; its practitioners come from many fields, including sociology, philosophy, women's studies, cultural studies, geography, anthropology, economics, social psychology, history. Even though the field embraces different theoretical positions, both concerning theory and methodology, all theoretical positions share a commitment to empirical studies, which challenge a *deterministic* and *essentialist* understanding of technology, i.e. they focus on socio-material practices.[9] In other words, artefacts and technologies are not understood as pre-existing entities but they are seen as coming into being in a particular socio-material practice. Artefacts and people are seen as being intertwined in heterogeneous, societal arrangements. In order to study what is at stake in a particular practice it is necessary to bring both humans and non-human items, i.e. artefacts and technologies, into the analysis. It is a central tenet of this approach that things are not as innocent as is often assumed in modern discourse, which typically describes artefacts and technologies as a neutral means to an end.

The French philosopher and sociologist Bruno Latour, the Dutch philosopher Annemarie Mol and the Dutch Philosopher of technology Peter-Paul Verbeek provide resources that can be used to describe the non-innocence of objects and technology. Latour describes the body,[10,11] and Mol[11,12] describes diseases as 'enacted'–i.e. coming into being as a consequence of a particular socio-material practice. This does not mean that these authors see the body and diseases as being constructed, rather than real, but rather they want to stress that all knowledge has a history and that materiality has an important role to play in the production of scientific knowledge.[11, 13] Latour, Mol and Verbeek all take an interest in materiality and artefacts[12-15] and they argue in favour of a *relational ontology*.[16] A relational ontology highlights the contributions that come from humans as well as *non-humans*; it strives to overcome the dichotomy between humans as intentional and active, and artefacts as mute and passive. The term 'non-humans' is often used in STS and refers to, among other things, concepts, artefacts, technologies and materiality.

What role do artefacts play in our technology culture? This is the question that Verbeek explores in his version of postphenomenology.[15] He strives to move beyond a commonsense approach to technology as either an *instrumentalist* approach in which technology is a neutral means to an end or the *substantivist* approach, which sees technology as a determining and controlling force.[15] He is also critical of philosophies of technology, such as those of Jaspers and Heidegger, who see technology as an alienating force. Drawing on resources from the philosophy of technology and newer strands of Science and Technology Studies, Verbeek develops resources which allow us to study the contributions of concrete artefacts to particular practices. Indeed, within postphenomenology a central concept is mediation, i.e. technologies are seen as being more than intermediaries; they are *mediators* because they shape the relationship between human beings and the world. In the same way, Verbeek argues that technologies relating to maternity care are not neutral since they help to shape the way in which we understand and 'enact' pregnancy and childbirth and they help to make us who we are. In other words, Verbeek explores what things do and who we become as we use them. To explore these questions, he focuses on nuchal translucency scans, among other things.[17]

His conclusion is that ultrasound scans, such as nuchal translucency scans, are not a neutral means to an end. They do more than simply measure the size of the clear (translucent) space at the back of the baby's neck. The very fact of carrying out a nuchal translucency scan affects the way in which a pregnancy is managed and affects who the users become. For this reason, Verbeek calls ultrasound a 'moral' technology. Nuchal translucency scans shape pregnancy as a *medical event* and Down's syndrome is framed as *preventable suffering*. In the same way, parents are made into *decisions makers*. This is an example of how technology and users are co-constituted in practice. However, such a non-essentialist understanding of technology comes with consequences. If we take a non-essentialist take on technology then it follows that we should not define technology *a priori*; we must inevitably study what the technology becomes in practice. In the following section I shall discuss the consequence of this kind of approach, using the Pinard as an example.

The Pinard in action

As all midwifery students know, it takes experience to use a Pinard; the midwife must learn how to place the Pinard on the stomach, she must learn to distinguish between sounds in the womb, and she must also learn to understand the sounds that she hears. How can we describe the relationship between a midwife and a Pinard? Verbeek describes the relationship between an experienced midwife and a Pinard as an *embodiment relation*,[15] i.e. she becomes a 'Pinardmidwife'. The experienced Pinardmidwife does not feel the Pinard; instead she focuses on the sounds that she hears. The Pinard is experienced as an extension of her body, in the same way as Merleau-Ponty's blind man (carrying a white cane) experiences the world, and not his cane. When a midwife joins up with a Pinard she is transformed into a 'Pinardmidwife', who is capable of listening to sounds inside a woman's body. (I use the term 'Pinardmidwife' to emphasise that the Pinard and midwife become a single entity.) I emphasised above that the midwife who experiences the Pinard as an extension of her body is an experienced midwife. It takes experience to learn to understand the sounds which are heard, i.e. it takes time to develop a midwifery ear. It is also important to note that a Pinard invites one and only one listener at a time. A Pinardmidwife is thus both privileged and responsible; she is the one who hears the sounds in the womb and at the same time she is responsible for making judgements about the well-being of the fetus. The fact that the midwife is the only person who hears the heart sound can sometimes make the midwife vulnerable. This is because if, for instance, the baby dies unexpectedly she cannot refer to any authority outside herself; she can only refer to her own embodied midwifery knowledge. This means that some midwives choose not to use the Pinard because they refuse to risk having their competence questioned.

Midwifery is *not* as monolithic and homogeneous as is often assumed—in fact, midwifery practices are best described as diverse and multiple. Apart from 'listening to the fetus' for diagnostic or screening purposes, many midwives also use 'listening to the stomach' as a way of bringing the mother and child *relationship* to the foreground. These practices are learned in the workplace, and there are very limited descriptions to be found in obstetrics and midwifery textbooks. Science & Technology Studies therefore offers a way of bringing these practices into the foreground.

An interesting picture emerges from a small booklet (used to inform pregnant families about maternity care), issued by the Danish Board of Health.[18] What is portrayed is an antenatal appointment that involves a pregnant woman, family members, a midwife and a Pinard. The woman is lying on a table, and several family members are standing around her. The midwife is placing her hand on the woman's stomach and she is watching a small boy, who is placing his ear at one end of a Pinard; the other end of the Pinard is placed on his mother's stomach. This is a difficult task so in order to accomplish it the boy needs help from his father. The sound that the little boy hears is *not* the same sound as the midwife hears. In fact, it is not even important whether he hears a sound or not; 'heart sound' is not what is enacted in this situation. What is enacted is in fact a future family member. In other words, the Pinard *invites* family members to relate to an unborn child, a (future) family member, and the midwife is constituted as a professional who acknowledges that being pregnant is a family event, not a medical event. The Pinard therefore appears to encourage family members to be *involved*, and it is used as a way of *connecting* the unborn baby to its significant others. In this particular socio-material practice, the Pinard is not a diagnostic instrument, it is a *connecting aid*. Therefore, a Pinard is a multiple entity: it can be a *screening device*, a *diagnostic device*, and a *connecting tool*. Meanwhile, the unborn baby is constituted either as a *fetus* or as a *family member*.

In fact, the Pinard can be more than a medical device or a connecting tool. Some midwives even use the *silence* of the Pinard to keep the unborn baby *inside* the woman's body, and at the same time assure her that she can trust her physical sensations. Whatever its real use at any one time, the midwife who uses a Pinard to listen to the unborn baby is constituted as 'she who can hear the child within'. The midwife has to perform an *act* in order to become a person who can listen to the child within. She cannot do this on her own; she has to join up with a Pinard. The midwife hears the sound of the heart but neither the woman nor anyone else who is present hears these sounds. After performing the listening act, midwives will sometimes tell the woman that she is in a *privileged* position; they will stress that being pregnant is a state that allows a woman to turn her attention to the 'child within' at *any* time. The woman does not need to be in a special place, such as a clinic or a hospital, and she doesn't need an instrument or a sound, as does the midwife, to know that the baby is well. The woman can trust her feeling of 'a moving baby', even though she does not *see* or *hear* it.

Tools that can be used to keep the baby inside the woman's body are rare in modern maternity care, and that's why it is important not to eradicate those that we do have too easily. Akrich and Pasveer[19] describe a set of *trajectories* in which ultrasound, triple tests, amniocentesis and a range of other technologies inform a woman about her body and the well-being of her unborn baby; of course, all of these are trajectories that are produced *outside and at a distance* from the embodied pregnancy. The Pinard is in this respect different because, as I explained before, in this particular social-material practice it can be used to keep the unborn baby inside the woman's body.

The Sonicaid, like the Pinard, can be used to connect the unborn baby to its significant others, but it does so in a slightly different way than the Pinard. The Pinard invokes a private and intimate connection to the unborn baby because only *one* person can hear the fetal heart sound, and the listener must make an effort to listen to the sound. It is not possible to listen to a Pinard and talk at the same time. A Pinard invites one listener at a time, whereas the Sonicaid invites multiple listeners to share the sound. And since the Sonicaid distributes the sound of the fetal heart to multiple listeners, it also produces witnesses to the fact that the fetus is alive and invites listeners to *share* the sound. What does it take to produce an audible representation that can be shared by multiple listeners? The audible representation is produced by ultrasound, and as the Sonicaid is used the unborn baby immediately becomes an 'unborn baby being exposed to ultrasound'. This is an important difference between Pinard and Sonicaids: Sonicaids expose the unborn to ultrasound, even though women are often not always aware of this... They simply see the Sonicaid as a loudspeaker.

Continuing our comparison between the Sonicaid and the Pinard, it is important to note that the Sonicaid is easier to use than the Pinard—it doesn't take much training. During the fieldwork I undertook as part of my PhD a nurse who worked outside the obstetrics department came to the labour ward one late afternoon, and asked if she could borrow a Sonicaid. She told us that she was taking care of a grandmother-to-be and that they expected her to die within hours. This woman had hoped to live to see her granddaughter. The birth was expected two weeks later, but it was quite clear now that the grandmother would not meet her grandchild. The daughter had asked the nurse if her mother could have a chance to hear the heart sound of the baby she was expecting and she wanted to be able to tell her child later that the grandmother had heard its heartbeat before it was born. The Sonicaid became a means to connect the grandmother to a child of the future. The account of this event would then travel with the child and connect it to a grandmother who had passed away before it was born. This incident made me realise that a Sonicaid is more than merely a medical device: it has the potential to act as a *connecting tool*. Therefore, it should not be taken for granted that 'listening to the stomach' is an act that simply involves a fetus and/or a fetal heart. Listening practices can constitute the unborn baby as *a fetus* and as *a family member*, as well as *enact pregnant bodies as bodies that can be trusted*.

In other words, it is clear that listening practices might very well be different from those described in obstetrics textbooks. If we want to know what goes on in antenatal care practices, we should not turn to randomised trials, but explore everyday practice instead. I previously said the recommendation from the Danish Board of Health produces 'noise' due to my position in STS and midwifery. I shall now discuss the argument the Board of Health presented in their guidelines so as to explain its 'noisiness'.

What is wrong with the Danish Board of Health's line of argument?

When the Danish Board of Health called for evidence-based guidelines, they also made a call for randomised trials and/or meta-analyses that documented the effect of 'listening to the fetus in pregnancy'. This kind of epistemology (a word derived from Greek, which means 'to stand upon') is at the core of evidence-based medicine. The epistemology of a discipline describes how practitioners know what they know and how they justify the methods they use to produce knowledge. Evidence-based medicine is concerned with questions such as how can we know that a treatment is effective. And it justifies the knowledge it produces by referring to the randomised trial.

The point of departure for the Danish Board of Health was the randomised trial. If it cannot be documented in a randomised trial that 'listening to the fetus' provides *valid knowledge,* expressed as a lowering of the perinatal mortality or morbidity rates, it follows from this that this practice should be discontinued. As I mentioned before, I take Stengers' suggestion seriously and I wonder whether questions about effects are the right questions to ask in relation to listening practices in antenatal care. I shall now argue that such a point of departure (which involves restricting ourselves to randomised trials) might silence productive practices.

The implicit line of argument put forward by the Danish Board of Health goes something like this: both Pinards and Sonicaids produce sound and they are both a neutral means (*listening devices*) to an end (*monitoring fetal heart sounds*). This line of argument takes it for granted that both Sonicaids and Pinards are listening devices that can be used for one and only one purpose. If we see these devices as sound-producing devices and devices that produce good experiences through sound, then the Sonicaid wins the game. However, it was only possible for the Danish Board of Health to appoint the Sonicaid as the winner because they chose not to take the question about ultrasound exposure into their analysis.

In fact, because 'diverse listening practices' had to be pushed and pulled in order to fit into the framework that an evidence-based method requires, a confused text was the result. I call it confused because it tried to submit to what was the right thing to do from an evidence-based position, i.e. stop listening to the fetus. But due to a sense that there 'is something more to it' this was quickly reframed as 'a good experience' and/or psychology. Abandoning the issue in a hurry, the working group left a confused text behind. In other words, the recommendation to use a Sonicaid comes with an implicit assumption that 'listening to the fetus' is a single, homogeneous practice, equivalent to what is described in obstetrics textbooks. Here, a Pinard or a Sonicaid are simply devices that can be used for screening or diagnostic purposes. The evidence-based framework to which the Danish Board of Health subscribed did not allow for an exploration of what Pinards and Sonicaids are in midwifery antenatal care practices. It also did not allow Pinards and Sonicaids to become anything more than a medical tool.

The Board of Health take for granted that the *sound* is what is important so the guideline text does not speak of the Pinard and Sonicaid as connecting tools or the Pinard as a tool to help women trust their bodies. These tools are invisible to people without an intimate experience of maternity care, and or to people who study antenatal care at a distance.

To a midwife, though, a Pinard is a multiple entity. Sometimes it is a diagnostic device, sometimes a screening device, sometimes a tool that can connect and sometimes a tool that can bring attention to the capacity of the pregnant body. In this way, the sound is secondary because the fetal heart sound is not an *end*; it becomes a *means* that a midwife can use to turn attention towards the woman's body, as well as a starting point for talking about the child and the experience of being pregnant.

A multiple entity does not fit well into the language that evidence-based medicine offers. The evidence-based framework does not provide us with language that can make sense of multiple entities, emergent bodies and acting artefacts. Evidence-based medicine subscribes to what Latour called a *diffusion model*.[14] Diffusion is what takes place when an order, claim or artefact travels *unchanged* through different practices. It is a central assumption in a randomised trial that an intervention can be tested in a trial and the result used to predict the effect in similar future practice. If this were not the case, it would not make sense to do trials. Those who subscribe to evidence-based medicine know perfectly well that technologies are often used differently in different contexts, but they (often) frame these differences as a problem of education or malpractice. The analysis that I have laid out here emphasises that objects can be *translated* as they are introduced into new socio-material practices; Pinards and Sonicaids become something different from what they were designed to be.

The Danish Board of Health recommends that midwives use the Sonicaid but, being unable to provide evidence-based arguments, how did they justify their statement? They did not look for theoretical resources outside the evidence-based framework so—if they could not argue from a technical rationale—what kind of argument remained? They turned to *psychology* and framed the practice as a way of shaping good feelings. If Pinards or Sonicaids were to have a place in Danish maternity care, the only place where reason could be safely parked would be 'the woman's experience of the listening act' and this is why the Danish Board of Health referred to it as 'a good experience'.

Why did the Danish Board of Health use 'a good experience' as an argument? Clearly, the epistemology of evidence-based medicine feeds on Cartesian dualism. The French Philosopher René Descartes said "Cogito, ergo sum" (I think, therefore I am), and thus he argued that knowledge precedes being. He framed the world in terms of two substances: an outside world that could be measured (*res extensa*) and the conscious human (*res cogitans*). The line of argument of the Danish Board of Health relates to this way of thinking: to justify its position it places reasons in either of Descartes' two boxes: *res extensa* (the measurable medical effects) or *res cogitans* (the conscious woman who experiences). Having found no reason that could be measured (perinatal mortality and morbidity), the Board framed the use of the Pinard or Sonicaid as being the creator of a good experience and it connected this experience to sound. In doing so the medical enactment of listening to the fetal heart was the one and only point of departure. There was no room for the multiple enactments of 'listening to the stomach' that take place in everyday midwifery practices, which I have detailed. These multiple enactments were stored in the term 'a good experience'. These three small words do not offer much space for talking about what is at stake in these listening practices. (Here, of course, in detailing what the Danish Board of Health's implicit line of argument was, I'm simply pointing out the probable sequence of thoughts, and not meaning to indicate any implicit ill will.) What it is important to understand is that the evidence-based framework sets the standard for how questions are asked and the solutions that we are allowed to imagine, and thus the world that we can speak of. In evidence-based vocabulary it is only possible to frame *the effect* of listening practices either in terms of *technical effects* (evidence), or *experience* (psychology and sociology). If effects are to be located outside these domains they are exiled from the guidelines. This is because randomised trials simply do not allow for the exploration of multiple devices or unexpected effects.

I have now illustrated the relationship between *everyday* midwifery practices and randomised trials. Randomised trials are not innocent experiments... They participate actively in shaping the treatments/interventions that are put to the test. The randomised trial does not leave room to explore unexpected effects and it assumes that technologies are stable and homogeneous. Clearly, those who subscribe to evidence-based methods can easily get themselves into trouble if they assume that the objects that are used in everyday practice *correspond* to the objects that are used in randomised trials. Since some randomised trials come to carry tremendous authority they carry the potential to destroy local productive practices, sometimes even without noticing them. And as one standard prevails, other standards cease to exist.[20]

Clearly, randomised trials are not without their shortcomings. Based on my examples of listening practices, I have shown how the use of randomised trials and the promotion of evidence-based midwifery come with a price. Evidence-based medicine is strongly connected to positivist science and within this framework, everyday midwifery practices can easily be framed as practices that are irrational and unfounded, or at best as practices that produce 'good experiences'. Furthermore, evidence-based medicine can produce an unhealthy division between those who know, and those who are ignorant, between those who adhere to evidence and those who are seen as working without evidence in everyday practice. It is time to give voice to those practices that an evidence-based framework silences, since it places the randomised trial at the top of the evidence hierarchy. It is time to acknowledge that other qualitative research methods can be productive for researchers who strive to describe and understand what goes on in everyday midwifery practices.

Jette Aaroe Clausen is a senior lecturer in midwifery in Copenhagen. She has qualifications in public health sciences, medical anthropology and health humanities and has a PhD from the Center for Science and Technology Studies at Aarhus University. For more than 20 years Jette has been involved in developing midwifery, i.e. changing episiotomy rates, introducing water births, promoting home births and working in other ways to reassess and reduce interventions in pregnancy and childbirth. She has also been involved in developing and implementing a bachelor's degree in midwifery. Her research interest is Science and Technology Studies (STS) and the philosophy of technology, particularly postphenomenology. Her focus area is how humans and technology become woven together in concrete everyday practices.

References

1 Chalmers I, Enkin M, Keirse M. *Effective Care in Pregnancy and Childbirth*. Oxford University Press 1989.

2 Jadad ER, Enkin M. *Randomized Controlled Trials. Questions, Answers and Musings*. Oxford. Blackwell Publishing 2007, p.129.

3 Stengers I. "The Cosmopolitical proposal" In *Making things Public. Atmospheres of Democracy.* MIT Press 2005.

4 Sundhedsstyrelsen. *Anbefalinger for Svangreomsorgen.* Copenhagen. Sundhedsstyrelsen 2005.

5 Aaroe Clausen Jette. 2010. *How does materiality shape childbirth. An explorative journey into evidence, childbirth practices and Science and Technology studies.* Ph.D. thesis. Centre for STS Studies, Faculty of Humanities. Aarhus University.

6 Reiser SJ. *Medicine and the Reign of Technology.* Cambridge: Cambridge University Press 1978.

7 Olesen F. Technological mediation and embodied health-care practices. In: Selinger E. *Postphenomenology. A critical companion to Ihde.* Albany. State University of New York Press 2006:231-245.

8 Lejumeau de Kergaradeck. *Uber die Auskultation (das Hören) in Beziehung auf die Schwangerschaft, oder Untersuchungen über zwei Zeichen, mittelst deren man mehrere Umstände des Schwangerschaftszustandes erkennen kann.* Weimar 1822.

9 Jasanoff S, Markle GE, Petersen JC, Pinch T (eds) *Handbook of Science and Technology Studies.* London. SAGE publication Ltd.1995.

10 Latour B. How to talk about the body? The normative dimension of Science Studies. *Body and Society* 2004:10:2-3:205-229.

11 Law J, J Hassard (eds) Actor Network Theory and after. Oxford. Blackwell Publishers 1999.

12 Mol A. The Body Multiple. Ontology in Medical Practice. Durham. Duke University Press 2002.

13 Latour B. *Science in Action. How to follow scientist and engineers though society.* Harvard University Press1987.

14 Latour B. Where are the missing masses? The sociology of a few mundane artefacts. In Bijker WE, Law J. *Shaping Technology / Building Society. Studies in Sociotechnical Change.* Mitt Press 1992.

15 Verbeek P *What things do. Philosophical reflections on Technology, Agency and design.* Pennsylvania. Pennsylvania State University Press 2005.

16 Ihde D, Selinger E. *Chasing Technoscience: Matrix for Materiality*. Bloomington. Indiana University Press 2003.

17 Verbeek, PP. (2008). Obstetric ultrasound and the technological mediation of morality: A postphenomenological analysis. *Human Studies* 2008:31:1:11-26

18 Sundhedsstyrelsen. *Barn i vente. Graviditet, fødsel, barselstid. Vejledning til gravide*. Copenhagen.Sundhedsstyrelsen 2005.

19 Akrich, M, Pasveer, B. Obstetrical trajectories. On training women's bodies for (home) birth. In *Birth by design.* DeVries, Benoit, Van Teijlingen & Wrede eds. London: Routledge 2001.

20 Berg M, Timmermanns S. "Order and their others. On the configurations of Universalities in medical work. *Configurations* 2000;8:31-61

The need to reconceptualise birth and harmonise the technological and biological models

Verena Schmid

The predominant conceptualisation of birth in contemporary society

The current paradigm of birth is medical. Birth is seen as a potential risk, so pregnancy and birth care are focused on the search for signs of risk. As a result, in any case of diagnosis and/or therapy the expectation is always that something could go wrong. At the centre of care are the professionals with their medical and technological knowledge. Around birth there is an atmosphere of emergency and excitement, the same atmosphere as is transmitted by films which include birth stories. Medicalisation is believed to be safe. The bigger the hospital, the safer the birth! Safety is measured in terms of survival rates: infant and maternal mortality. In the name of safety (survival) women become easily blackmailed and deliver themselves, their body and their child into the hands of the experts, giving up any control they might have over the process and their body.

While there is some call for this model in the rare case of pathology in pregnancy and birth, it is not appropriate for healthy women and babies. Medicalisation for all women and babies has created a rise in pathology and interventions. Normal pregnancies and births are decreasing. Surgical birth is becoming normal. According to the World Health Organization (WHO) normal pregnancies and birth should be between 90% and 95%, while today only about 40% of pregnancies and only 6% to 7% of births are normal without any intervention.[1]

In industrialised societies technology represents progress and liberation from trouble, hard work and suffering

The medical model of birth has developed since the 18th/19th century together with industrialisation. In industrialised societies technology represents the idea of progress and of liberation from trouble, hard work and suffering. A society of 'well-being' has emerged, which is based on the belief that disease, problems and pain can be completely eradicated thanks to drugs and technology. Therefore, the medical paradigm of birth is coherent with this new lifestyle[2] and pain management in childbirth satisfies the need to be only ever 'well', avoiding experiences which take women deep into themselves, which could also uncover unpleasant feelings. It is little wonder that modern women living this techno-lifestyle want a fast, easy 'techno-birth'.

Pain management in birth helps women avoid experiences which take them deep into themselves

The need to reconceptualise birth

At the peak of medicalisation in the 1980s the medical model came under some criticism. Birth had become dehumanised and violent, and women often had a traumatic experience of birth. Rates of caesarean section, induction and episiotomy were so high that morbidity of mothers rose to an unacceptable level. As a result, some researchers started to challenge these medical practices. With the advent of obstetric epidemiology[3] medical routine practice was questioned and most of the normally performed interventions were found to be obsolete and dangerous; the recommendation was for them to be abandoned. Obstetric epidemiology recommended that healthy women should receive more effective care in small centres with lower levels of intervention, staffed with non-specialised professionals.[4] The most effective approach for healthy women was found to involve continuity of care by a midwife and empathetic support during pregnancy, labour and postpartum,[5,6] exactly the opposite of what is carried out according to modern healthcare policies. One of the interesting conclusions of this research related to the pain paradigm: after years of epidurals and other painkillers, research revealed that women who gave birth with painkillers and epidurals were not more satisfied than women who gave birth without these forms of pain relief, with their own hormones and experiencing labour pain.[7,8,5]

This new evidence from research together with reports of traumatic experiences of childbirth led to the need for a new paradigm of birth. This involved humanising the experience and improving the quality of care. The humanisation of birth movement, which started in the 1980s, is still based on the medical model, but integrates some ideas about interpersonal relations. However, as long as the focus in pregnancy, labour and birth is on risks with the inevitable fear that involves, and as long as it is on survival (with the idea of death which that implies), true quality cannot be achieved.

We have to move beyond this paradigm, based solely on survival, towards a new paradigm which recognises the other basic need of pregnant and labouring women and newborns (beyond survival): the need for health and well-being.

The German gynaecologist Sven Hildebrandt defines healthy birth as follows:

> *A healthy birth is a birth in which both mother and baby can live birth as a positive moment in their life story; it is a birth in which their needs are completely satisfied and which they can integrate into their future psychosocial development.*[9]

Focusing on health and well-being leads caregivers away from fear, towards trust and hope. Hope is a belief in a positive outcome; it means optimism—a feeling that what is wanted can be achieved and that things will turn out for the best (not for the worst, as is assumed when fear is the overriding emotion). Hope activates people's motivation and inner resources. Hope can improve the outcomes in terms of health and well-being.[10]

Focusing on health and well-being leads practitioners away from fear, towards trust and hope

This new paradigm involves a different theoretical basis and a different approach to care. To move beyond the medical paradigm and its negative impact on healthy women and babies, the focus has to switch from pathology to health; from professional-centred care to women- and baby-centred care; from diagnosis and therapy to the activation of resources; from the search for signs of pathology to the search for signs of health, from control to relationship and support.

A PROFESSIONAL-CENTRED APPROACH...	A PERSON-CENTRED APPROACH...
is scientific, quantitative, abstract, numerical, mechanical	is scientific, qualitative, experiential, concrete, global and holistic
over-simplifies issues	views issues as complex
applies standardised, protocols	uses individualised, personalised procedures
is dominated by political health systems (i.e. it is institutionalised)	is based around the 'system' which is a person
is based on ideology (i.e. it implies "I believe in...")	involves an open-minded approach
is rigidly aligned with beliefs and prejudices	involves a dialogue and an integrative approach
involves control over the 'patient'	involves empowering the woman who is receiving care
makes use of technological and surgical tools	makes use of empirical, manual, relational tools
implies an authoritative relationship	implies empathic relationship and support

The health paradigm is based on women's potential

The health paradigm is based on women's potential and on her inner resources. Of course, it entails putting the woman at the centre of care and implies acceptance of the idea that she knows about her body and her child and an acknowledgement of the professional's need to ask, listen and explore the woman's resources. This can be achieved with continuity of care.

The salutogenic caregiver searches first for signs of health, and she or he seeks out both the women's and baby's resources. If some of these are missing, the caregiver, together with the woman, activates more resources using non-medical tools (e.g. communication, touch, interventions against stress, problem-solving, social adaptation, education and manual treatments). Only if these resources are insufficient is appropriate medical care used, based on the woman's needs and the choices she makes. In this way the caregiver is able to generate health and keep pregnancy and birth healthy in most cases.

Of course, this approach requires completely different tools from the medical approach. Priority is given to tools relating to relationships, communication, education, observation, clinical reasoning with the woman and manual treatments. A therapeutic—or 'maieutic'—relationship sees the woman as an equal partner and involves an exchange of knowledge and experience. This kind of therapeutic relationship also means that the caregiver respects the woman's choices and provides support for these.[11] Continuity of care one-to-one or with a small team (three or four people) constitutes an adequate setting for this approach.

The need to harmonise the technological and biological models

The practical implications of the new paradigm are that basic, continuous midwifery care will be provided and that there will be *integration* at every level. This means integration of professionals, of systems; integration between the community and hospitals; and integration of resources and knowledge! It also means integrating the old model with the new, so that the new health paradigm predominates, while the advantages of the old paradigm, which is capable of dealing with pathology, is not lost.

The theory of salutogenesis,[12] which is a model of applied physiology, offers theoretical support for this new, holistic approach to person-centred care. Stress management is crucial within this integrated model of care. According to Aaron Antonowsky, stress can be activating (rather than debilitating) if it is alternated with relaxation. Relaxation alternated with activation can harmonise the physiological adaptation systems such as the fight-and-flight response[13] and lifestyle and rhythms are also crucial for coping positively with life events. [12,11]

A person's basic stress tolerance levels are determined in the early period of life. The primary system of adaptation (which involves cooperation between the hormonal, immune and autonomic nervous systems) builds up with homeostatic competencies, provided there is not too much stress during this early period. During pregnancy, if the mother often experiences distress, the primary adaptation of the baby can settle at a high level of receptivity to stress factors (involving high levels of cortisol) and the growing baby can then lose some of his or her capacity to respond to stress in an adequate way.[14-16]

The role of adaptation in the integrative process

Adaptation (to stress) is therefore the key word in an integrated physiological model of care and it involves the following:

- ·*physiological adaptation* based on a person's biological resources, and
- ·*psycho-social adaptation* based on a person's psychic and social resources

Physiological adaptation involves working with biological resources within the physiological systems, so as to facilitate homeostasis. Women's physical perceptions and intuitions are the key for accessing their inner resources. Hormones and emotions are an expression of the body-mind unity and they can be harmonised through communication and relationships. Verbal and nonverbal communication between the midwife and the woman, between the woman and her partner and the woman and her growing child also facilitate inner communication between physiological systems. Cyclic adaptation to physiological rhythms also supports the changing processes of motherhood. Holistic observation on every level (physical, emotional and behavioral), holistic interventions and health education (salutogenesis) relating to the woman's physical experiences are the midwife's main tools for supporting physiological adaptation. Mother-baby attachment is considered here in its biological aspect where mother and baby are understood as a unit from conception up to the first months after birth.

Psycho-social adaptation involves cultural deconditioning, positive communication with an optimistic view, and the activation of social, psychological and cultural resources. The 'system' which relates a person to his or her environment (the 'person-environment system') demands psycho-social adaptation. Body and environment are an open system. A positive environment also supports effective physiological adaptation. Bio-social systems of adaptation find a basis in Antonowsky's theory of salutogenesis and his 'sense of coherence'.[12] This sense of coherence, which is built up in the early period of life, determines a person's coping capacity. This coping capacity in turn depends on a *person's level of orientation and knowledge*, on the possession of *specific tools to face an event*, and on the *personal meaningfulness of life events*. The main tools for activating a person's psycho-social resources involve a person's lifestyle, behaviour, the modulation of behavioural rhythms, the expression of emotions and feelings, support, communication with other women, relationships, problem-solving, information and choices. Communication within the person-environment system reduces the inner conflict which exists between self realisation and social adaptation and belonging. Mother-baby and father-baby attachment here are considered in a social and psychological light. The baby is seen as an individual, as are the mother and the father. Every individual has his or her specific needs.

Person-environment adaptation

This holistic approach is supported by the theory of psychoneuro-endocryno-immunology (PNEI).[16] This theory explains how the context around a person has a direct influence on physiological dynamics. It shows how there is a direct exchange between a person and his or her environment. For example, aggression coming from the environment triggers the release of adrenaline and this in turn activates the sympathetic nervous system. An environment of intimacy triggers the release of oxytocin (engendering feelings of trust) and endorphins (which result in feelings of joy and facilitates bonding). Hormones and reactions from the autonomic nervous system create behaviour and this behaviour has an influence on the physiological systems.[11] The main dynamic is a movement between contraction and expansion. The context of any situation can therefore improve both contraction and expansion, but since pregnancy and birth require expansion, expansion is needed specifically. The sexual hormones produced during pregnancy, birth, breastfeeding and sexual activity result in expansion. The production of these hormones can be stimulated by an atmosphere of intimacy and safety and in the context of good interpersonal relationships. Stress hormones, on the other hand, lead towards contraction and are stimulated by an atmosphere which is stressful, unsafe and/or aggressive and in an atmosphere where interpersonal relationships are strained.

By facilitating physiological and social adaptation and a positive context for pregnancy, labour and birth, caregivers–particularly midwives–can influence these basic movements (of contraction and expansion) so as to favour homeostasis, i.e. the maintenance of a stable environment. This approach requires the active participation of the woman during pregnancy so as to optimise her health.

The challenge of promoting normal birth in a technological world

In the current climate it is not easy to propose normal birth, as a means of getting 'back to nature and strong emotional experiences' and there is insufficient information available about it to help women obtain this choice.[17] I think the reason for this is that our current lifestyle has become too remote from natural experiences. Today, lifestyles are mostly unhealthy, virtual, divorced from both nature in general and physical experiences in particular. Technology, medicine (drugs) and processed food are a ubiquitous part of our daily lives. Moreover, an individualised, personalised way of giving birth is strongly associated with an individualised lifestyle and system of beliefs, which is uncommon in our postmodern society. Social messages support the view that birth needs to be medicalised and depersonalised (because of the emphasis only on 'survival') and these social messages about birth also condition women's views and beliefs. Therefore, interventions in promoting normal birth need to focus on women's personal lifestyles and wishes as well as on the wider social context of birth and on what needs to be changed in this context to make normal birth possible. A health-oriented paradigm needs to have an ecological context (involving interaction and interdependency), in which quality of life is linked to a relationship with nature and the highs and lows of nature.

The upcoming model of normalising birth, where everything is normal, is as dangerous as the medical model, where everything is at risk or pathological. It is just a mirroring of an approach through schemes, protocols and guidelines. What is needed is an approach which involves relating to the individual woman.

Barriers to change

One of the main reasons it is difficult to change the 'survival' paradigm is because of midwifery education: as long as midwives study and work in a medical context and use the medical paradigm which is focused on risks, women will not be considered 'healthy enough' to have a normal birth. Women today need to learn about maternity, because after two generations of strong medicalisation and women's 'emancipation' this feminine wisdom is no longer innate. The learning which needs to take place involves 'body learning', i.e. women need to learn about their bodies and the cyclical nature of their body. They also need to do some 'social study' in that they need to relearn how to become and be a mother in contemporary society, which has become distanced from the stereotypes of the past.[18] Midwives also need to learn about these things. According to Walsh, midwifery education should provide a political reflection of the position in which midwives find themselves between the medical and the health paradigm in a system of patriarchal power.

As I've explained, in my view midwives need to learn a new paradigm of care, which is independent from the medical model and suitable for healthy women based on salutogenesis, coping strategies and applied physiology (the laws of nature). Education and interpersonal relationships are a central part of the health paradigm. Women in pregnancy basically need someone who will listen to them, explain things, accompany them on their path to transformation with empathy, and lead them closer to themselves, offering them choices, not only relating to birth but also about the kind of woman and mother they want to be.

Women need empathy and support: physical support, informational support, practical support, emotional support, and advocacy. They need to learn. Their partners need to be welcomed and involved. Pre- and postnatal classes for women and partners should be led by midwives with a salutogenic and physiological focus. These classes are an important way of preventing problems during pregnancy, birth and the time afterwards and promoting salutogenesis. They are a kind of investment.

In such a context women would be able to open up to pregnancy and birth and their bodies would be able to work properly. They would experience birth as an empowering event in their lives. As you read this, do you perhaps consider that it is not your job to facilitate these processes? Actually, I think it is because through your knowledge of physiology, you will be able to support homeostatic function of the physiological systems. Helping the woman to open up, you can prevent many obstetric complications and caesarean sections. This is the art of being an effective caregiver.

But why is it so difficult to effect the change towards a 'health' paradigm? One key reason is that our system is patriarchal in terms of economy and politics. Over the centuries men and doctors have taken control over women, their bodies and childbirth.[19] Contemporary society and politics are still oriented towards patriarchy. Our medical system is male-dominated, abstract, linear and mechanical, and distanced from women's experience. It has taken control over women's bodies. Women's bodies are also a field of financial speculation (drugs, interventions, surgery). Anthropologist and midwifery advocate, Robbie Davis Floyd, expresses it as follows: "Western society's core value system is strongly oriented toward science, high technology, economic profit, and patriarchally governed institutions."[20] The need of the patriarchal system to control birth and women is based on a deep fear: a fear of the fundamental events of life, which are birth, sexual acts and death and which are all associated with the act of giving birth. The strong power of these events transcends our civilised nature and lets the force of our incontrollable instinctive and savage nature emerge.[21] The incontrollable aspects of life and the fact that we depend on nature creates fear in both men and women. Women today are fragmented, and the aspects of their personalities compartmentalised, and this condition improves fear more and more. This fear and these conditions are to be taken into account when we promote any change in the paradigm under which we operate. To give control back to women and midwives is a step which involves a multi-gender approach and the integration of female values into the patriarchal world view. We are far from this goal, far from the kind of social homeostasis (i.e. balance) it would involve. At the moment, men will not so easily give up control over women and over financial speculation on women's bodies.

In recent years, many of the conquests achieved by midwives working within the health paradigm during the last 15 to 20 years (like teamwork; caseload midwifery; birth centres; homebirth, and continuity of care), have been attacked by politicians and destroyed all over the world. This emerged clearly at the international Strasbourg conference 2010 organised by *Midwifery Today*. Last year in Germany, the country with more then 100 birth centres and many independent midwives, insurance premiums were increased to 10 times their former level and no midwife or birth centre can afford insurance any more. In Japan, a country with a tradition of small birthing houses, these houses are being closed down. In England a very effective group called 'Albany Midwifery' was closed for political reasons; another very effective project 'Sure Start' is now being downsized; and many caseload practices in London has been dissolved. In Italy, where legislation until now has given a lot of freedom to midwives' autonomy in pregnancy and childbirth, fundamental decisions about maternity care for each individual woman (made at the first antenatal appointment) now need to be taken by doctors, instead of midwives.

In Mexico, where traditional midwives had started a journey of education and integration of knowledge, these traditional midwives have now been stopped by the government. There are many other similar changes occurring around the world.

The social conditions of women and midwives are strongly interconnected. Midwives who work within the health paradigm and empower women in birth are marginalised in the same way as women who take their own women-friendly decisions. They are a minority in a technocratic society and are perceived as dangerous, but very vital. It is clear that women and midwives will have to fight together as allies so as to establish a new space and culture for birth.

Strategies for facilitating change effectively

In order to facilitate change successfully, we need to do the following:

- Change the context of childbirth (by reorganising midwifery care in schemes of continuity).
- Change the culture and patriarchal politics of childbirth.
- Offer and actively promote the option of giving birth in small maternity units, birth centres and at home as the most effective places for birth for healthy women.
- Bond with women and other midwives.
- Offer women in pregnancy learning opportunities.
- Provide pregnant women with a social network in which they can activate their social and biological resources (i.e. engage in psycho-social adaptation).
- Offer specific body work (physical exercises) and relaxation opportunities, so as to help women activate their own inner resources (i.e. encourage physiological adaptation).

- Tune into women's lifestyles and provide appropriate care.
- Develop an empathic, symmetrical relationship with clients so as to provide effective midwifery care.
- Abandon standards, schemes, protocols and guidelines which are ineffective for the complex process of birth.
- Change basic midwifery education from the medical into the health paradigm and encourage a personal approach.
- Undertake qualitative research into questions which are relevant to midwifery.
- Work towards accepting and practising care (within an integrated paradigm), which combines the physiological systems with appropriate medical care and which honours women's needs and choices.

Integration in practice

Considering the link between lifestyles and models of birth, between the social view of birth and women's choices, and considering the fears that arise within the technocratic model of birth, integration is the key to making progress and evolving towards improved birth models. Integration of the two paradigms, when guided by appropriate reasons, offers the highest level of safety for both women and their babies.

When practising in an integrative way, we also need to bear in mind that all women are different, that individuals have different belief systems and varying perceptions of security. Technology, used as a resource and not as a means of controlling women, can be a precious tool in childbirth, nevertheless it should only be used in rare cases. The key to using it effectively is to respect women's choices and to solve problems creatively in a woman-centred approach. True choices are based on honest and complete information, which explains the pros and cons of every option; it is also based on a learning process which touches a woman's mind, heart and body; it is based on cultural exchange; it involves learning about new experiences. Problem-solving leads to choices and compromises which are feasible for an individual woman and appropriate in terms of her state of mind and situation at any one point in time. Integration allows every individual woman to find her own way of giving birth, which corresponds as closely as possible to her own way of being. The midwife's task is to lead every woman as close as possible to health and to help her *back* to health if she has lost touch with it. In short, the midwife's task is to find compromises within the two paradigms.

The health paradigm should be promoted on a political level because it is effective in creating health and well-being and it is cost effective. But together with political pressure midwives, women and fathers should promote a different culture of lifestyle and parenting. This should be offered to women as the first choice, alongside medical options, when appropriate. The word 'appropriate' is significant because a medical intervention is only appropriate when there is a specific indication for it to take place. The indication could be medical, but also psycho-biosocial. For example, a woman who has experienced abuse in her past may not be able to give birth normally because it might traumatise her all over again (because it revives memories). If her pelvis cannot open up, or if pain is too traumatic for a woman like this she should have the option of an epidural or a caesarean section. This is a good use of progress.

However, the possibility that a physiological vaginal birth might help a woman like this to work through her past trauma and become empowered through birth should also not be overlooked... Alternatively, a woman who believes in technology and only feels safe in a large hospital with many doctors around her should have the option of giving birth in that context, with the interventions she chooses—after her complete situation has been assessed.

For all women, the humanisation of hospital birth with appropriate care, which is not based on routines but on scientific evidence (relating to each individual woman's situation), empathic relationship and support, is possible only when midwifery care and the health paradigm are integrated into the medical model. This is because midwifery care provides information, choice, support, empathy and the possibility of relationships... all aspects which are missing from the medical model.

I would like to end with a quote from Robbie Davis-Floyd:

> *"Adjusting our critical lens to see birth within the larger and more holistic contexts of cross-cultural and evolutionary perspectives, we can combine the best of what technological innovations have to offer, while also embracing the wild beauty and instinctive power of the big bad wolf in the birthplace" (Davis Floyd 2009)*

Verena Schmid is an independent midwife with independent thoughts. She assisted home births and offered continuity of care for 25 years. She has integrated her practical experience with research from physiology and other disciplines and has organised this knowledge into a new model of care, a teaching model and a professional magazine for midwives. Author, teacher and lecturer nationwide and in Europe she promotes midwifery within a health and normal birth paradigm on different levels: practical, political, cultural and professional. For this work she was awarded the international Astrid Limburg award in 2000.

References

1 Schwarz, Clarissa (2009): Entwicklung der geburtshilflichen Versorgung—am Beispiel geburtshilflicher Interventionsraten 1984-1999 in Niedersachsen. Development of obstetrical care in Germany—based on obstetrical intervention rates in Lower Saxony 1984-1999, Hebammenzeitung 15.JG, AUSG. 1/09, Jänner 2009

2 Davis-Floyd RE. Doctoral thesis: The Technocratic, Humanistic, and Holistic Paradigms of Childbirth. International Journal of Gynecology and Obstetrics, Vol 75, Supplement No. 1, pp. S5-S23, November 2001.

3 Enkin M, Chalmers I, eds. Effectiveness and satisfaction in antenatal care. Clinics in developmental medicine nos. 81/82. London, UK: Spastics International Medical Publications; 1982

4 Enkin M, Keirse M, Neilson J, Crowther C, Duley L, Hodnett E, *et al.* A guide to effective care in pregnancy and childbirth. 3rd edition. Oxford: Oxford University Press, 2000.

5 Walsh D, 2007: Evidence based care in normal labour and birth, a guide for midwives, Routledge pub, London and New York

6 Hodnett E, Gates S, Hofmeyr G, Sakala C (2006): Continous support for women during childbirth,The Cochrane database of Systematic reviews, Issue 2

7 Morgan BM, Bulpitt CJ, Clifton P, Lewis PJ. Analgesia and satisfaction in childbirth (the Queen Charlotte's 1000 mother survey) Lancet 1982; 2 (Oct 9) 808-810

8 Buckley Sarah (2009), Gentle Birth, gentle Mothering, One Moon Press, Brisbane Australia

9 Hildebrandt S, (2008): Zurueckhaltung ueben, Deutsche Hebammenzeitschrift 12/2008, pp 22-25

10 Walsh D (2010) Models of Care that Work: Evidence Base of Midwifery Led Care, presentation at the conference “Il parto è un’altra cosa”, Florence 29/10/2010

11 Schmid V. (2007) Salute e Nascita, la salutogenesi in gravidanza, Apogeo ed. Milano

12 Antonowsky A (1987): Un raveling the mystery of health, how people manage stress and stay well, Jossey-Bass Publishers, San Francisco

13 Rockenschaub A (1996/2002): Gebären ohne Aberglauben, eine Fibel der Hebammenkunst, Aleanor Verlag, Wien

14 Gerhardt S (2004): Why love matters, Routledge, London and New York

15 Bauer J (2005): Warum ich fuehle was du fuehlst, Heyne Verlag Muenchen

16 Bottaccioli F (2005): Psiconeuroimmunologia, la grande connessione tra psiche, sistema nervoso, sistema endocrino e sistema immunitario, L'altra medicina studio/51, red, Como

17 Davis-Floyd RE, Cheyneythis M. ‘Birth And The Big Bad Wolf: An Evolutionary Perspective’. In *Childbirth Across Cultures* by Selin H, Springer 2009.

18 Schmid V. (2010): Apprendere la maternità , le nuove sfide di oggi tra natura e cultura, APOGEO ed. Milano

19 Duden B (1991)Der Frauenleib als öffentlicher Ort. Vom Mißbrauch des Begriffs Leben. In: *Luchterhand Essay* Band 9, Luchterhand, Hamburg 1991 (in english: Disembodying Women. Perspectives on pregnancy and the unborn, Harvard University Press, Cambridge, MA / London 1993

20 Davis-Floyd RE, 1992. Birth as an American Rite of Passage. Berkeley: University of California Press.

21 Richards H. Cultural Messages of Childbirth: The Perpetration of Fear," ICEA Journal 7(3):28, May 1993.

Power and professionalism in midwifery practice: impediment or precursor to normal birth?

Trudy Stevens

Changing centres of control

During the previous century in many countries around the world there has been a radical shift of control over childbirth, transferring from the family to the state, which has assumed responsibility. This movement has facilitated the development of a strong medical hegemony and the demise of midwifery knowledge and authority. However, whilst maternal mortality may have diminished so, apparently, has women's ability to birth without assistance.

In England, dissatisfaction with the maternity services was addressed by both the Winterton Report[1] and *Changing Childbirth*[2] and both reports sought to give power back to women. Changes in the organisation of midwifery practice, with the development of caseload midwifery, was seen as a possible solution to the widespread dissatisfaction (which involved fragmentary care). However, the reports' recommendations also allowed for the possibility of power shifting *between* professionals rather than simply devolving to childbearing women. The question remained, after these reports were published, as to how improvements could be made and–if appropriate–how midwives could once more have higher levels of responsibility, as had been the case in earlier decades.

Caseload midwifery: a new form of more egalitarian professionalism

In my own ethnographic doctoral study of the implementation of caseload midwifery[3], an analysis of power relationships within institutions suggested that hospital midwives were effectively being disempowered and that–through the internalisation of values–they actually ended up supporting the medical model to the detriment of normal birth. Interestingly, though, new knowledge and power were seen to develop within caseholding practice, whose particular organisational features facilitated this development. Changes were not immediate or inevitable but took time, as practitioners gained confidence in themselves and the women they cared for.

Based on this research, my conclusion is that caseload midwifery engenders a new form of professionalism which is founded on positions of equality. It acknowledges client participation as integral to a relationship that promotes the sharing of knowledge, and theoretical perspectives no longer dominate but support this relationship. The ways in which such a relationship between midwife and mother-to-be may impact on the physiology of labour will be considered in the light of the potential this relationship has for being an effective precursor to normal birth.

A particular case...

Following Kirkham's suggestion that midwives learn well by storytelling, I shall use a true story to illustrate the issues I explore throughout this chapter:[4]

Mary was a para 1+0 at 40 weeks gestation. She had had a previous emergency C/S at 9cm for fetal distress and was now aiming for a vaginal birth (VBAC). She presented with irregular contractions and cervical dilatation of 3cm. The midwives in the consultant-led unit admitted her and, deeming her within the 'high risk' category, said she should have no food by mouth. However, a student midwife in her third year of training took over the case with her mentor and questioned this decision. The issue was resolved when the consultant obstetrician undertook a ward round and, considering Mary not yet to be in established labour, 'allowed' her to eat as she wished.

Let's unpack this story to consider the position of the main players and how the issues of power and professionalism might have been influencing this situation... Undoubtedly, Mary was encouraged to have a hospital birth because of the dangers considered inherent in a 'trial of scar'. Also, her previous experience indicated that the baby might again have difficulty and need assistance for delivery. Thus, it is likely that issues of safety, expertise and trust predominated in Mary's agreement to follow the advice to have no food by mouth. (After all, there are few mothers who do not want the safest birth for their babies.) With a reduction in the number of births for each woman and births predominantly taking place in hospitals, women lack birth experience. Therefore, as with most elements of their complex post-industrial lives, they rely on recognised experts to advise and guide them appropriately.

Women are particularly vulnerable during their childbearing experiences and, with little specific knowledge, are almost forced to trust the expertise of the caregivers they meet; a good reputation, education and interpersonal skills further promote such trust. It is likely that these considerations would initially have a positive influence on Mary's levels of confidence... but would they be sufficient to sustain the delicate orchestration of hormones that she needed to experience birth naturally?[5]

Women are particularly vulnerable during their childbearing experiences and are almost forced to trust the expertise of the caregivers they meet

In general, midwives working in a consultant-led unit are caring individuals and their work is demanding in personal terms because it involves staffing the unit 24 hours a day. Undoubtedly, they would have initially spoken to Mary when she telephoned the unit once she had started contracting. Following the unit guidelines for VBAC, they would have advised her to come in and they would have welcomed her when she arrived. Nevertheless, the midwives did not know Mary and any knowledge of her was through the medical notes, so this knowledge would have been limited and clinically orientated. Admitting her part way through their 'shift' (a time-limited period of duty—for example, eight hours) they would have been able to spend only a few hours with her and take responsibility for a time-limited part of her birthing experience (unless she'd had a particularly short labour). Their care of Mary would have been managed alongside other commitments on the unit so their main aim would have been to concentrate on the safety of all birthing women admitted to the unit, providing the best possible care for their period of responsibility. The unintended consequences of this focus (in this case and others) results in both a task-orientation, and a time-orientation to work, neither of which support the physiology of labour. After all, physiological labour is a process-driven phenomenon, which requires skilful 'presencing' as opposed to simply a monitoring of progress.

A system which promotes inequality and hierarchical decision-making

- **Limited freedom for the mother**

  Considerable inequality of power is displayed in situations where midwives act as 'hosts' to women who are admitted as 'guests' in an environment which is strange to them. The manner in which midwives (who are relative strangers to the women) exercise power means that women end up being controlled: they are confined to a specific area (their room), their movements are curtailed by the limited space and equipment used, and normal acts such as eating and drinking are disallowed if starvation is considered necessary for 'safety' reasons. All this curtailment of freedom is undertaken in the name of good midwifery and guidelines are adhered to with a view to ensuring consistency in safety and quality of care.

- **Limited freedom for the midwife**

  Deeper consideration must force us to conclude that the midwives themselves are also confined, controlled, and starved by strangers when working in a system like this. The requirement to staff a unit limits midwives' movements for the duration of their shift and ties them to weekly patterns of work that frame their whole existence. Policies, guidelines and protocols control how they work—and the busyness of the unit all too frequently prevents midwives from taking designated meal breaks and even comfort breaks on many occasions! The whole system is sustained with the objective of meeting the needs of women who are not personally known to the professionals, so that "Who am I working with?" becomes "What will walk through the door next?" Women are reduced to clinical cases and midwives to the "*caring robots*" that the institution requires.[3,6] Indeed midwives working in this kind of system may be likened to Weber's 'agents of bureaucratic power', which he described as:

  > *a small cog in a ceaselessly moving mechanism,*
  > *which prescribes to him an essentially fixed route of march.*[7]

A system which is not conducive to good decision-making

The possible consequences of this situation have long been recognised. From the midwives' point of view the development and maintenance of their skills of judgement and decision-making are inhibited.[8, 9] Such a system also stifles any creative and imaginative thought[10] and encourages a dependence relationship between midwives and the institution within which they work.[3] In other words, midwives are effectively disempowered. Link this situation to the complex physiology of birth and it becomes apparent that *robots*, however caring, are unlikely to be able to offer the protective relationship that is fundamental to the facilitation of 'undisturbed birth' as defined by Buckley,[11] which many writers consider 'normal', since it is the physiological default.

The consequences (in terms of behaviour) of this kind of system are the unintended result of maintaining an *institutional* model of childbirth... but it does not have to be this way. My study of caseload midwifery, which embodies the principles set out within *Changing Childbirth*,[2] made me conclude that very different consequences result from a caseload model. Many of the issues identified in my analysis were illustrated in the following quote from a midwife who had moved from hospital work to caseholding:

> *I was stagnating there completely—whereas at least this job you're continually meeting new challenges all the time in your daily round. Just different sort of pregnancies, different sort of people, different social backgrounds. You know, you get involved with many more disciplines—like social workers, health visitors and doctors. It's a far more professional way to work.* [2nd interview with caseload midwife 23][3]

Observing how caseholding midwifery worked in practice, in my analysis I identified a number of probable consequences of this model of care.[3] Most importantly, according to my data, it appeared to stimulate the development and maintenance of skills of judgement and decision-making, as well as clinical expertise. Without the constant presence of colleagues to seek advice from, the midwives working this way learnt to become autonomous practitioners and to accept responsibility for the care they provided. No longer constrained by the confines of the institution, this model of practising really encouraged creative and imaginative thought, adaptability and flexibility because seeing each woman through the entire process of pregnancy and birth appeared to make them attempt to really meet individual women's needs, within a diverse population. Most importantly, the continuity of caring seemed to facilitate the development of a reciprocal relationship between midwives and mothers, and this offered immense satisfaction to both parties. Working in a caseloading model resulted in a rebalancing of the power relationship so that both midwives and mothers ended up seeming effectively empowered.

In Mary's situation, thinking back to our specific story, the hospital midwives were reacting to Mary not as an individual, but as a 'case'. Following what was deemed an appropriate plan of care, they had somehow 'lost the plot' and had failed to recognise the latent phase of Mary's labour. (If they had done so, starvation would surely not have seemed necessary.) The lack of knowledge about Mary's labour effectively disempowered both Mary and the midwives who provided her care.

Knowledge as power

Knowledge has long been recognised as an important source of power. Drawing on some fairly generic thinking on the subject, Parsons saw functionally specific knowledge, with controlled access, as forming a major contribution to professional authority[12] whilst Foucault highlighted the role discourse plays in the distribution and control of power by shaping attitudes towards phenomena, with 'experts' defining the agenda.[13] Thus, in Foucault's interpretation, when one student midwife dared to ask the question *"WHY should Mary be restricted in eating?"* this posed a challenge to the 'system', which her 'disempowered' mentors felt unable to address.

Training to facilitate decision-making

Degree-level midwifery training was introduced in recognition of the importance of education in helping individuals to 'think outside the box' and be confident in challenging a system in any case where accepted care might be inappropriate. As a midwifery lecturer on such courses I remain disturbed by the power of the institutional model, which apparently converts passionate new midwives into clones of the system within months of qualification. The speed with which new midwives are seen to internalise a whole new set of values, which they would not have accepted only months before, is indicative of the power of this model of practice.

In Mary's case, the student midwife felt able to question the care provision, but unfortunately (perhaps) she was not yet qualified to alter it; although challenged, her mentors were unable to endorse the student midwife's view, and they relied on the obstetrician to verify that Mary could indeed have something to eat. What had happened to their own powers of judgement and decision-making?

Models of care influencing knowledge-generation

In my ethnographic study it became apparent that different models of care had contrasting influences on the use and generation of knowledge. In the institutional model, the requirement was for 'instant' knowledge; situations needed to be dealt with immediately, with minimal forewarning of specifics that would come from knowing the individual. However, with the movement into university- rather than hospital-based midwifery training, a wide separation of midwifery knowledge and clinical skills took place, with the traditional theory-practice gap being widened by geographical as well as ideological space. Midwifery tutors and midwifery-specific reference books were no longer available in the clinical setting as a source of knowledge for students or practitioners, because they had both been moved to the relevant university. Instead, the main quick source of knowledge was books which focused primarily on medical issues as hospital libraries were medically orientated. In this situation, midwives automatically turned to doctors as the easiest source of advice.

Midwives automatically turned to doctors...

Less obvious were the effects of the temporary nature of care provision. The data I collected revealed that short hospital stays and shift patterns of work meant that advice offered could not be followed through. Not only did this result in conflicting advice, which confused women, it also precluded midwives' abilities to assess suggestions and learn what worked in particular situations. Also, the women's movement through different wards and midwives' shift work enforced a compartmentalised, segmented form of care, with midwives rarely seeing a woman through her entire birth experience. My analysis of this data made me conclude that childbirth was being understood in specific, task-orientated sections.

In my data this contrasted with the clear generation of knowledge that ensued through the continuity of care provided in the caseholding model of midwifery practice. In this model, individual midwives generally had a sense of ownership of their work and they accepted responsibility for care, which was seen as an investment for the new mother's subsequent care. For example, discussions undertaken during the antenatal period could inform care provided during labour when it was inappropriate to be determining the mother's wishes. Midwives were able to see the results of their advice and care, and modify it accordingly. In following the complete childbirth episode, they developed a deep understanding of childbirth and spoke of learning from their women. Moreover, the constant use of all aspects of midwifery care (antenatal, intrapartum and postnatal) forced midwives' knowledge and skills to be honed on a daily basis as they were constantly resituating and adapting their knowledge and skills to specific situations and needs. When unusual or more complex situations arose, midwives had the freedom to seek out new knowledge or expert advice from a variety of sources, as needed, as they were not tied to specific times and places. Whilst they all noted a very steep learning curve when they started working within a caseloading model, the caseload midwives seemed to have developed confidence and maturity in their work as their knowledge base had grown, which ultimately made them empowered professionals.

Different relationships within the two care models affecting care

In my ethnographic study trust emerged as a vital lubricant which enabled the smooth working of a complex maternity care system involving a number of practitioners. Within the institutional model, by contrast, this trust seemed to be absent because obstetricians admitted to 'testing' midwives and indeed they were seen doing this during the observational study of the doctors' ward round. In caseloading practice on the other hand, after a midwife had presented a succinct and relevant summary of a particular case, outlining a clear plan of action, there was often just a cursory visit, after which the midwife and mother were left alone. Within both models of care, inappropriate or lack of response on the part of the midwife resulted in the midwife being watched with care and medical involvement in the case was likely. In other words, it was clear that the caseload midwives, who knew their women well, fared considerably better than midwives who had recently taken over the care of an unknown woman.

Over time, the obstetricians got to know the caseload midwives well and they reported that they quickly decided who to trust; several noted how they modified their treatment, 'pushing the boundaries' for appropriate care. For example, if a rise in blood pressure developed they might decide not to bring the woman in for frequent hospital visits as they knew the woman and caseload midwife were in close communication and that the midwife would swiftly report anything adverse. The senior obstetricians also noted their growth of respect for and recognition of maturity in the caseload midwives–something which was not seen in the majority of hospital midwives with similar years of experience.

As highlighted in the quote presented previously, the midwives commented on how carrying a caseload was "a far more professional way to work". They clearly appreciated the respect their work engendered and enjoyed the sense of equality they experienced as respected members of the care provision team. It is perhaps not difficult to argue that being professional must be a prerequisite for providing good care, so must be in the best interests of pregnant and labouring women.

Midwifery as a profession

Although midwifery has been conceived of as 'the oldest profession', emerging as an essential occupation that developed as bipedalism evolved,[14] many would argue that the institutionalisation of childbirth has diminished its status. Indeed, the traditional model of a profession which encompasses expert, objective knowledge,[12,15] which promotes the mystification of such 'esoteric' knowledge,[16,17] and which encourages the development of social distancing[18,19] (whereby the client is dependent on and subservient to the professional) sits ill with any concept of midwifery being 'with woman'.

As Buckley has so authoritatively detailed,[11] the mammalian need for safety and privacy are paramount if women are to be able to 'let down their guard' and allow their hormones to flow; only then can they reap the rewards of the 'hormonal ecstasy' that has such beneficial effects on mother and baby in terms of safety as well as bonding and maternal satisfaction. Odent drew the parallel between orgasm and birthing, noting that both resulted from the same hormonal processes.[20] However, whilst support is deemed so important for birth, the characteristic of the professional detailed above would surely prove to be an impediment to orgasm, or indeed to the facilitation of undisturbed birth. The shift in consciousness and sense of submission and surrender that is integral to birthing needs a very different sort of professional companion.

The potential for the development of a different professional paradigm did emerge from my analysis of caseload midwifery because I identified a new model of midwifery professionalism. This encompasses the development of implicit knowledge or *'connoisseurship'*, as identified by Polanyi[21] and Benner[22] and the recognition of a more democratic relationship, whereby a partnership develops from the synthesis of the practitioner's knowledge and the client's 'lay expertise'.[23] This does not mean that midwives abdicate responsibility but that they develop the additional skill involved in identifying and utilising the resources available from the women themselves. The professional relationship which I saw to evolve in my study, acknowledges and honours both parties equally and respects the different forms of knowledge which both parties bring to the situation.

Perhaps most important for the promotion of normal birth in my study was the emergence of the reciprocal nature of this mother–midwife relationship.[24,3,25] The power of this was most clearly demonstrated by the number of mothers who managed to delay birthing their baby until 'their' caseload midwife returned from a planned absence of a weekend off duty or a holiday. Clearly, this was neither universal nor automatic but it proved a significant factor that has been anecdotally confirmed by a number of midwives who work within a caseloading practice.

A model which promotes better outcomes

To summarise the advantages of caseload midwifery, it means that midwives provide continuity of care and that both midwife and mother can regain the power accorded to them by the experience of normal birth. Within an institutional model, relationships, decision-making and practices work to the detriment of the women cared for because the values of an institution are internalised and hospital midwives support the medical hegemony, even in cases where additional information would otherwise result in entirely different decisions being made.

Caseload midwifery means that midwives provide continuity of care and that both midwife and mother can regain the power accorded to them by the experience of normal birth

Mary, the mother whose case we have been following, laboured within an institutional model and it was only chance which allowed an unhelpful (and potentially misguided decision about the withholding of food during the latent phase) to be reversed. If Mary had experienced continuity of carer it is likely that the latent phase of her labour would have been recognised and admission to hospital delayed. Any anxiety she experienced could have been minimised by the reassuring presence of a known 'professional' operating in familiar surroundings and with familiar behaviour. Since hospital birth had been Mary's preference, offering her a 'safety net' should her baby need it (since she was having a VBAC), the question of interventions is also relevant. In cases where women labour in hospital within an institutional model of care the cascade of interventions so frequently generated by unnecessary or inappropriate care that results from client and practitioner being strangers to each other might more often be avoided with continuity of carer. As I have tried to explain, it is not the actual place of birth that necessarily inhibits normal birth but the dynamics of power and the relationships which develop within whichever setting is chosen.

Fortunately, Mary's story does have a happy ending. Having been given permission to eat, she walked across to the hospital canteen with her partner and enjoyed a large fried breakfast! She then birthed four hours later, having had no interventions or analgesia. Unhappily, because of the too frequent cascade of interventions which takes place within an institutional model of care, other mothers may not have similar outcomes. My research led me to conclude that this need not be the case if more midwives could work within a model of care which facilitated the development of trust (between mother and midwife and her colleagues) and less hierarchical decision-making processes.

... if more midwives could work within a model of care which facilitated the development of trust and if decisions were less hierarchical...

Trudy Stevens has been a practising midwife for 35 years, 10 of which were spent working in remote and resource-poor countries. She returned to England to read anthropology at the University of Cambridge and has subsequently been involved in both research and teaching. She has a Master's degree in social research methods and her PhD was an ethnographic study of the implementation of caseloading midwifery practice. Considering she learnt the meaning of true midwífery from the traditional birth attendants she has worked with, Trudy is passionate about the development of a more humane maternity service—which she considers would benefit midwives as much as mothers.

References

1 House of Commons, 1992. *Maternity Services: Second Report to the Health Services Select Committee* (Winterton report). London, HMSO.

2 Department of Health, 1993. *Changing Childbirth. Report of the Expert Maternity Group Part 1.* London, HMSO.

3 Stevens T, 2003. *Midwife to Mid wif: a study of caseload midwifery.* PhD thesis (unpublished). London, Thames Valley University. P.195.

4 Kirkham K, 1997. Stories and Childbirth. In Kirkham K, and Perkins E, (eds). *Reflections of Midwifery Practice.* London, Balliere Tindal. Pp.183-204.l

5 Schmid V, 2007. *About Physiology in Pregnancy and Childbirth.* 2nd ed. Translated from Italian by Manca Anna Lou. Florence Italy, Litografia LP.

6 Stevens T, 2009. Time and Caseload Midwifery. In McCourt C, (ed). *Childbirth, Midwifery and Concepts of Time.* Oxford, Berghahn Books.104-126.

7 Weber M, 1978. *Economy and Society* Vols. 1 & 2. Berkeley, University of California Press. pp.987-8.

8 Robinson S, 1989. The role of the midwife: opportunities and constraints. In: Chalmers I, Enkin M and Keirse MJNC (eds). *Effective Care in Pregnancy and Childbirth.* Oxford, Oxford University Press, pp. 162-180.

9 Chamberlain M. 1996. The clinical education of student midwives. In: Robinson S, Thomson A (eds). *Midwives, Research and Childbirth* Vol. 4. London, Chapman & Hall, pp 108-131.

10 Kirkham M, 1999. The culture of midwifery in the National Health Service in England. *Journal of Advanced Nursing* 30(3): 732-739.

11 Buckley S, 2009. *Gentle Birth, Gentle Mothering.* Berkeley, Celestial Arts.

12 Parsons T, 1949. *Essays in Social Theory: pure and applied.* Glencoe Illinois, The Free Press.

13 Foucault M, 1980. *Power/knowledge: Selected interviews and other writings 1972-1977.* Brighton, Harvester.

14 Trevathan WR, 1997. An evolutionary perspective on authoritative knowledge about birth. In: Davis-Floyd RE, Sargent CF (eds). *Childbirth and Authoritative Knowledge.* Berkeley: University of California Press, pp.80-88.

15 Popper K, 1972. *Objective Knowledge.* Oxford, Oxford University Press.

16 Freidson E, 1977. The future of professionalisation. In: Stacey M, Reid M, Heath C, and Dingwell R, (eds). *Health and the Division of Labour.* London, Croom Helm. pp.14-38.

17 Williams J, 1993. What is a Profession? Experience versus expertise. In: Walmsley, J, Reynolds J, Shakespeare P, and Woolfe R, (eds). *Health, Welfare & Practice. Reflecting on roles and relationships.* London, Sage Publications. pp.8-15.

18 Johnson T, 1989. *Professionals and Power.* London, Macmillan.

19 Atkinson P, 1995. *Medical Talk and Medical Work; the liturgy of the clinic.* London, Sage Publications.

20 Odent M, 2009. *The Functions of the Orgasms: the highways to transcendence.* London, Pinter & Martin

21 Polanyi M, 1958. *Personal Knowledge.* London, Routledge & Kegan Paul.

22 Benner P, 1984. *From Novice to Expert.* Menlo Park California, Addison-Wesley Publishing Company.

23 Bloor M, 2001. On the Consulting Room Couch with Citizen Science: a consideration of the sociology of scientific knowledge perspective on practitioner-patient relationships. Keynote paper. *British Sociological Association Medical Sociology Annual Conference*, University of York. September 2001.

24 Guilland K, and Pairman S, 1994. The Midwifery Partnership: model for practice. *New Zealand College of Midwives* 11(October): 5-9.

25 McCourt C,. & Stevens T, 2009. Relationship and Reciprocity in Caseload Midwifery. In Hunter B, & Deery R, (eds). *Emotions in Midwifery and Reproduction.* Basingstoke, Palgrave Macmillan. pp.17-35.

Embedding normality within the midwifery education curriculum

Linda Wylie, Karen McDonald, Evelyn Mohammed and Madge Russell

The role of normality within midwifery education in the UK has changed greatly within the past 50 years from being a traditional midwifery philosophy in the 1950s and 1960s to one in which there has been increasing pathology throughout the 1980s and 1990s to a recent return to an emphasis on normality over the past 10 years. This has been paralleled by the increasing medicalisation of childbirth and the attempt to return to normality within midwifery practice as a whole. Within the University of the West of Scotland lecturers have planned the most recent curricula around the concept of normality, balanced with appropriate high risk care. This chapter looks at the driving forces, influences and barriers to this process.

Driving forces

Within the UK as a whole, the increasing medicalisation of childbirth was a result of publications such as the Tennant Report[1] and the Peel Report[2] which led to a move towards consultant-led care in large obstetric units. Many maternity homes and GP units, where the care of the majority of women was based, closed with a loss of the concept of normal, physiological, midwifery-led care, where this had been focused on.[3] Medicalisation and intervention became the norm in the 1970s and 1980s, with increases in induction and operative delivery rates accompanied by a perceived loss of choice and control by women and decreased autonomy for the midwife.[4]

In the early 1990s, the Winterton Report, *Changing Childbirth* brought about a change in focus.[5] Its themes of choice, continuity and control[6] highlighted a possible change in care strategy. Pioneering initiatives encompassed the demands and desires of childbearing women and midwives who wished to reclaim autonomy and partnership between women and medical staff. The Scottish equivalent document *Provision of Maternity Services in Scotland*[7] brought about initial changes in approaches to services, with midwives providing an all-encompassing pattern of care. However, it was not until the publication of the report *A Framework for Maternity Services*[8] and the subsequent *Expert Group on Acute Maternity Services (EGAMS)* report[9] that there was a move towards a radical change in the maternity services in Scotland. This change involved services being categorised according to the number of births, facilities available and obstetric and paediatric staffing levels.

This Scottish Executive report also reiterated that pregnancy and childbirth are normal physiological processes.[9] It was at this point that the emphasis on a return to promoting normality began to show a significant impact on the way in which midwives, as well as obstetricians, cared for women. This led to greater training needs at all levels.

Influences

In parallel with and in association with the above initiatives, a number of key influences resulted in a change in the way obstetricians and midwives worked, both separately and together. The European Working Hours' directive and the reduction in junior doctors' hours meant that a change in working practices was required.[10] The role of the supervisor of midwives was key within these changes with her or his primary role being protection of the public. The emergence of the lecturer-practitioner and consultant midwife roles within the field of education (as well as practice) were pivotal in the changes proposed.

The supervisor of midwives

In the UK, the midwifery profession is arguably the most securely regulated profession amongst healthcare professionals.[11] Since the 1902 Midwives' Act statutory supervision of midwives has been in place and this Act was viewed as a means of regulating midwives by ensuring that they were appropriately educated. In the 21st century education continues to be a central aspect of the supervisor of midwives' (SOM) role. The Nursing and Midwifery Council (NMC)[12] supports this by stating that:

"Education programmes are designed to prepare students to practise safely and effectively so that, on registration, they can assume full responsibility and accountability for their practice as midwives."[13]

The responsibility of the supervisor of midwives to protect the public by empowering midwives and student midwives to practise safely and effectively is therefore a vital aspect of their role.[14] Part of this role is to ensure that the quality of care given in a professional capacity to women and their babies is constantly improving. The influence of the supervisor of midwives is seen as vital in the development and support of all programmes of midwifery education and her or his input is a necessary part of any programmes or modules developed, both in terms of planning and deciding how programmes or modules ought to be taught.

The lecturer practitioner

During the 1990s, in an endeavour to improve nursing and midwifery care and the education of practitioners, the role of the lecturer practitioner (LP) emerged. The aim was to embed the LPs into the organisation of nursing and midwifery services so as to promote greater links between education and clinical practice, as well as to promote the education of practitioners through an undergraduate and post-registration programme. Hart *et al* highlight that:

"A recurring issue in midwifery education is the perceived, and sometimes actual, lack of integration between classroom and practice settings, which can undermine the effective implementation of innovative teaching and learning."[15]

An issue is lack of integration between class and practice

Part of the LP's role within the University of the West of Scotland was to engage with mentors, managers and supervisors of midwives, and to work alongside student midwives during their clinical placement, particularly in the latter part of the student midwifery programme and upon qualification, so as to ensure that teaching matched reality. Before the LP post was phased out of midwifery in the West of Scotland they also supported mentors, who were responsible for confirming that students had met the necessary standards of proficiency to progress through their training. Anecdotally, student midwives certainly seemed to value the clinical teaching opportunities and discussions on reflective practice which were facilitated by the LP. This appeared to increase the harmonisation of clinicians and educationalists, working together across the spectrum of midwifery care from promoting normality to managing complex, high risk care. Due to financial constraints, these posts were phased out. Although a challenging position for those in post, the lecturer practitioner role went some way towards lessening the theory-practice gap.

The consultant midwife

One of the responsibilities of the consultant midwife is the promotion of normality. In Scotland the consultant midwife was instrumental in developing the initiative Keeping Childbirth Natural and Dynamic (KCND).[16] KCND was developed to help the multi-professional team implement the principles outlined in the *Framework for Maternity Services* report.[8] The ethos of this programme is that childbirth is a normal physiological process and that unnecessary intervention should be avoided. One of the key principles of KCND is the right of pregnant women to be provided with current, evidenced-based information and to be involved in decisions regarding their care and that of their baby. For low risk women midwives were to be the lead professional in their care.

The education of midwives

As a result of the reports *A Framework for Maternity Services*[8] and *EGAMS*[9] it became apparent that there were two patterns of practice arising at opposite ends of the care spectrum for childbearing women—consultant-led units for those perceived as high risk (linked also to the growing numbers of assisted conceptions and an aging childbearing population) and community midwifery units (CMU) for those women deemed low risk. In the CMU midwives could work totally autonomously.

EGAMS challenged midwives to regain their role in childbirth and provide women with a better birthing experience.[9] With the emergence of CMU it was recognised that midwives required a range of additional theoretical and practice initiatives to enable them to work autonomously and flexibly so as to ensure safe practice for women and their babies. A training needs analysis identified a need for both high and low risk education and Scottish universities were asked to develop modules to meet these needs. The University of the West of Scotland was charged with the responsibility to run a module nationwide to promote normality and have led the way subsequently in offering modules at all levels in this field.

A new module: Promoting Normality in Childbirth

This module was intended to develop core midwifery competencies. It was felt that midwives should be...

- confident about providing intrapartum care in a low-technology setting
- comfortable about using embodied knowledge and skills to assess a woman and her baby, as opposed to using technology
- able to let labour 'be' and not interfere unnecessarily
- confident to avert or manage problems that might arise
- willing to employ other options to manage pain without access to epidurals
- responsible for outcomes, without access to on-site specialist assistance
- confident to trust the process of labour, being flexible with respect to time

The module was designed for Level 9 of the Scottish Credit and Qualifications Framework and intended to run over one semester. It aimed to build upon existing knowledge, experience and competence in dealing with normality and to facilitate the further development and implementation of evidence-based practice within a low-technological setting.[17] The underlying philosophy of the module was to provide a supportive teaching and learning strategy and an environment which is sensitive to the individual needs of midwives. A key aim of the module was to enhance the midwife's own awareness of abilities and limitations. The module focused on self-directed learning and also provided up-to-date, evidence-based knowledge and theory so as to inform safe, effective and appropriate practice and promote the reappraisal of core skill competencies.

The underlying philosophy was to provide a supportive teaching and learning strategy and an environment which is sensitive to the individual needs of midwives

A variety of teaching and learning strategies were utilised to meet the learning requirements of the module. Core lectures, tutorials, practical sessions utilising the skills laboratories (which include the latest simulation models) and online discussions were all designed to encourage lifelong learning appropriate to the new situations in which many midwives were finding themselves.

The module was also recognised as being very relevant to student midwives and thus was incorporated into their three-year programme, which was initially shared with the qualified midwives. This, however, proved challenging to all participants and it was quickly recognised that the needs of the two groups were very different so the module was subsequently taught separately.

The needs of the two groups were very different

Educating pre-registration student midwives

Within the UK, midwifery pre-registration education programmes are required to meet the NMC standards for pre-registration midwifery education.[12] A close look at these standards identifies that midwifery education must be carefully balanced to give student midwives experience in caring for women within a variety of settings. The NMC stipulates that students must demonstrate competence in:

> *'being autonomous practitioners and lead carers to women experiencing normal childbirth and being able to support women throughout their pregnancy, labour, birth and postnatal period, in all settings including midwife-led units, birthing centres and the homes".*[18]

The NMC also identifies that the primary focus of pre-registration midwifery programmes is to ensure that student midwives are safe and effective in practice when supporting women who are experiencing normal childbirth. The NMC therefore firmly sets the foundations for promoting normality in midwifery practice. To what extent a midwifery curriculum meets this standard depends very much on the philosophies and experiences of the midwifery lecturers who are delivering the curriculum.

The primary focus should be to ensure that student midwives are safe and effective in practice when supporting women experiencing a normal form of birth

At the University of the West of Scotland the promotion of normality is clearly evident both at programme and at module level. The three-year programme is designed to move from an emphasis on normality in the first year, to one of high risk in the second year but to then firmly re-establish the midwife's role in promoting normality towards the end of the second year through a module currently named 'Managing Midwifery Care'. This module is the successor to the module 'Promoting Normality in Childbirth'. The module explores the concept of salutogenesis (health promotion) and revisits pregnancy and birth. Reflective discussion of experiences already gained within the programme is encouraged so as to promote normality.

During the third year of the programme student midwives consolidate skills in all areas and have the opportunity to experience the childbearing continuum by supporting a small caseload of women. Caseload holding enables the student midwife to plan, deliver and evaluate a programme of midwifery care, while developing skills in problem recognition, risk assessment and decision making. In the third year, placements are also offered across a range of areas, including community midwifery units and, where possible, midwifery in remote rural communities (where midwives tend to actively promote normal midwifery practice). Home births are on the increase and the student midwives are encouraged to go on call for these whenever possible.

Similar initiatives are evident in most pre-registration midwifery programmes but the emphasis on normality continues in the detail of the curriculum. Lecturers teach normal physiology and management before introducing an intervention, irrespective of whether the intervention in question is common or not. A good example of this involves management of the third stage of labour. Physiological management is taught first as the 'norm' with active management considered an intervention to be used only when required. Another example is that equal time is spent considering methods of managing pain with massage, water and complementary therapies as on pharmacological methods. Vaginal breech birth is taught utilising evidence from acknowledged experts in promoting normality, such as Mary Cronk and Jane Evans.[19] Local advocates of promoting and supporting normal midwifery practice such as hypnobirthing trainers, independent midwives and consultant midwives are regular contributors to the teaching programme. Skills simulation sessions are set up with equal emphasis on the use of high risk computerised models as on the home birth / pool room.

Assessment strategies are also geared towards encouraging normal midwifery practice, where appropriate. In one module in which the legal, ethical and professional responsibilities of the midwife are explored, a scenario is utilised in which an area of potential conflict between a medicalised and a midwifery model of care highlights the rights of a pregnant woman and the role of the midwife in dealing with the situation. One example of this is the potential conflict when a woman identifies her intention to have a Vaginal Birth After a Caesarean (VBAC) at home in a pool. Another module utilises online discussions to challenge the student midwife to risk assess and debate evidence-based practice.[20]

Of course, the midwifery lecturers recognise that these challenges to student midwives to promote normality often contrast with the experiences the students have in practice. This too is discussed at length within the classroom. The student midwives are encouraged to explore this dichotomy and this occurs spontaneously as their experiences vary considerably across the obstetric units and community areas in which they are placed. This has led to an increase in the number of students who request a placement outside their local area despite the time and financial consequences that result and the stress of moving out of their comfort zone of the known protocols and procedures of the unit in which they have been placed for the previous two years, so that they can experience something different. These students recognise the very real benefits of a broader experience within their midwifery programme and wish a greater exposure to a more 'normal' experience. The programme team would like the students to spend more time working within the CMUs but these placements could potentially detract from their need to develop competence in caring for high risk women, which is a practical requirement in today's complex society. Working with the expert in promoting normality, the independent midwife (IM), would also be invaluable but placing students with IMs leads to inequity of student experience due to the small numbers of IMs.

Barriers to promoting normality in midwifery education

Midwifery education has evolved over the past 20 years and now involves curricula which are evidence-based. The process of developing appropriate, evidence-based curricula has been not been easy. It is a challenge to merge theory and practice when delivering midwifery education and to support student midwives in clinical placements while competently delivering care to women and their families.[21] In the UK midwifery education programmes are required by the NMC to be 50% theory-based in a university and 50% practice-based.[12] This will ensure that the students will integrate the theory learnt in university within their clinical practice. Thomas however highlighted that the NHS did not consistently provide strong and positive role models for student midwives and this therefore could be considered a barrier to learning.[22] With the majority of mentors working in high risk units this limits the student midwives' opportunities to see and participate in promoting normality in practice. In addition, CEMACH identified that members of the multi-agency team failed to identify and act on critical situations in a timely fashion.[23] This has led to considerable media attention about substandard health care.[24] The repercussions of this has led to questions being raised in both political and public arenas regarding the education of student midwives and their ability to promote normality whilst balancing this with the knowledge of how to recognise and act when deviations from the normal occur.[25]

For practitioners, the gap exists because real practice works and theory is based on obscure research ideals

The theory-practice gap has been of concern for many years. Rolfe suggests there are two aspects to the gap.[26] For theorists, the gap is between that which is evidence-based, theoretical knowledge and what is actually happening in clinical areas.[21] For practitioners, the gap exists because real practice works and theory is based on obscure research ideals. However, the promotion and support of normality in the childbearing experience is high on the political and professional agendas.[27,28] Nevertheless, there is a resistance from many midwives to change traditional practice and it is unfortunate that many newly qualified midwives who are more familiar with the concepts of promoting normality are leaving the profession and thus hindering change and preventing the promotion of normality from being seen as an accepted principle.[29] Hospital policies and procedures that restrict the practice of midwives are two of the reasons cited for leaving the profession.

Politically, despite government recognition that midwives are the most suitable lead professionals to care for low risk women, funding cuts have led to the closure of community midwifery units, despite evidence identifying the high quality of midwifery care offered. This also restricts the opportunities available for the education of midwives in promoting normality.

Closures have taken place despite evidence of quality

Addressing the challenges

Recent developments such as the Scottish Maternity Multidisciplinary Programme (SMMDP)[30]—a response to issues raised in CEMACH[23]—have enhanced and encouraged a unified national approach to care delivery by bringing together all parties involved in maternity care such as midwives, medical practitioners and allied health professionals. Student midwives reap the benefits of midwifery lecturers' involvement in the delivery of the SMMDP programmes as the ethos and pattern of management presented in simulated practice mirrors real-life clinical situations.

A foundation for future progress

The promotion of normality is now firmly embedded within the midwifery curricula. The majority of women are at low risk of complications and it is widely accepted (in the UK) that midwives should be the lead professionals in their care. It is therefore vital that midwives, mentors, student midwives, lecturing staff and supervisors of midwives learn to promote normality, be inspirational and embrace their role as advocates for women so as to empower each woman to take holistic control over the birth of her child. The collaborative effort of a number of health professionals may not only ensure high quality care for women in pregnancy, childbirth and the postnatal period but it may also mean that women leave maternity care with fantastic memories of childbirth.

Linda Wylie has been a midwife for over 30 years with experience in both community and hospital practice. A lecturer since 1994, previous publications include *Essential Life Sciences for Maternity Care* (2005) and The *Midwives' Guide to Key Medical Conditions* (2008). Linda has a particular interest in promoting normality and is an active member of the Association of Radical Midwives. Originally born and bred in England, Linda has four delightful grown up children, three of whom were born in Scotland.

Karen McDonald works at the University of the West of Scotland. She teaches on both undergraduate and postgraduate midwifery programmes and is a strong supporter of non-intervention and normal births within rural community settings. Karen has four children, all normal births with no intervention other than TENS, and was a 'very elderly' primigravida

Evelyn Mohammed has a varied clinical background, having practised as a registered nurse and midwife. Her midwifery experience has mainly been in the community setting. Throughout her career Evelyn has developed an interest in public health issues. She has previously been employed as lead research midwife on an RCT study which aimed to establish whether the use of motivational counselling during pregnancy would help pregnant women to stop smoking. Evelyn is currently working as a midwifery lecturer at the University of the West of Scotland.

Madge Russell works at the University of the West of Scotland. A midwife for 34 years, she has an extensive background of working in maternity hospitals in both the highlands and lowlands of Scotland as a practitioner and a manager prior to entering education. Madge was the first midwifery lecturer practitioner in Scotland. Her passion is educating the future generation of midwives about normal birth and as a supervisor of midwives she strives to ensure that the quality of care to women and their babies is constantly improving.

References

1 Scottish Home and Health Dept *1973 Maternity services: Integration of maternity work (Tennant Report)* HMSO Edinburgh

2 Department of Health (DOH) 1970 *The Peel Report* HMSO London

3 Reid L 2005 Midwifery in Scotland 3: intranatal practices *British Journal of Midwifery* 13(7): 426-431

4 Reid L 2000 *Scottish Midwives: Twentieth Century voices*. Tuckwell Press, East Lothian

5 DOH 1992 *Second report on the Maternity services (Winterton report)* HMSO London

6 Sandall J1995 Choice, continuity and control: changing midwifery, towards a sociological perspective. *Midwifery* 11(4): 201-209

7 SHHD 1993 *Provision on Maternity Services in Scotland –a policy review* HMSO Edinburgh

8 Scottish Executive 2001 *A Framework for Maternity Services in Scotland*. SEHD, Edinburgh

9 Scottish Executive 2002 *Expert Group on Acute Maternity Services (EGAMS)* SEHD, Edinburgh

10 DOH 1993 *Hospital doctors; training for the future. The report of the workgroup on specialist medical training (Calman Report)* DOH, London

11 Donnison, J. (1988) *Midwives and Medical Men: A History of the Struggle for the Control of Childbirth*, Historical Publications, London.

12 Nursing and Midwifery Council (NMC) 2009 *Standards for pre-registration midwifery education.* NMC, London

13 NMC 2009 p3.

14 Carr NJ 2008 Midwifery supervision and home birth against conventional advice *British Journal of Midwifery* 16(11); 743-745

15 Hart A, Lockey R, Henwood F, Pankhurst F, Hall V, Sommerville F (2001) *Researching professional education*. E.N.B. London. See http://www.rcm.org.uk/midwives/in-depth-papers/the-midwifery-lecturer-practitioner-in-practice

16 NHS QIS 2009 *Pathways for Maternity Care (KCND)*, NHS Scotland

17 Cummings M 2006 Can education programmes 'promote normality in childbirth?' *Midwifery Matters* Winter (111): 11-12

18 *NMC 2009 p4*

19 Price L 2010 Out on her own. *Midwives* 13(7):16-17

20 Wylie L 2006 Debating 'normality'. *Midwifery Matters* Winter (111); 13-14

21 Lange G, Kennedy H 2006 Student perceptions of ideal and actual midwifery practice. *Journal of Midwifery and Women's Health* 51(2):71-77

22 Thomas BG 2006 Making a difference: midwives' experiences of caring for women. *Evidence Based Midwifery* 4(3): 83-88

23 Lewis G (ed) 2007 The confidential enquiry into maternal and child health (CEMACH): Saving Mothers' Lives; reviewing maternal deaths to make motherhood safer 2003-2005. *The seventh report on confidential enquiries into maternal deaths in the UK*. CEMACH, London

24 Findlay N , James C, Irwin J 2006 Nursing education changes and reduced standards of quality care. *British Journal of Nursing* 15(13):700-702

25 Kenny G 2004 The origins of current nurse education policy and its implications for nurse ducators. *Nurse Education Today* 24 p84-90

26 Rolfe 1995 Linking care to excellence *Elderly Care* 7(1): 16-17

27 International Confederation of Midwives (ICM) 2010 *Mission statement* www.internationalmidwives.org

28 Royal College of Midwives 2010 Campaign for Normal Birth www.rcmnormalbirth.org.uk

29 Ball L, Curtis P, Kirkham M 2002 Why do midwives leave? *The Royal College of Midwives*, London

30 SMMDP 2010 Scottish Multiprofessional Maternity Development. www.scottishmaternity.org

Reclaiming meanings for birth, pain and risk within the home setting

Céline Lemay

It is "...about space, about language, and about death ; it is about the act of seeing, the gaze."[1]

Biomedical research convincingly supports the idea of normal birth but studies from various disciplines are essential if a subject as fundamental as birth is to be understood and if we want normal birth to become a reality in practical settings. Home birth has become an essential focus of research because although there is only a negligible amount of quantitative research data, giving birth within the home has enormous value in socio-symbolic terms. What has the phenomenon of home birth got to say to us today in our culture of technocratic care, where we constantly hear the background music of fear? To answer this question, I used a methodology rooted in hermeneutic phenomenology because this methodology allows us to come to a greater understanding of this profound human experience and explore the questions of meaning and being, which go beyond a consideration of mere facts. The knowledge generated can only enrich our biomedical knowledge on childbirth. Anthropological work I carried out on women's experience of home birth[2] serves as my point of departure for exploring the meaning of childbirth, pain and risk. At various points in this paper I shall also quote from interviews I conducted during my research.

First of all, we need to understand to what extent home birth is imbued with the semiotic value of the home i.e. to what extent it has symbolic significance. It is important to mention and learn from the representations of the home in order understand the impact the context of birth has on the process itself as well as on the lived experience.

The home—more than a mere location

The home is not only the place where we live, but also the place in which we feel alive... "It's my living space; it's my world."[3] The home is an intimate space of our 'being-in-the-world', as Heidegger would say. It is a place where there is coherence, where the different aspects of its inhabitants' lives are held together. Women suggest various analogies... They liken the concept of home to a nest, a refuge, a cocoon, a den. It's easy to see how the home can evoke strong images of protection and intimacy.

Women talk about the comfort that is associated with their home: "It has nothing to do with the physical space... my house gives me a kind of internal comfort. That's where I feel good."[4] It is the comfort which comes from living in accordance with one's beliefs and one's habits... It is the comfort which comes from not having to change 'culture', when moving from one place to another.

A home is more than a simple place: it is territory in which our control over our environment gives us a sense of security. "At home I'm the one who makes the rules."

When we consider the concept of control, it becomes obvious that a home is more than a simple place: it is territory in which our control over our environment gives us a sense of security: "At home there is nothing I dislike. I'm the one who makes the rules. I don't need to fit around anyone else."[5] This feeling is associated with a woman being able to be herself and being able to let herself go when the time to give birth comes. By contrast, an institution is a place where behaviour is strongly codified and a hospital is seen as a territory where the medical world (the biopower) expects 'docile bodies'.[6]

At home, timeframes are different. "Here, time is *my* time."[7] Women claim ownership of the complex and unique rhythm of their bodies. According to Ricoeur,[8] there are two different types of time: 'time of the soul' (human, lived time), and 'time of the world' (objective, linear succession). Women who give birth at home tune in to 'time of the soul' and want to distance themselves from 'time of the world'.

As a result, the home can be considered to be a true *monad* (Leibniz), i.e. a unit where a woman can tune into herself and cope with the enormous unheaval and powerful movement of emergence that is the arrival of a new being.

Reclaiming meanings for birth, pain and risk

Accounts I collected from women who gave birth at home shed light on how these women assigned meaning to birth and to two main issues frequently raised by women around birth outside hospital: pain and risk.

Meaning of birth for women

For the women I interviewed, giving birth was closely bound up with a sense of the space in which they wanted to experience this event: they wanted it to take place in their home. The use of key metaphors can help us to understand the meanings of the lived experience of giving birth.

- **Opening up**

  For these women, birth was, above all, a process of physical opening up, but at the same time it was seen as a psychic unfolding, an opening up. Although the women felt the uncertainty of the event, giving birth meant that they were opening up to another person and, in doing so, they reported they were experiencing facets of themselves, which they had not previously been aware of. "Birth is about moving into the unknown... Life is coming, but how is this going to happen? It is a moment in which a woman opens herself up to her strength and tenderness..."[9]

- **Emanating strength**

  Some women experienced and described birth as being an incredible energy, experienced inside themselves. They said this energy was certainly physical but they also reported it as being the experience of power (not power *over* but power from *within*)—a force, a capacity: the capacity to bring their own children into the world... Rabbuzzi described it as being the experience of "being swept up in a force of nature so powerful that your ordinary experience of yourself is gone."[10] Khan used a poetic expression of the birthing energy, describing it as an 'oceanic feeling'.[11] It is the act of giving birth that makes a woman feel strong and capable. "After I gave birth, I felt as if I would be able to do anything at all in my life... I felt I would be capable."[12]

- **Going within**

  The women saw birth as a process which took place within themselves, on the inside, at the depths of their being. They saw it as very personal and intimate. Sharing this intimate event with friends and family helped the women to strengthen family and social bonds. One woman said: "I felt that I was part of a community."[13] Being conscious of the unique experience of the feminine space experienced by some women was a way of feeling deeply connected to all other women-mothers on the planet.

- **Instinct**

  Unlike a mental or rational process, they said that childbirth was instinctual. They felt this instinct needed to be protected because any interference seemed to have an adverse effect on the process.

- **Transition**

  Women said that they experienced childbirth as a passage, a transition from the time when they were carrying their child inside themselves to the time when this child had come out into the world. They reported that both they and their babies experienced this transition, which caused "a kind of imprinting... for both me and my baby."[14] Socially, the woman who gives birth moves from the state of being a daughter to being a mother and, as a result, has to reorganise her identity, so that she is transformed for the rest of her life. This 'total social fact'[15] has become a medicalized rite of passage[16] in Western societies.

- **Occasion**

  Women saw childbirth as an opportunity to move something forward in their lives, to feel stronger and more capable. They see childbirth as an enlightening event that revealed the woman to herself and also taught her something about life. "When you give birth, it is Life itself that is taking shape in the most eloquent way."[17]

- **Story**

  They saw birth as an event which marks time, as an event which is part of a woman's history, part of the history of a family, and even generations. Women who gave birth at home were more interested in recording this event in the family annals, than in a hospital register, as part of statistical records. One woman said: "This is where my own life took place... This is my history... My baby was made here."[18]

- **Whole**

  Birth was considered a 'whole' event, which embraced elements which are frequently contrasted and even opposed: body *and* mind, head and heart, strength and weakness, pain and joy, inside and outside, the 'yes' and the 'no', life and death...

  From an ecological perspective, social, biological, psychological and spiritual dimensions of the process are clearly all linked together in a complex and profound way. This seems to be precisely the perspective of Suzanne Arms when she criticised the system of obstetrics saying that: "today childbirth and parenting may be the worst ecological disaster area of all."[19]

Meaning of pain for women

In the world of home birth, the word 'pain' does not appear to have just one single meaning—it is not just a physical experience. It has several, which are intimately linked to the way in which women see childbirth.

- **Part of normality**

  The pain of childbirth was reported as being different from the pain which occurs after an injury or when any kind of pathology is present. If childbirth is a normal process of the female body, the pain involved is therefore *normal pain*. If birth is not a disease, most pain associated with it is not considered to be something that needs to be 'cured'. It is simply a part of the *gestalt* of childbirth. One woman commented: "In birth, there is pain, but that is not all there is."[20]

- **A signal**

  The pain a woman experiences at the end of her pregnancy usually signals to her that her labour is about to begin. The process of childbirth without any sensations of pain would probably be risky and even dangerous for any women in a public space or alone at this major and delicate moment in her life and in the life of her child. In all cultures women have precise instructions about what they should do when they start to feel some pain. This is not an alarm call, but a signal for most women to seek out support and a place where they feel safe.

- **Part of the whole experience of birth**

  Labour and birth pain seem to be as intimate and personal as the process of childbirth itself. Wanting to fully live the natural process seems to involve living the reality of pain as part of the overall experience. As one woman explained it: "It is part of the event and I can't detach myself from it. If someone were to do something about the pain, that would change the experience as a whole. That would be like going to a concert and taking the sound away, or going into the garden and making all the smells of the flowers vanish."[21] Giving birth without pain would be like living with a sensory handicap at a moment when all a woman's senses need to be available so that she can meet and welcome her new baby. Therefore, pain should not be a focus of care, separated from the person who is experiencing it. Wanting to manipulate the pain would mean risking disturbing the action of birth itself, which is a total experience of opening up.

- **A way of being with the baby**

  While pain is taking place, the baby and mother are still a biological and psychic unit. Removing the pain for the mother doesn't have the same effect on the baby. So, experiencing pain could be a way for a woman to experience something intense with her baby. Referring to pain, one woman commented: "It created a kind of complicity with my baby."[22]

- **Part of the 'letting go' of the process of childbirth**

  When a woman is not required to move to another place during her labour she can put all her efforts into concentrating on going deep within herself and adapting in an optimal way to her situation. Having complete freedom to move around is seen as being a way of coping with pain, of making it manageable (and less dramatic). Labour pain is not seen as something which needs to be controlled. It is considered to be part of the 'letting go' process which women seem to perceive as necessary to the experience of birth. One woman said: "The pain touched something in me. I went deep inside myself."[23] A midwife once wrote: "In the final analysis, the best way of dealing with the pain is to go deep into it!"[24]

- **Part of the sense of achievement**

  Accepting the pain means taking charge of birth, which is perceived as a thing that has to be accepted by the woman. Another woman explained: "When I am in pain, I am all alone. It is *my* labour and I'm the one who has to go through it. Nobody can experience this in my place."[25] Integrating pain into the experience is then considered as part of the achievement of giving birth itself. One midwife understood this perspective precisely when she wrote an article on labour pain with the title: "Don't touch my pain!"[26]

- **Part of the power of birth**

  For some women, labour pain is a pain of effort. People generally consider it normal for there to be pain when they work hard or when they take part in a sporting competition. In the same way, it is normal for it to hurt when a woman gives birth. There is no need for the woman to be afraid of that pain and that power. If we refer to contractions as 'waves', the labouring woman may be afraid of capsising or sometimes of drowning if the waves seems too big or too strong. The woman needs to be reminded that she is also the *water.* She is also the ocean.

- **A sign of our humanity**

  Pain is not just normal... it is part of being human. Here, we are not talking about the idea of humanising birth, which is commonly interpreted as offering pain relief. The pain of labour and birth has an effect which it is important to understand. Le Breton reminds us that: "In a human world, that is to say, in a world which is full of meaning and values which prompt action, pain is without doubt a fundamental given... It is definitely an experience which all humans share, just as they share the experience of death."[27] Admitting that pain is *part* of childbirth also means recognising that we are human beings.

- **Part of the intensity of childbirth**

  If birth is a process which is intense and profound, pain is certainly part of that. One woman I interviewed said that pain "constitutes *the* intensity of childbirth. It is like a musical piece. There is always a crescendo at the end. At the end of pregnancy, when you give birth, there is a big crescendo. It is intense and loud!"[28]

- **Part of the depth of birth**

  Labour pain is closely connected with birth and is as deep as the experience—it is at its very foundation. Yet, in the intimacy and profundity of childbirth, the sensations are not necessarily interpreted as being painful. One woman reported: "The pain affected me somewhere... in my soul... Because I was very focused inside myself... it came as waves. It wasn't pain exactly. At a certain moment, you don't even need the word 'pain'."[29]

Meanings of pain for midwives

For midwives, childbirth is conceived as a process of creation, of transformation, of separation, and of initiation. According to their perspective, pain is a sign of these processes taking place. It is also...

For midwives childbirth is a process of creation, of transformation, of separation, and of initiation

- **A sign of creation**

  Labour pain is so much part of birth, it is considered part of the process of creation. Ontologically speaking, pain is different from the mechanical concept of process involved in industrialised manufacturing. The process of creation is often painful. All artists know that.

- **A sign of transformation**

  Many midwives see birth as a process of transformation on several levels, and pain is a sign that this transformation is taking place. However, in cultures in the modern, so-called developed world "... the pain we have been told we feel when we give birth has been constructed as anything but self transformative."[30] For midwives, the pain of birth cannot be reduced to a single element which needs to be endured.

- **A sign of transition**

  Bringing a child into the world involves moving from the state of being a maiden to being a mother. Birth is therefore a rite of passage where pain and ordeal are present. Nevertheless, Davis-Floyd convincingly demonstrated how the medical culture uses interventions on women to encapsulate birth in a mechanical and technocratic model and mostly to hide the threatening effect of natural childbirth which is essentially feminine, powerful and creative.[31]

- **A sign of separation**

  Pain is also considered to be an expression of the process whereby the mother separates from her baby, from a biological and symbiotic relationship. "It is impossible for them to continue living together. Only focusing on the physical experience disregards the symbolic, emotional and psychic aspects of what it means to open oneself up so as to let a child emerge."[32] This inevitable separation is painful in itself.

- **Part of the initiation process**

  To some midwives, labour pain has the power to initiate women into a new life and a new self. Like any other initiation, birth becomes a way of measuring oneself, of feeling one's strength and one's limits, of showing one's ability to cope with difficulties in life and to experience the sacred. The fact of having to pass through the process of childbirth seems to have the effect of *empowering* women.

Finally, midwives recognise that painful experiences in life (related to solitude, depression, anxiety, past experiences, family problems, marital problems, etc) can also be real and important and cannot be separated from a woman's experience of giving birth. Making the body silent will not necessarily silence the crying inside.

Risk

An obsession with safety has become a characteristic of our age[33] and concerns about risk are omnipresent in pregnancy and motherhood, particularly when birth takes place at home. In my research, when I asked people who had faced risks what they thought about them, they usually began by repositioning birth within a global context and defined childbirth as being something which is a "major event, which is not just medical."[34]

An obsession with safety is a characteristic of our age

Moreover, women considered birth outside their home to be a risk factor which interfered with the women's ability to give birth successfully. Their fears were not connected to biomedical risks but to factors which would inhibit their capacity to let themselves go, so as to give birth "somewhere else... there are many things which stop me from letting go and there will be censorship... and there are too many people around."[35] For a woman who chooses to be at home, it seems that childbirth is not just a question of having a beautiful, healthy baby. For her, it is about opening up. The feeling of being in control of her environment becomes an element that creates a feeling of security. "... it makes me feel safer. Having nurses there for eight hours doesn't give me a sense of security."[36]

After all, feeling safe is more to do with interior norms. And birthing is not about satisfaction or comfort. "Here... I can live life to the full and experience joy..."[37]

For some midwives risk is a way of perceiving reality. It is one perspective, but not to do with reality or the facts. One woman commented: "Risk is not reality, it is a mathematical calculation, a statistical calculation. And numbers are a way of seeing things... There are other ways."[38]

Confidence

Home birth reveals another perspective on risk. While caregivers talk about risks relating to birth, women talk about their confidence in *themselves* and in life itself. A feeling of safety does not preclude uncertainty, though. But while the system of biomedicine is based on the potential pathology of pregnancy and birth, home birth makes midwives see the process of giving birth as something which is full of *possibilities,* as an opportunity. It makes them see the glass as half full, not half empty.

In the 21st century, the concepts of risk and safety are strongly defined in biological terms. Exploring the world of home birth allows us to extend our understanding of risk and safety in terms of their emotional and even spiritual dimensions.

Exploring the world of home birth allows us to extend our understanding of risk and safety

Conclusion

Home birth can be seen as a text which can be analysed and interpreted.[39] While the humanisation of birth is associated with the right to consumer choice and the availability of pain relief, home birth reminds us that humanisation is also about having the power to name, define and assign meanings to birth, pain and risk. Giving birth at home is a way of asserting another way of being in the world.

Homebirth emphasises the importance of the process of birth

Home birth emphasises the importance of the process and not only the outcome. Without being a goal in itself, it would seem to be a way of affirming that birth remains an entirely unique process. Giving birth at home can be seen as a way of 're-enchanting' the world–referring to Gauchet's expression 'the disenchantment of the world'[35] when he was talking about the 'invisible' aspects of life becoming depleted.

In the 21st century when people promote normal birth they usually concentrate on promoting physiological birth. Although this is important, it is necessary to realise that focusing on this tethers us to the biological dimension of birth and makes us tend to forget that a normal birth is also a highly social and spiritual event. Isn't it surprising that physiology is being seen as a goal, when in fact these are the processes which had the basic role of maintaining life in the human body and ensuring the survival of *homo sapiens* for millennia?

In a cultural context where women's bodies, pregnancy and birth have all been 'normalised' and defined in a reductionist way, home birth can remind us of the richness of meanings and the complexity of the process which is childbirth. When birth happens outside the dominant context of a hospital, interdisciplinary research has the potential to expand our conception, knowledge, and especially our perspective on birth. Finally, perhaps it is time to explore childbirth from a transdisciplinary perspective[40,41] and then expand our ways of knowing the complexity and wonder of birth. The actual problem with biomedical knowledge about pregnancy and birth is not that it is dominant... it is the fact that it is insufficient.

Céline Lemay started serving women as a midwife 20 years before midwifery became legal in Quebec. She was one of the founders of a midwifery association which organised practice and worked for solidarity between midwives. She was politically active so as to ensure that midwifery became recognised as a profession which is distinct from nursing and medicine, in 1999. She did an MA in Anthropology and a PhD in Applied Human Sciences at the University of Montreal. She is now a board member of the Association for Public Health in Québec and has spent years considering the role of midwifery and birthing centres as part of the state's overall public health strategy. She has three children and four grandchildren.

References

1 Foucault M, 1994. The Birth of the Clinic: an Archaeology of Medical Perception. New York: Vintage Books, p ix. This sentence is the first of the book. It is a key to understanding major issues around birth. The historical construction of clinical medicine is, for Foucault, a question of space, language, death, and fundamentally about the particular 'gaze' of medicine, constructed from reading death (pathology). Very differently, midwifery evolved around the space of home and constructs its 'gaze' and knowledge by seeing birth in the broadest sense of the word.

2 Lemay C, 1998. *L'accouchement à la maison au Québec: les voix du dedans.* Master thesis in anthropology, University of Montréal.

3 Lemay C, 1998, p 39.

4 Lemay C, 1998, p 42.

5 Lemay C, 1998, p 42.

6 In Petersen A, Bunton R (ed), 1997. Foucault, health and medicine, New York: Routledge.

7 Lemay C, 1998, p 43.

8 Ricoeur P,(1988) *Time and Narrative*, translated by Blamey K, Pellauer D, Vol 3, Chicago: University of Chicago Press.

9 Lemay C, 1998, p 48.

10 Rabuzzi KA, 1994. *Mother with child. Transformations through Childbirth*, Indianapolis: Indiana University Press, p ix.

11 Khan RP, 1995. *Bearing Meaning: The Language of Birth*. Urbana: University of Illinois Press.

12 Lemay C, 1998, p 49.

13 Lemay C, 1998, p 50.

14 Lemay C, 1998, p 51.

15 In relation to the expression coined by Mauss. The consideration of the body, the spirit and the social context have to be hand in hand.

16 Davis-Floyd RE, 1992. *Birth as an American Rite of Passage*. Berkeley: University of California Press.

17 Lemay C, 1998, p 68.

18 Lemay C, 1998, p 54.

19 Arms S, 1994. *Immaculate Deception II*. Berkeley: Celestial Arts, p 170.

20 Lemay C, 1998, p 68.

21 Lemay C, 1998, p 69.

22 Lemay C, 1998, p 71.

23 Lemay C, 1998, p 71.

24 Brabant I, 1987. Ne touchez pas à ma douleur. *L'une à l'autre,* Winter 1987.

25 Lemay C, 1998, p 72.

26 Brabant I, 1987. Ne touchez pas à ma douleur. *L'une à l'autre,* Winter, 1987.

27 Le Breton D, 1995. *Anthropologie de la douleur*. Paris: Métailié, p 15.

28 Lemay C, 1998, p 73.

29 Lemay C, 1998, p 74.

30 Rabuzzi, KA, 1994. *Mother with Child. Transformations Through Childbirth.* Indianapolis: Indiana University Press, p 101.

31 Davis-Floyd RE, 1992. Birth as an American Rite of Passage. Berkeley: University of California Press.

32 Lemay C, 1998, p 76.

33 See Foucault.

34 Lemay C, 1998, p 93.

35 Lemay C, 1998, p 93.

36 Lemay C, 1998, p 93.

37 Lemay C, 1998, p 94.

38 Lemay C, 1998, p 95.

39 Ricoeur P, 1986. *Du Texte à l'Action: Essais d'Herméneutique II.* Paris: Seuil.

40 Nicolescu B, 2002. Manifesto of Transdisciplinarity. State University of New York Press. Translation from the French by Karen-Claire Voss.

41 Max-Neef MA, 2005. Foundations of transdisciplinarity. *Ecological Economics*, 53: 5-16.

What can we learn from traditional cultures in the promotion of normal birth?

Mandy Forrester

Like many other newly developed countries around the world, the United Arab Emirates (UAE) has seen a change in childbirth practices, from a traditional model to a more technological one, meaning that the country now has a 98% hospital birth rate.[1] The UAE, formed in 1971, is typical of the Gulf region, where rapid social changes over the past 50 years have occurred, thanks to a shift from a traditional society to an industrial society, based on oil revenues. However, an ethnographic study I conducted of Emirati women in 2006 revealed that, despite the transfer from traditional practices to a more technological approach to childbirth, traditional practices and beliefs prevail.[2] In this chapter I shall reflect upon such practices and beliefs, consider how they influence childbirth in the UAE today and also consider what we can learn from practices and attitudes in terms of promoting normal birth.

Life before oil

Little evidence exists to reveal what women's lives were like in the era before oil was discovered in the UAE. We do know a few things, though... The economy was based around agriculture, fishing and pearling. Society was tribal, some tribes being nomadic or Bedouin, and all were patriarchal. Homes were primitive and lacked sanitation or clean water; people's diet was limited to local produce of fish, rice and dates. A Western doctor was not present in the area until 1960, which was also when the first hospital was built. Clearly, women's lives must have been hard, and made worse by the harshness and aridity of the climate. However, although the common perception of women in the Middle East is perhaps of disempowered individuals, women did have a role in tribal affairs, but only behind the scenes. In fact, the tribal matriarch was an important woman in tribal society.[3]

Like records in general for this newly developed area, statistics were also not routinely kept until the formation of the country in 1971. No figures exist regarding maternal mortality, although in 2004 Heard-Bey estimated that rates were around 40% before modern medical facilities were introduced.[4] According to the UAE Ministry of Information and Culture (writing in 2001), infant mortality rates have fallen from 145 per 1000 in 1960 to 10 per 1000 in 1998.[1] Typically, women died from infection and complications of vaginal atresia [constriction of the vaginal opening] following vaginal packing. It was not that no treatments were available before recent developments; an informal system of health care based on folk medicine and religious beliefs did indeed exist in nomadic life.[5] The *daya* (the Arabic word for 'midwife'), like the British handywoman[6] not only cared for pregnant women but also laid out the dead.

Usually older women, they learnt their practice from other women, gaining experience of being with women in labour and becoming skilled in traditional midwifery skills, such as massage. It was the responsibility of the *daya* to escort the bride to the marital bed, most probably to open the vagina after female genital mutilation, which was also a common practice in the Gulf region. However, despite the existence of *dayas,* relatives would often deliver women in their family without a midwife being present.[7] This was not considered unusual and Doumato has argued that this custom may have resulted in fewer complications than unskilled midwives may have caused.[8]

Childbirth practices before 'development'

Before the advent of the first Western medical team in 1960, women in the UAE delivered squatting over a pile of sand, supported by other women, frequently also using a rope tied to the main tent pole or a pole in the sand outside for additional support. Holton records an older *sheika* (daughter or wife of a sheik) recalling birth:

> *'It was not as it is now. There was a pole, a thick strong pole put in the ground. When the pains come you squat down and hold the pole. Then you push your head against the pole. There are some women to help. One held down one leg at the heel and another held down the other leg. The third held up the back. The bottom. This way the child was born. But no sound ... You cannot make a sound. It is not polite. Only like this: [soft grunt].'*[9]

Labour and birth were treated with caution, privacy and secrecy.[10] Elderly women supported the woman by offering prayers and encouragement as well as herbs, massage and readings from the *Qur'an* to provide comfort. Since it was not possible to call for medical help until 1960 the journey to find any help needed would have been long and difficult, on camel back, over sand.

The actual birth was completely unaided because it was considered impolite to ask for help. In my study a woman described her birth as follows:

> *'I was sitting when I delivered the baby. I didn't move a lot, someone held me at the back. No help, I just pushed it out myself. Only the daya, she cut the cord.'*

Even today, over 40 years later, the placenta and cord are surrounded by deeply rooted beliefs.[5] Viewed as the 'secret cord', the midwife has the responsibility for cutting it. It is believed that the baby is spiritually and physically linked to the placenta and cord so they are (usually still) treated as a living soul, and buried accordingly.

In traditional practice, immediately after the birth the mother and baby would be washed with hot water, salt and herbs. The birth would have been announced, prayers whispered into the baby's right ear and a sheep slaughtered in thanksgiving for the safety of the mother and child.[5]

The placenta and cord are surrounded by beliefs

Surprisingly, the belief is that once a woman has had a baby without intervention, she may go to hospital

My own study found that since hospitals have been available, women still do not go in until they want to push, or after the membranes have ruptured. Surprisingly perhaps, the belief is that once a woman has had a baby *without* intervention, she may then go into the hospital for subsequent labours and births. This practice was, and still is, encouraged by older women and results in women arriving at hospital in the second stage of labour. A young woman I interviewed told me:

> *"My mother, she said she didn't go until she wanted to push. Even for us they tell us not to go until the waters break or they will give you injections and that is happening up till now. If you want to go, they wouldn't take, they wouldn't take'"* [i.e. the relatives wouldn't take the woman in].

From the context above and from the next two quotes, I deduce that the 'injection' referred to is actually an IV containing syntocinon:

> *"Because in the hospital, they think that they will get you and give you the injection immediately you get into the hospital. And that's what they are saying, they will deliver you before your time. They will come and give you the injection."*

This fear was also found in my own study, which was confirmed in a study of Egyptian women. In both studies women spoke of the 'injection' with fear.[19]

> *"I waited until 42 weeks until I deliver and they [my relatives] won't let me go. They say 'Oh my God, they will give you the injection!' But if the baby is pushing, it is alright because it is more clean and they have everything."*

It would appear that women are prepared to go to hospital for the benefits of cleanliness and safety but only once they are thought to be past the stage of labour when interference is anticipated. This may be attributed to the fact that in the past, maternal and infant mortality rates were high. (Other researchers recorded women in Afghanistan describing the fear of death which prevailed.)[11] Considering that infant mortality rates in 1960 were estimated to be 149 per 1000 (Ministry of Information and Culture, 2001),[1] it is not surprising that women welcomed an alternative system of care.

Privacy

The pay-off for safer, cleaner birth resulted in diminished privacy when women went into hospitals. Traditionally, birth had been a quiet and very private event to the extent that one of the oldest women I interviewed, reported that she kept her *abayah* [long, black 'outer-garment'] over her until the baby was born.

Before modernisation not even the *daya* handled either woman or baby until she had cut the cord:

> *'And also they used to cover.* [Grandmother shows her abayah over her body.] *Yes, everything covered. I don't know all of them or not but my grandmother because she is so private. I don't know if all them like this. And she is saying she is covered'* [referring to another woman present].

In the past, women in labour even faced the wall and did not have other women with them while they were in labour so that they could increase their privacy.[2,8,13]

All this means that women experienced a dramatic shift from an intensely private experience (where they were protected and nurtured by a few close relatives and the *daya*, who respected their privacy and modesty), to a less private experience in hospital. One woman described having to 'fight' with hospital staff so as to be able to cover herself:

> *'You cover yourself, they uncover you. I had to [be uncovered], I didn't have any choice.'*

The women I interviewed also reported that care has become more invasive over time, since birth moved into hospitals:

> *'In the old days in the hospital, there was only the doctor and the nurse. Not like now when they let anyone in. She* [a relative] *stood on the door not to let anyone in.'*

In contrast there was also the complaint that companions the women wanted were not permitted into the delivery room:

> *'No only the midwife in the hospital. They don't allow anyone to go inside. Nothing changes from the first to the last baby. No one went inside except my grandmother when she was alive. Now they* [midwives] *say no one inside, not even mother.'*

More disturbing was the loss of control felt by one woman:

> *'I felt bad because when I had my baby they kept coming in.*
> *(Me) 'They didn't ask?'*
> *'NO they didn't ask.'*

It appears that the women have to trade their feelings about privacy or modesty, or having any control of the situation, against the feeling that they will be helped more if something goes wrong; this was a constant thread throughout my findings. Nevertheless, despite their desire for safe and effective care, the women I interviewed all mentioned a lack of privacy as the most negative aspect of hospital birth.

Women have to trade their feelings about privacy or control against the feeling that they will be helped more

Salt packing

Some traditional practices employed were harmful—for example the practice of packing the vagina with rock salt, which resulted in vaginal atresia and death in subsequent pregnancies.[8,14]

The practice of salt packing is, in fact, widely documented in research conducted over the last few decades.[15-17] Damp rock salt was moulded into a banana shape and inserted into the vagina after the birth.[13] The *daya* might insert the salt or the mother would insert it herself. It was a painful procedure which was repeated every day for 20 days for a first baby and 15 for a second.[2] And the practice was not restricted to the UAE: it was also witnessed in Kuwait, Bahrain and Saudi Arabia by missionaries in the 1930s.[8] Various authors[8,13] report seeing women with vaginal and cervical atresia following salt packing, and in some instances seeing this result in fetal and maternal death. The high maternal mortality rates are also offered by some as an explanation for men taking more wives, because a man *expected* his wife to be able to bear children and obviously a dead wife would be unable to do so.[4,16] Boersma[16] gives a personal account of women from Oman using salt. Apparently, Omani women believed that the mother would live if salt was used, and that—if it was not used—she would die. All researchers looking into this practice also report the perceived advantage of salt packing in terms of reducing the incidence of infection. This is clearly the main reason Middle Eastern women see it as being a useful practice. One woman, who clearly had erroneous notions about the rationale for IVs and injections, told me:

> *'You use the salt. It was used to avoid inflammation and to stop it going mouldy. Today you get an injection* [antibiotics via injection] *but we didn't have. So we used salt to keep clean. Women who didn't use the salt died. Yes they had smell if they didn't use salt.'*

In Oman, education programmes caused the practice to stop[16] and the introduction of birthing in hospitals is cited as the reason for the practice becoming obsolete in other parts of the Gulf.[18]

Nowadays, while salt packing is rarely seen, a reliance on salt water for washing the perineum remains, probably because of the widespread fear of infection. Clearly, women still resort to their own methods when their fear of infection is stronger than their belief in a doctor's advice:

> *'They think that even with stitches the area will be bigger. They were told to wash the area with salt and water. The doctors said don't use Dettol or salt, just water. But they used to mix Dettol and salt and water to avoid infection.'*

Other researchers portrayed the family as a source of knowledge (particularly El-Memer, *et al* and Green and Small).[19,20] While it was the mother in particular who gave advice in these studies, in my own research I found it was older family members who were seen as the trusted informants. However, like El-Memer *et al*,[19] I found a conflict between experiential knowledge which was handed on by the family and the authoritative knowledge of medicine.

Religious beliefs

The ways in which Allah's (God's) help is sought has not changed since early missionaries' reports.[8,13] Prayers were offered by whispering into water and then drinking the water:

> *'When it is hard they just read the Holy Qur'an* [the religious book of Muslims] *and drink the water. They whisper the words into the water and then drink.'*

Qur'anic verses were written on paper and washed off with rose water; the woman would then drink the rose water. Through many discussions with Emirati women, it became apparent that there is a high level of trust in Allah. When discussing coping with labour one woman said:

> *My aunt, she said they trust in God. Yes it hurts but when it comes it comes. Allah will look after me. I trust God if I will die.....'*

However, although a certain amount of fatalism appears to be associated with cultural and religious beliefs, medical expertise does also seem to be accepted. Although doctors know about technology, the belief is that Allah gave them this knowledge. This in turn allows Arab women to accept medical intervention:

> *'You believe in God and God gives them* [doctors] *the knowledge.'*

Despite fatalism, medical expertise seems to be accepted

The 'evil eye'

Another important concept is that of the 'evil eye'. There is a strong belief, which prevails today, about this and also about the power of envy.[2] The mother is considered very vulnerable to evil powers in the postnatal period. Ghubash[21] reports nine names to describe a state experienced in the first few weeks of the postnatal period in which the woman suffers emotional and psychological disturbance, which is characterised by fever, fear and unrest. While, in terms of Western medicine, this may be seen as being puerperal psychosis or delirium associated with puerperal fever, in the Arab world the cause of this condition is believed to be the evil eye or envy from another person.

In 1919, missionary observer Eleanor Claverley recorded that the women of Arabia not only have faith in God but also in "jinns, demon possession, enchantment and all kinds of charms and magic".[22] (This was also recounted by Holton.)[23] Amulets or charms were traditionally used to protect a person who had been affected by the evil eye.[24] I have data in my own research which suggests that these beliefs are still prevalent. The children of one family slave I interviewed died of fever, one when it was 14 years old, the other at 10 days. The slave believed the cause of infection was that "someone gave it the eye" [evil eye]. This belief still holds fear for women so they cover their baby's cot with a white *shailah* (head cover); the idea is that if the baby is seen, people will give it the evil eye and then misfortune will affect the child.

A mix of old and new: lessons to be learnt and points for reflection

In conclusion, although the availability of skilled midwifery and obstetric care and free access to hospitals has undoubtedly improved maternal and infant mortality rates, traditional culture is still very much in evidence in birth practices in the UAE.

Rather than dismissing the 'old' practices out of hand, I would suggest that it is useful to consider what lessons can be learnt from the traditional culture of the Emiratis and other people in the Arab world. Clearly, while practices such as salt packing have no place in modern birth, the wisdom of older women is worthy of reflection. They know the value of avoiding intervention and even today they encourage younger women to avoid this by keeping them at home until they are in advanced labour.

It is particularly interesting that these 'wise women' look positively on hospital birth once a woman has had a first normal labour and birth there and that they are less reluctant to take their kin to hospital in subsequent labours. (When their first experience ends with a good outcome, they are understandably more positively predisposed to submit to care in later pregnancies.) However, the comments made by interviewees about the labouring and birthing woman's need for privacy and the need for a quiet, safe environment in which the woman can go into herself supported by other women are interesting... These 'wise women' clearly understand that privacy and lack of disturbance is fundamental to the normal birthing process.

Finally, the positive belief Arab women have in a higher power is clearly helpful to them; we should perhaps ask whether beliefs of a religious or cultural nature give women strength and a focus during childbirth in other cultures.

Overall, it is clear that the attitudes of Emirati women, which have remained over generations—the awareness of risk, as well as the deep understanding of the labouring woman's needs—reflect an implicit knowledge and understanding of the process of birth. Perhaps there are things we can learn from this so that traditional approaches are not thrown out completely when birth becomes medicalised in other contexts, or when medicalised contexts attempt a return to more human values when considering the personal aspects of the experience of birth.

Mandy Forrester has worked as clinical midwife in hospital and community settings, education and research. In 1997, Mandy joined the Ministry of Health, Abu Dhabi and was appointed as Chair of the newly formed Midwifery Committee in December 1998. During this time, the Midwifery Committee strategically planned midwifery regulation and registration; developed Scope of Practice and midwifery competencies; and wrote, prepared and supervised registration exams. Mandy initiated the inauguration, and was an ex-officio member, of the Midwifery Professional Practice Group. Since returning to the UK in 2004, Mandy has worked as a community Matron, project midwife and community midwife. She is currently a midwifery adviser at the Nursing and Midwifery Council.

References

1 Ministry of Information and Culture, 2001. *United Arab Emirates Year Book 2000/2001.* London: Trident Press.

2 Forrester MJ, 2006. Changing Maternity in the Face of Modernity: An exploration of the factors that influenced the move from home to hospital birth in the indigenous population of the United Arab Emirates between 1960 and 1975. Unpublished.

3 United Nations Development Fund for Women, undated. Women in the UAE. Available from: http://www.unifem.org. [accessed on 15/05/2003]

4 Heard-Bey F, 2004. *From Trucial States to United Arab Emirates Dubai.* Motivate Publishing, p 148.

5 Hurriez SH, 2002. *Folklore and Folklife in the United Arab Emirates: Cultivation and Culture in the Middle East.* London: Routledge Curzon.

6 Leap N, Hunter B, 1993. *The Midwife's Tale. An oral history from handywoman to professional midwife.* London: Scarlet Press.

7 Green KE, 2003. Change in the Desert: Parenting Practices Across Three Generations of Arab Women. Unpublished. Abu Dhabi: Zayed University.

8 Doumato EA, 2000. *Getting God's Ear Women, Islam and Healing in Saudi Arabia and the Gulf.* New York: Columbia University Press.

9 Holton P, 1991. *Mother Without a Mask.* Dubai: Motivate Publishing, p 212.

10 Hurriez SH, 2002. *Folklore and Folklife in the United Arab Emirates: Cultivation and Culture in the Middle East.* London: Routledge Curzon, p 88.

11 Kaartinen L, Diwan V, 2005. Mother and child healthcare in Kabul, Afghanistan with focus on the mother: women's own perspective. *Acta Obstetrica and Gynecologica Scandinavica.* 81(6) pp 491-501.

12 Purkiss J, 1998. The medicalisation of childbirth. *MIDIRS Midwifery Digest.* 8:1 pp 110-112.

13 Boersma J, 1991. *Grace in the Gulf. The Historical Series of the Reformed Church in America.* No 20. Primary Mission Sources. Michigan: Eerdmans Publishing Company.

14 Personal communication Gertrude Dyck, 1999.

15 Doumato EA, 2000. *Getting God's Ear Women, Islam and Healing in Saudi Arabia and the Gulf.* New York: Columbia University Press, p 189.

16 Boersma J, 1991. *Grace in the Gulf. The Historical Series of the Reformed Church in America.* No 20. Primary Mission Sources. Michigan: Eerdmans Publishing Company, pp 114-116.

17 Doorenbos H, 1976. *Postpartum salt packing and other medical practices: Oman, South Arabia Medical Anthropology.* pp 109-111. Paris: Mouton Publishers, p 109.

18 Doumato EA, 2000. *Getting God's Ear Women, Islam and Healing in Saudi Arabia and the Gulf.* New York: Columbia University Press, p 191.

19 El Nemer A, Downe S, Small N, 2006. 'She would help me from the heart': An ethnography of Egyptian women in labour. *Social Science and Medicine* 62 p 81-92.

20 Green KE, Smith DE, 2006. Change and continuity: childbirth and parenting across three generations of women in the United Arab Emirates. *Childcare, Health and Development* 33:3 p 266-274.

21 Ghubash, 1998, cited by Hurriez SH, 2002. *Folklore and Folklife in the United Arab Emirates: Cultivation and Culture in the Middle East.* London: Routledge Curzon, 2002, p 89.

22 Claverley E, cited in Doumato EA, 2000. *Getting God's Ear Women, Islam and Healing in Saudi Arabia and the Gulf.* New York: Columbia University Press, p 147.

23 Holton P, 1991. *Mother Without a Mask*. Dubai: Motivate Publishing, p 78-84.

24 Heard-Bey F, 2004. *From Trucial States to United Arab Emirates*. Dubai: Motivate Publishing, p 139.

The challenge of promoting normality and midwifery in China

Anshi Pan and Ngai Fen Cheung

The history

When we talk about China today, we are talking about a population of 1.3 billion, of whom 610-630 million are women.[1] Even under the one-child policy that has lasted for three decades, in which the fertility rate has dropped from 7.50 in the 1960s to the current 1.79,[2] it is still a great challenge to promote normal childbirth and labour in an increasingly industrialised China, where any medical technology used in childbearing is seen as modern and progressive. However, our evaluation of the challenge will depend on what is meant by 'normality' in childbirth and labour, to be meaningful in the Chinese context.

The Chinese developed theories of health and illness in the first millennium BC. It was not until the 12th century that women's problems in relation to childbearing were comprehensively discussed and written about by medicine men.[3] Maternity care in general was very rarely recorded, but was certainly an indispensable social undertaking in a society where continuity of the ancestral line was always central to the concerns of family groups. Important as they were, however, childbirth caregivers, always women of a certain age and experience (mostly) in the local community, were on the edges of society, ranking lowest in types of women practitioners.[4] They were collectively referred to by a word which had even become an idiom（三姑六婆, which was used in literary works, as well as in daily jibes to mean 'people engaging in trivial door-to-door selling and gossiping'. The historical credit for ensuring that childbirth was safe was given to medicine men, who were able to administer herbal remedies to women (including herbal oxytocin), irrespective of whether these remedies were effective, ineffective or even bizarre.

In those days, knowledge of childbearing physiology was not developed, although it was not entirely absent. The age-old Chinese theories of health and illness, based on certain anatomical knowledge and ideas,[5] were not religious wizardry, but quasi-scientific in some correct but still inaccurate ways and these theories were closely associated with nature. Even this knowledge was not within the grasp of traditional midwives, though, because most of them were illiterate.[6] High maternal mortality could be expected, so although it might be an exaggeration it is not a surprise to read in Chinese historical records of the 1st century AD about a duchess who made a strong appeal for people to take childbirth seriously, saying that it was a life-and-death event in which "10 out of 11 women would die".[7] Dangers of childbirth had certainly been an obsessive focus for women, at least in central China, for millennia. Therefore, childbirth was necessarily, and still is, seen as dangerous, weakening women's bodies and making them susceptible to disease, although it was not seen as being entirely pathological.

The high mortality rate in China was certainly the reason why the European medical model of childbirth, including hospitalised care, was so readily adopted, first by the elite population of China around the turn of 20th century, then as a new method of giving birth, which was promoted throughout the country. The medicalisation of childbirth and the improvement in living conditions did indeed reduce both maternal and infant mortality rates. Chinese maternal mortality dropped from 1,500 per 100,000 live births after World War II to 36.6 per 100,000 in 2008.[8] Although the country still had quite a way to go to reach the maternal mortality level achieved by many European countries—e.g. Italy: 3.9, Sweden: 4.6, UK: 8[9]—and to reach the UN Millennium Development Goal (MDG) by 2015 that China's maternal mortality rate should decline by three quarters from its 1990 level, which was 88 per 100,000,[10] it looked like the age-old battle against maternal and infant death could be won, thanks to the progress made by modern medicine and the scientific world generally. In fact, the latest investigation in China into causes of maternal and infant mortality revealed that over 75% of deaths could be prevented.[10] This is the case because although China theoretically has the obstetric capability to solve the problem of high mortality rates, obstetric help is not accessible to many women and it is wrongly used in many cases. In fact, it seems that medicine itself actually claims some lives, instead of preventing deaths. Moreover, despite increasing management of birth it is recognised that since the 1990s, the decline in both maternal and infant mortality rates has slowed down,[11] so the earlier positive trend is not continuing.

Overall, maternal health in modern China does seem to be improving, but with underlying problems. One problem is that obstetric medicine is under-used in the places where it is needed most, while it is over-used in other (wealthy, urban) areas. This is due to developments in the capitalist economy: as China has been actively engaged in a market economy for the past four decades, the gap between the rich and the poor becomes ever more widened. With medical resources increasingly concentrating in large cities and becoming highly priced, few can afford the care. A 75% preventable maternal mortality rate is then not a surprising outcome for the whole country. (This means that three quarters of women who die in childbirth, need not have died, if care had been available to them, or if they had not had unnecessary and/or inappropriate interventions.) On the other hand, obstetric medicine is over-used, with both economic and political agendas, similar to what has happened in industrialised societies in Europe, where feminist writers have observed that the arrival of obstetric technology provided man-doctors with the opportunity to control female bodies.[12] In China in recent decades, when it also became industrialised, the fast-increasing caesarean rate in cities, from 34% up to 100% in some city hospitals[13] is a testimonial to the medical power that has been unleashed with the mistaken intention of modernising maternity care. As a result, more obstetricians were trained than midwives, who were seen as obsolete in the industrial era. In a major policy shake-up in the last decade of the 20th century, midwifery as an important subject was erased from the curriculum of the educational institutions in China and childbirth became 100% hospitalised, with obstetric care or treatment.[14] Medical science not only has the power to control women's bodies, but also the power to profit from such control.

As healthcare is not an exception to the market forces principle in China's economic growth, medicine is becoming the very means for profiteering so as to increase hospital and caregivers' income.[15] There seem to be good reasons for medicine to be used more, only these reasons do not have anything to do with improving women's health in childbirth.

> *Medicine is becoming the means for profiteering so as to increase hospital and caregivers' income*

Childbirth is in fact a physiological, social and cultural cycle in human life which is in need of care but not manipulation. In bearing a child, a woman undergoes an enormous physiological, social and cultural change. These changes constitute a brand new life experience for the woman and her immediate community. The experience no doubt has the most profound effects on women and the people around her. It is this experience that should be at the centre of care. Since childbirth is a natural, healthy process in human life, medicine, apart from treating occasional abnormal or pathological conditions in births, obviously has no other role. It is not very hard to find evidence that shows the enormous feeling of change women experience when they have a baby. Women in the UK said that childbirth experiences "strike at the very heart and soul," "touch new emotions not experienced before and bring a whole new perspective to life" and that "nothing can compare to the experience of giving birth and holding your child for the first time. It definitely altered (our) relationships."[16] Chinese women describe their birthing experience as worthier than anything. An invasive way of managing a childbirth, such as using medicine or medical instruments to speed up a birth, will certainly have a negative effect on these feelings.

There is no doubt that childbirth is not pathogenic. Childbirth is not even simply a physiological process, but it involves what is socially and culturally important. Therefore, it is more useful to see the social and cultural values of childbirth and to see what is meaningful in childbirth to women and to society as a whole. The social and cultural values, in which women's important feelings about giving birth are respected, are the very bases for making childbirth normal. In some cultures around the world, such as in Northern India and Tibet (further discussed in a section below), childbirth may be seen as devalued.[17] In these cultures, because of the idea of 'pollution', women giving birth are often left alone and do not receive the proper care that they need. High maternal mortality and morbidity are found in these areas.[18] In these cases, healthy, physiological births easily become affected by disease. These births are not normal. In the same way, both under- or over-use of medical resources in childbirth in industrial societies, for money and power, can also be seen as devaluing childbirth, making childbirth abnormal. We see these as presenting major challenges to the normality of childbirth in China. To further understand these challenges, we shall first look at some statistics which emerged from some recent research carried out in China.

Untangling the statistics

In China, over the last 30 years of its fast economic development, in the field of childbirth, as happened in many societies in Europe during their industrialisation, modern medical science has quickly replaced midwifery care. As the new millennium began, it became state health policy that childbirth should become totally hospitalised.[19] This policy was in effect a political statement that childbirth could only become safer under obstetric care. Papers attributing the reduction in maternal mortality rates to institutional birth[20] mostly referred to obstetric, technological care so this further promoted the idea that obstetric care was the only way forward.

However, one problem which was implicitly recognised is the connection between the increased use of surgery and *increased* (not reduced) mortality and morbidity. One important report did, in fact, concede that caesareans might have been responsible for some avoidable maternal deaths and morbidity.[21] We can surmise that hospitalisation must have encouraged caregivers to overuse caesareans.

The rise in caesarean rates around the country does, in fact, seem to be a generalised problem. Around the country, between 1993 and 2003, rates rose from 6.7% to 20.6%, on average. This would perhaps not seem too dramatic, but the statistics revealed that the trend for caesarean birth was much more marked in big cities, where it rose from 18.1% to 34.7% in the same period, reaching 50% to 100% in some cities.[22] Some researchers laid the blame for the rising caesarean rate, even if only partly, on women's increasing preference for caesareans.[23] The other reason, however, which was somehow omitted from the research papers, must surely have been exactly what the research was trying to convince people of: the importance of hospitalisation and obstetric technology in childbirth.

In China now people generally believe that the prerequisite for good maternity care is enjoying good economic circumstances.[24] This is because if there is more money, there are more hospitals, more obstetric equipment and more drugs. As a result, it has been claimed that the reason maternal mortality rates were high in economically underdeveloped areas was because in these places the per capita income was low. While it cannot be denied that a certain standard of living is necessary for mothers to have babies successfully (good hygiene and physical care being among the most important factors), logic based on finances can, in fact, be dangerous logic, and sometimes completely fallacious. It is easy to see where this logic comes from, although figures suggesting the opposite also appeared in the same papers. In the research, figures show that from the year 2000 to 2007 per capita income increased 120% in urban China, compared to 84% in rural areas, but figures also show that in the same period, while rural areas had a 38.5% drop in maternal mortality rates, (from 67.2/100 000 in 2000 to 41.3/100 000 in 2007), urban areas only had a 12.8% drop (28.9/100 000 to 25.2/100 000).[25] This suggests there is no direct correlation between increased wealth and improved statistics.

In China today, 80% of health resources–involving high quality facilities, human resources and services–are concentrated in large and medium-sized cities, but these centres provide care for no more than 10% of live births in China. Meanwhile, in rural areas, which include small cities, residents have access to only 20% of healthcare resources but these facilities provide care for at least 90% of live births. The fact that money is provided primarily for cities is recognised as being far from ideal.[26] That money logic is on the wrong side of arguments can be further illustrated in other respects. For example, in China, attempts to deal with maternal and infant mortality rates have so far lagged far behind some other developing countries, which operate at or below China's level of economic development.[27] Furthermore, in coastal provinces, which include capital cities and economic centres such as Beijing, Shanghai and Guangdong (Canton), where China has experienced the most economic success and where most of the country's wealth is generated and concentrated, maternal mortality has increased by 5.7%.[28] The fallacy that money is the solution can also be seen in the USA, one of the wealthiest nations, but where the maternal mortality rate increased from 11.5 in 1990 to 16.7/100 000 in 2008.[29] It seems there is much left to be explained.

In 2005, the Chinese Ministry of Health, jointly with WHO, UNICEF and UNFPA, carried out a large study on the conditions of maternal and infant survival in China.[30] This study also showed that in Chinese cities, the maternal mortality rate increased in the period 1996-2004 and while generally noting some positive developments in maternity services in China since 1990, identified the challenges ahead. Inadequate government funding for maternity services was seen as the first of the problems and challenges. The researchers concluded that the government could have had enough money available, but for some reason the money was not made available. In fact, China has experienced a higher level of economic development since the 1990s than countries like Sri Lanka and Vietnam, but these countries have achieved a higher reduction in maternal and infant mortality rates than China.[31]

As part of China's industrial development, by 2005, as many as 150 million peasants had migrated to cities to find work.[32] This figure was to rise to 229 million by 2009.[33] The UN-China joint study attributed the rise in the maternal mortality rate in cities to the large number of migrant workers, who had put a strain on urban maternity care resources, but other facts seemed to repudiate such a claim. After all, the study also found that according to surveys in cities, such as Beijing, Wuhan and Shenzhen, the rate of antenatal checkups in the migrant population was only 50-70% and only around 50% of migrant workers gave birth in hospitals.[34] It is therefore clear that it was not because the migrant population put a strain on hospital facilities that there were so many more deaths, because they simply did not make use of them. Furthermore, among migrant workers in China now only 34.1% are women[35] and not all of them would have had babies in a place where they did not have permanent residence. We did, in fact, collect some evidence (in face-to-face interviews) which indicated that quite a few female migrant workers chose not to give birth away from their own village. Although this needs to be further verified, the figure about maternity care among migrants as produced above in the official study of UN-China would still not square with other figures about maternity services in the cities. For example, urban antenatal care in 2002 was estimated at 96% by the same study and active management of labour in Chinese large cities in 2006 was said by WHO to be 95%.[36] Other studies reported that in 2004 hospitalised births in the city of Tianjing had risen to 99.7% (see below). These statistics, obviously, did not include migrant workers' births.

There was a big increase in the rate of maternal deaths between 2002 and 2003 in the country as a whole, in both rural and urban areas.[37] We may note that this was when the policy for total hospitalisation of childbirth was being promoted.[38] Even more interesting is the fact that, in the first decade of the new millennium, maternal mortality rates in provincial city hospitals accounted for 24.3% of the country total in 2006, increasing from 19.9% in 2000, and in regional hospitals this rate rose from 20.8% in 2000 to 35.1% in 2007, while the maternal mortality rate when births took place in women's homes dropped from 40.7% in 2000 to 17.6% in 2007.[39] These figures do not seem to totally support the claim that the policy for total hospitalisation of childbirth was a major contribution to the reduction in maternal mortality rates, particularly since the referral system (when mothers birthing at home needed to be transferred to hospital) had not been very good.[40]

The policy of total hospitalisation of childbirth was, in fact, a very ambitious plan in such a big developing country like China, with varying degrees of development in different regions. By 2004, in highly developed coastal cities such as Tianjing (a major port municipality east of Beijing), the total hospitalisation of childbirth had nearly become a reality because 99.7% of births was already taking place in hospitals. By contrast, in remote and mountainous provinces such as Tibet and Guizhou in south west China, only 34.1% (2005) and 48.7% (2005) respectively of births were hospitalised.[41] This meant that an average of 67% of births took place in hospitals, accounting for 57.4% of the total maternal mortality rate of the country, while 33% of births which took place in other places (i.e. the home, the village midwifery room, or en route to this facility) accounted for 43.6% of the total maternal mortality. This means hospitals may just look slightly better than other places. However, while the maternal mortality rate in rural areas on the whole was twice as high as that in urban areas (with the rate in remote rural areas being seven times higher), we should bear in mind the fact that 80% of all the quality care facilities, human resources and services were only available in large and intermediate cities. All quality care facilities in the country are concentrated in hospitals. Seen in this light, if basic birthing care expertise had been available around the corner, home births would not have been as horrific and it is likely they would not have resulted in such poor outcomes.

So far, we seem to have had all the numbers, but what has happened qualitatively in maternity services in this vast country, which constitutes one fifth of the world's population? In 2004, we visited the southern Chinese village where we had worked 34 years before. The houses built of loamy soil (an architectural practice which is usual in this part of the country) were still there, and only the old barn house in front of the village was now made from red brick. Little seemed to have changed to the village but the same could not be said for the inhabitants. One man, who had been a toddler 34 years before, was now an adult with two children. When asked about his wife's experience of birth, this man said that in his village consisting of 37 households, while not a single woman had had a caesarean during childbirth (although he said there was one woman who'd had a caesarean in a neighbouring village), no one nowadays gave birth at home. There were hospitals in two small towns about 5km away and in a bigger town, now a small city, which was about 15km away. Hospitals were apparently more welcoming now than in the past, since it used to be the case that a person needed to have connections to be treated well. Total hospitalisation seemed to be working in this part of China, but medication and technological births seemed to be a luxury because 80% of care resources were concentrated in large and medium-sized cities; in those larger cities caesarean sections were often carried out.

If we had gone to other parts of China, to the south west, to the west and to the mountainous areas of the north west plateau, where people like the Tibetans have a much more varied social and cultural life than the Chinese living in central and eastern China, we would have seen something different. Those areas are the least developed in financial and material terms. With a population of around 20 million and a human density of only 15 people per square km (compared with 277 per square km in central and eastern China), these areas have the highest maternal mortality rates and the highest rates of children dying under the age of five in the whole country–96/100 000 compared to 76/1000 in 2004.[42] Rates in some of these areas can be as high as 500/100 000.[43] Perhaps this is because people in these areas believe that childbirth is impure, so Tibetan women in many areas today are still expected to give birth outside the home, out in the open or in a structure where animals are kept.[44] As we have noted before, births in these areas can be seen as devalued from other cultural points of view. More research is needed in these areas to understand Tibetan values regarding birth before we can decide with Tibetans what can be seen as normal and appropriate care for women giving birth in Tibet.

Normal childbirth as an indicator of health

Maternal and infant mortality has long been the principal problem in childbirth throughout the ages around the world, alongside other complications which are mostly preventable and curable using the skills and technology available today. However, the obsession with the dangers of childbearing is still very much with us, so much so that at the beginning of the third millennium, leaders of the world gathered to sign a 'Millennium Declaration' which committed individual nations to 'Millennium Development Goals' (MDGs). One of these goals was for each nation to reduce its maternal mortality rates (Goal 5) and mortality rates in children under five years of age (Goal 4) by 2015.[45] Maternal and child survival is regarded as the most important indicator of the development of a particular country.[46]

These goals would further suggest that good maternal and infant mortality rates are indicators of a nation's health. While maternal and infant survival rates can be very specific goals in the maternity care provision of a particular nation, they do not necessarily indicate the well-being of women and infants during childbirth. As we have pointed out before, under China's fast economic development, medicine became part of the market economy and was over-used in childbirth in large cities, because it brought some people money and power. Under such circumstances, even when maternal and infant mortality is reduced, it could hardly be said that women and newborns are well cared for. The over-use of medicine and obstetric technology in childbirth can have a negative effect on women's general well-being, especially when we argue that childbirth is not only a natural physiological process, but more importantly a social and cultural process in which profound social and cultural values exist. These values should be respected and it should be remembered that they can be disturbed through the use of medical procedures, particularly when they are unnecessary.

The goal to achieve the MDGs by reducing maternal and infant mortality might have encouraged China's policy for the total hospitalisation of childbirth (which effectively meant medicalising it). Maternal and child survival was seen to reflect the country's developmental level, image and stature.[47] Nevertheless, the idea of total hospitalisation and the promotion of obstetric medical technology so as to reduce maternal mortality rates must have seemed a good way of placating the market-oriented healthcare system of China and it may also have allowed the government to feel it was meeting its responsibilities.[48] After all, the prevailing view was that science and technology were the hardware of modernisation and development, which were generated by money, and which also generated money effectively.

Under the influence of the UN MDGs, the well-meaning UN-China investigation a few years later, in 2005, into the condition of maternity services in China emphasised the need to reduce maternal mortality rates even more. The study produced some very important data concerning maternal and infant mortality in China, which might just have shown the tip of the iceberg as regards maternity services, but this data certainly needs to be reinterpreted. For example, if no women (or almost no women) in Chinese villages were having caesareans, and if they had not even heard about caesareans, the rate in cities must have been far higher than 50% (judging by the overall average), and if many minorities from different cultural backgrounds on the Chinese borders (such as the Tibetans) were still having babies in the wild, what challenges were the maternity services in China actually facing? It seems that Chinese maternity services are really facing an ideological crisis at the current time, and there certainly also seems to be an absence of understanding of the basic concepts underpinning maternity care. This lack of understanding of basic principles seems to have been exacerbated by the disparities generated by the country's extremely fast economic development, which, ironically, it was hoped would improve the situation, not make it worse. Money has been used where it should not have been used. And while both maternal and infant mortality rates may indeed have been greatly reduced, whether maternity services have improved is another question altogether.

Among the most important recommendations and proposed strategic directions for maternity services in the 2005 UN-China study entitled 'A Review of Maternal and Child Survival Strategy' was the call for the government to ensure universal provision of essential maternity services, which was mostly referred to as the provision of 'obstetric care', since the report concluded that maternity services should now focus on key problems "such as interventions for congenital malformations, reduction of child malnutrition and injuries, delivery safety, prevention and treatment of common women's diseases and HIV/AIDS prevention and control".[49]

Although the study touched upon important issues such as the government's role in dealing with increasing social disparities in Chinese society, the need for essential maternity care provision, systemic reforms in human resources development and surveillance systems, as well as the need to improve funding efficacy, the emphasis seemed to be inappropriate in terms of overall strategy. The word 'intervention' was used quite frequently, as in the phrases 'preventive interventions' and 'effective interventions', amongst others[50] and this emphasis on intervention would seem to encourage the overuse of obstetric interventionist measures in care.

Perhaps the MDGs, which focused on reducing maternal and infant mortality rates as a starting point, caused this misplaced emphasis? After all, the authors of the report seemed to misunderstand what maternity care is all about... If the majority of women, who enjoy healthy living conditions, could have a normal experience of childbirth and if resources for intervention were directed at only the women who needed them, this could result in still greater decreases in mortality rates. In this way, promoting normal childbirth might just be the strategic goal necessary for improving Chinese maternity services. However, achieving this is impossible if an interventionist ideology is the foundation of all maternity care. In China, as elsewhere, in order to improve mortality (and also morbidity) statistics the main challenge is to change the underlying ideology of caregivers and establish a new foundation for maternity care which values normality. Normal childbirth is therefore indeed the health indicator of the nation's health and current trends indicate a low level of health in this respect.

The challenge for the midwifery profession

Midwives have provided essential maternity care to birthing women since the dawn of civilisation. There were indications that the profession was being hijacked by obstetric medicine in modern times, especially in China, as well as in many other industrialised countries. The vision discussed above by the UN-China joint study for the development of maternity services in China failed to acknowledge midwives as the most important human resource in maternity care provision. Since the need to reduce maternal and infant mortality rates was seen as strategically important, the science of obstetrics rose to a prominent position in discussions about maternity care. Another reason that midwives were overlooked is because, historically, midwives have had low intellectual status, and they were simply seen as people with manual skills which were not really relevant for reproductive health. As Confucius used to say: "Those who think rule; those who do are ruled"; from our perspective today, those who think and those who do can by no means be separate. With normal childbirth and labour established as the ideology for the development of maternity services, midwives would end up engaging in complex work which would be comparable to the work undertaken in any other area of medicine.

The discontinuance of midwifery education proved to be a disproportionate move, which led to the inappropriate or excessive provision of obstetric medicine and technology

In fact, though, China discontinued midwifery education in 1993, replacing midwifery with obstetric services.[51] This proved to be an unfortunate move, which led to the inappropriate or excessive provision of obstetric medicine and technology. The UN-China study also called to establish maternity care as a separate discipline in higher education so as to train high-level maternity personnel,[52] but this recommendation was not justified or explicitly substantiated in any way by data. In our view, midwives are just the right people to provide high-level maternity care. However, since no programme of midwifery education exists any longer, Chinese midwifery now faces a challenge. It urgently needs to establish itself as an academic discipline in Chinese universities.

Conclusion

Maternity services are indeed quite a good indicator of the health and development of societies, as has been generally recognised, but it is vital that people consider not only technical issues, but also ideological issues if this indicator is to be properly assessed. Ideological problems are indeed seen to be in evidence in the Chinese system because it is not promoting normal childbirth and labour. This is problematic because the aggressive promotion of technological 'solutions' does not appear to have led to an improvement in maternity and infant mortality rates.

Following reviews of maternity services in China over recent years, we have come to the conclusion that, if maternity care is to be successful (in terms of reducing morbidity, as well as mortality), normal childbirth needs to be re-established as the theoretical and ideological basis for healthcare provision. Care providers need to see birth not only as a natural process within the human life cycle, but also as cultural and social processes, which are interrelated, which influence society. The tasks of anyone wishing to promote normal birth in China or elsewhere are to explain the connection between birth, culture and society and to promote maternity services which reflect a more holistic understanding of what it means for a family to have a baby.

To improve statistics normal birth needs to be re-established

Anshi Pan is a researcher in social anthropology and other subjects in social sciences. He is now interested in learning about childbirth and maternity care from a social and cultural perspective, associating with the Midwifery Research Unit in the Nursing College of Hangzhou University in China. He co-authored the paper 'Childbirth across societies and cultures: a continuous reconstruction of our normalities' presented at the 5th Research Conference on Normal Childbirth and Labour in Vancouver in 2010. His previous studies include English linguistics, the theories of social and cultural anthropology and the interpretation of the pictographic culture and religion of the Naxi people in south west China.

Ngai Fen Cheung teaches research methodology to postgraduate nursing and midwifery students at Hangzhou Normal University. She is the first author of the groundbreaking bilingual research book *The Development of Chinese Midwifery and the Modernisation of Childbirth* [forthcoming] and she is particularly interested in the area of childbearing women's well-being, theorising normality of childbirth as an approach to developing midwifery and midwifery education in higher education in China. Her research aims to document and explain the practices of midwifery both in China and abroad, promoting normal birth and modern maternity care in China.

References

1 Chinese Ministry of Health (MoH), UN Children's Fund/WHO UN Population Fund/UNFPA, 2006. Joint review of the maternal and child survival strategy in China. See http://www.wpro.who.int/NR/rdonlyres/E6C29183-BC8E-4DEF-9A50-3606032E8CB4/0/MaternalandChildSurvivalStrategyin ChinaENG.pdf, accessed 16/10/2010; China Daily 2010 China's Population (1949-2000). See http://www.chinadaily.com.cn/china/2010 census/2010-08/20/content_11182379.htm, accessed 05/10/2010.

2 China Daily,2010 China's Population (1949-2000). See http://www.chinadaily.com.cn/china/2010 census/2010-08/20/content_11182379.htm, accessed 05/10/2010; CIA the World Factbook: Country comparison: total fertility rate 2010. See https://www.cia.gov/library/publications/the-world-factbook/randorder/2127rank.html, accessed 05/10/2010.

3 der Lee J, 2008 (in Chinese). *Nvren de Zhongguo Yiliao Shi: A Chinese Women's History of Medicine—Gender and Healthcare in the Han and Tang China.* Taipei: Sanmin Shuju, p 7.

4 Leung AKC, 1999. Women practicing medicine in premodern China. In Zurndorfer HT (ed.), *Chinese Women in the Imperial Past: New Perspectives.* Brill, p 102; Cheung NF, 2011 (forthcoming, in Chinese & English). *Zhongguo Zhuchan he Fenmian Xiandaihua: The Development of Chinese Midwifery and Modernization of Childbirth.* Beijing: People's Medical Publishing House, pp 229-235.

5 Veith I, 1949. *Huang Ti Nei Ching Su Wen: The Yellow Emperor's Classic of Internal Medicine.* Berkley & London: University of California Press.

6 Cheung NF, 2011 (forthcoming, in Chinese & English). *Zhongguo Zhuchan he Fenmian Xiandaihua: The Development of Chinese Midwifery and Modernization of Childbirth.* Beijing: People's Medical Publishing House, pp 6, 7, 19.

7 der Lee J, 2008 (in Chinese). *Nvren de Zhongguo Yiliao Shi: A Chinese Women's History of Medicine—Gender and Healthcare in the Han and Tang China.* Taipei: Sanmin Shuju, p 13.

8 UN ESCAP, 2008. Multi-sectoral determinants of maternal mortality in Anhui Province, China. See http://www.unescap.org/esid/psis/meetings/MMR/China.pdf, accessed 12/10/2010; Gao Y, Ronsmans C, Lin A, 2009. Time trends and regional differences in maternal mortality in China from 2000 to 2005. In WHO: *Bulletin of World Health Organization,* 2009; Vol. 87, No. 12, pp 913-920. See http://www.who.int/bulletin/volumes/87/12/08-060426.pdf, accessed 13/10/2010; *The Guardian* 2008: Maternal mortality by country. See http://www.guardian.co.uk/news/datablog/2010/apr/12/maternal-mortality-rates-millennium-development-goals#data, accessed 26/10/2010.

9 *The Guardian,* 2008: Maternal mortality by country. See http://www.guardian.co.uk/news/datablog/2010/apr/12/maternal-mortality-rates-millennnium-development-goals#data, accessed 26/10/2010.

10 Chinese Ministry of Health (MoH), 2006, p 6.

11 Chinese MoH, 2006, pp 4, 30.

12 Annandale E, 2009. *Women's Health and Social Change.* London: Routledge, pp 68-88.

13 Cheung NF, Mander R, Cheng L, Chen VY, Yang X, 2006. Caesarean decision-making: negotiation between Chinese women and healthcare professionals. In *Evidence Based Midwifery,* Vol. 4, No 3, pp 24-30.

14 Cheung NF, Mander R, Cheng L, 2005. The 'doula-midwives' in Shanghai. In *Evidence Based Midwifery.* Royal College of Midwives, December 2005, Vol. 3 No.2, pp 73-79.

15 Cheung NF, Mander R, Cheng L, Yang XQ, Chen VY, 2005. 'Informed choice' in the context of caesarean decision-making in China. In *Evidence Based Midwifery.* Royal College of Midwives, December 2005, Vol. 3 No.1, pp 33-38.

16 Beech BAL, Phipps B. Normal birth: women's stories. In Downe S, 2008 (2004) (ed.). *Normal Birth: Evidence and Debate.* Edinburgh: Churchill Livingstone, p 68.

17 Davis-Floyd RE, Sargent CF, 1997 *Childbirth and Authoritative Knowledge, Cross-cultural Perspectives* Berkeley & London: University of California Press, p 14.

18 *The Guardian* 2008: Maternal mortality by country. See http://www.guardian.co.uk/news/datablog/2010/apr/12/maternal-mortality-rates-millenium-development-goals#data, accessed 26/10/2010; Chinese Ministry of Health (MoH), UN Children's Fund/WHO UN Population Fund/UNFPA, 2006. Joint review of the maternal and child survival strategy in China. See http://www.wpro.who.int/NR/rdonlyres/E6C29183-BC8E-4DEF-9A50-3606032E8CB4/0/MaternalandChildSurvivalStrategyin ChinaENG.pdf, accessed 16/10/2010

19 Cheung NF, Mander R, Cheng L, 2005. The 'doula-midwives' in Shanghai. In *Evidence Based Midwifery.* Royal College of Midwives, December 2005, Vol 3 No 2, pp 73-79.

20 UN ESCAP, 2008. Multi-sectoral determinants of maternal mortality in Anhui Province, China. See http://www.unescap.org/esid/psis/meetings/MMR/China.pdf, accessed 12/10/2010. Page 10; Gao, *et al.* 2009, p 918.

21 UN ESCAP, 2008. Page 13. Gao, *et al,* 2009, p 918.

22 UN ESCAP, 2008, page 13; Cheung, *et al*, 2006, p 24.

23 Gao, *et al*, 2009.

24 UN ESCAP, 2008, p 8.

25 UN ESCAP, 2008, pp 2 and 8.

26 Chinese Ministry of Health (MoH), 2006, pp 6, 52, 79.

27 Chinese Ministry of Health (MoH), 2006, p 8.

28 UN ESCAP, 2008, p 2.

29 *The Guardian*, 2008; BBC News, Health reporter Helen Briggs. 12 April 2010. Maternal deaths 'fall worldwide'. http://news.bbc.co.uk/1/hi/8616250.stm, accessed 26/10/2010.

30 Chinese Ministry of Health (MoH), 2006.

31 Chinese Ministry of Health (MoH), 2006, p 22; *The Guardian* 2008; Google Public Data: World Bank, world development indicators. 2010. See http://www.google.com/publicdata?ds=wb-wdi&met=sh_dyn_mort&idim=country:GBR&dl=en&hl=en&q=u5mr#met=sh_dyn_mort&idim=country:CHN:BGD:DNK:AFG, accessed 28/10/2010

32 Chinese Ministry of Health (MoH), 2006, p 37.

33 Hangzhou Daily Press, 12/08/2010 (in Chinese). Show concern to our new generation of peasant workers. See http://hzdaily.hangzhou.com.cn/hzrb/html/2010-08/12/content_918463.htm, accessed 28/10/2010

34 Chinese Ministry of Health (MoH), 2006, pp 26, 27.

35 Sina.com, 08/03/2010 (in Chinese). People's Representative Zhang Xiaomei said we should help women migrant workers to integrate into the city. See http://video.sina.com.cn/p.news/c/v/2010-03-08/143906496286.html, accessed 28/10/2010.

36 Chinese Ministry of Health (MoH), 2006, p 60; WHO Department of Making Pregnancy Safer. 2005. China Country Profile. See http://www.who.int/making_pregnancy_safer/countries/chn.pdf, accessed 22/10/2010.

37 UN ESCAP, 2008, p 2; Chinese Ministry of Health (MoH), 2006, p 49.

38 Cheung, NF. 2009. Chinese midwifery: the history and modernity. In *Midwifery*, June 2009, Vol. 25, Issue 3, pp. 228-241.

39 UN ESCAP, 2008, p 4.

40 Gao, *et al*, 2009, p 913.

41 Gao, *et al*, 2009, p 915.

42 Chinese Ministry of Health (MoH), 2006, pp 51, 53.

43 Wu B, Logan P, 2009. Midwife training in Tibetan Sichuan lessons learned from a successful program. Kham Aid Foundation. See http://www.khamaid.org/IATS/midwife.pdf, accessed 29/10/2010, p 3.

44 Wu and Logan, 2009, p 4.

45 The United Nations, 2002. UN Millennium Project. See http://www.unmillenniumproject.org/index.htm, accessed 28/10/2010.

46 Chinese Ministry of Health (MoH), 2006, p 12.

47 Chinese Ministry of Health (MoH), 2006, p 33.

48 Chinese Ministry of Health (MoH), 2006, p 34.

49 Chinese Ministry of Health (MoH), 2006, pp 34-39.

50 Chinese Ministry of Health (MoH), 2006, pp 35, 78.

51 Cheung NF, Mander R, Cheng L, 2005. The 'doula-midwives' in Shanghai. In *Evidence Based Midwifery.* Royal College of Midwives, December 2005, Vol. 3 No.2, pp. 73-79.

52 Chinese Ministry of Health (MoH), 2006, p 10.

Reflections on general principles for promoting normal birth in 'developing' countries

Trudy Stevens

A personal perspective, informed by experience

Unlike my previous chapter, which was based on a significant study, in this section I am proposing ideas based on personal experience and a deeply held belief that history can be a wise teacher if only we are prepared to recognise the lessons.

Reflecting on the development of maternity services in the UK and my knowledge of working in resource poor countries (Nepal, the Maldives and Nigeria), I shall question whether the current strategies for the development of maternity services promoted by international organisations and various NGOs [non-government organisations] are necessarily in the best interests of the majority of birthing women. The reality of maternal mortality and morbidity rates cannot engender any complacency. Nevertheless, the millions more who could successfully birth normally should not be put at risk from inappropriate developments to their services and care.

The millions who could successfully birth normally should not be put at risk from inappropriate developments to their services and care

Thirty-five years ago, as a very newly qualified midwife I was posted as a volunteer to work in Nepal. The experiences I gained over three years undertaking both community-based and hospital-based 'midwifery' proved formative in my appreciation of midwifery as fundamentally a primary healthcare issue. Many times I was called to assist home births only when things had gone wrong (for example, the 'retained placenta' that proved to be an inverted uterus) and hospital births were only ever disaster situations in cases when we were fighting to save the mother. Working in that context I became skilled in procedures such as destructive operations on babies in utero (in cases where the mother's life was threatened) that no longer appear in modern obstetric textbooks. Slowly, the perception dawned on me that none of this was 'rocket science'; the disaster situations we dealt with on a daily basis did not have to have occurred if only we had been involved before it had all gone wrong. I experienced the harsh reality of the WHO statistics of a woman dying every minute from a childbirth-related cause and, even then, I knew we only saw the tip of the iceberg because we recognised that many women who experienced problems were never brought to us. Also, while the job clearly needed doing, I questioned where the 'midwifery' was in all that was being done...

Some years later, with this question still in my mind, I went back to Asia to work in the Republic of Maldives training traditional birth attendants (TBAs) and spent four years living and working with them in their remote communities. Despite the research indicating that TBAs' work is useful, TBAs have fallen into disrepute and their training has been suspended, since many consider it a waste of limited resources. Nevertheless, some years after money stopped being invested in this area of training, many people in the field are again questioning the wisdom of this strategy. Where I worked the World Health Organization had been supporting the training of TBAs for many years, but when I found out more about the courses I felt they were disturbingly inappropriate for the situation. The trainees gained hospital-based experience and they were then expected to replicate their practice in women's homes; fortunately many of those trained were women of status (e.g. the community chief's aunt, etc) rather than TBAs, whose service was deemed too important for the community to lose for the duration of training, so they had not been sent for training. To me, it was no surprise that such courses had little effect on maternal mortality and morbidity rates. It also seemed sad that TBAs were subsequently being sidelined and disregarded in favour of care, which was in effect inappropriate and unsuccessful.

In fact, it was in working with TBAs—'granny midwives'—that I truly learnt the meaning of being a 'mid wíf'. Perhaps I did successfully help these TBAs to understand the purpose and procedures of antenatal care, and the need for hygienic birth practices, and perhaps I did succeed in teaching them how to recognise possible complications needing referral, but in working alongside them and studying their practices I learnt something from these TBAs about the essence of 'being with woman'. I also learnt to appreciate how little power they had in influencing situations when transfer to medical help was indicated. Although illiterate, these wise women had keen empirical skills and learnt to recognise complications such as anaemia, oedema, dangerous fetal position and delay in labours... but persuading the woman's family to act on their advice proved more complicated. Birth was clearly socially situated and that proved to be its most defining characteristic; clinical issues were almost irrelevant in terms of what the family considered to be appropriate action—which was understandable when death posed less of a drain on very limited economic resources than hospital treatment.

Although I was trained in an era when the hospitalisation of birth was advanced and active management of labour was promoted as the 'way forward', my return to British midwifery coincided with the then widespread appreciation within and outside of the profession that all was not well. The outcome was the radical changes proposed in *Changing Childbirth*[1] Being involved in the evaluation of the implementation of caseload midwifery, I soon saw distinct parallels between the work of caseload midwives and TBAs. Had we indeed come full circle? Or was it more of a spiral, in which we were seeking to incorporate the positive benefits of advances in clinical knowledge with the relationships which were formed in more traditional situations?

A deeper perspective, informed by the academic literature

Since working with TBAs, my forays into academia—I'm now a Senior Lecturer of Midwifery—have led me to a deeper understanding of the situations I experienced. However, my reading and research have also caused me to question why, in the thinking and planning of maternity services in developing countries, there is such a strong drive towards an industrial model of childbirth. Surely common sense should force policy-makers to appreciate the lessons that can be learnt, as well as recognise the benefits that industrialised countries have enjoyed after developing their services? Should the recent widespread dissatisfaction in the UK and US not be a danger signal for policy-makers following a similar trajectory of early development? There is widespread recognition that the pendulum of hospital birth has swung too far because we now not only have increasing intervention rates, we also have a culture which increasingly believes that women can no longer birth naturally. If we are now attempting to regain a more balanced approach, why are hospital births being promoted so widely elsewhere?

Should the recent widespread dissatisfaction in the UK and US not be a danger signal for policy-makers following a similar trajectory of early development?

In fact, in industrialised countries such as the UK and US progress in maternal and child health has been strongly linked to public health issues. Improvements in water and sanitation supplies and transportation, clean environments and housing, better nutrition, and economically and geographically accessible healthcare provision have made an enormous difference to mortality and morbidity statistics. The unintended iatrogenic consequences of hospitalising birth, which have been widely recognised in the UK and US, have had very little influence on policy-makers' decisions in developing countries.

In England, the movement from private to public responsibility for birth that has occurred over the last century appears to have resulted in a litigious culture. (In 1902 the Midwives Act regulated birth attendants; then there was the development of the welfare state and the NHS specifically, which made hospital birth a reality for even the poorest families.) In the USA a similar trend towards litigiousness has occurred, albeit for different reasons. Clearly, whether the state or private hospitals are responsible for care, there is the likelihood that clients will want to sue when something goes wrong. When the family and dedicated caregivers take responsibility (under a caseload model of care) there is far less likelihood that anyone will want to resort to the legal system.

Clearly, whether the State or private hospitals are responsible for care, there is the likelihood that clients will want to sue when something goes wrong

An inappropriate focus for development

Recently, when attending an event in support of The White Ribbon Alliance, an excellent charity seeking to address safe motherhood issues, I was distressed to witness one of their promotional DVDs. Filmed in Africa, it contained graphic sequences of women labouring in circumstances that made me cringe. No, these were not situations related to impoverished families in remote communities, but hospitals where women shared mattresses, laboured in pubic wards without family supporters or the constant attention of a midwife—the very limited number of trained staff had to concentrate on actual births—and delivered on metal beds, generally in the lithotomy position. I had witnessed identical situations when undertaking a training course in Nigeria 13 years before. The aim of this film was to generate funds to improve the hospital service so that all women could birth in safety, but I seriously questioned whether this would be in the best interests of the women concerned.

Our understanding of the physiology of labour and the delicate nature of the successful orchestration of hormones essential for undisturbed birth, the significance of continuous support during labour and the dangers of the cascade of interventions that occur once we begin to interfere must surely cause us to question the promotion of hospital birth for low risk women. Where very limited healthcare budgets result in inadequate resources surely it is highly inappropriate, if not dangerous, to seek to normalise hospital birth—precisely because the hospitalisation of birth tends to make birth *less normal* not more. The infection risk alone from the sharing of mattresses is unwarranted, particularly given the problems with HIV and AIDS in many developing countries. The irony is that by disturbing rather than supporting the natural physiology it is likely that interventions will prove necessary and this will then 'confirm' the importance of being in hospital, where help is at hand.

A misunderstood reluctance

Sadly, increased hospitalisation is the focus for development and this development usually takes place to the detriment of indigenous birth attendants. While some TBAs might be less than ideal, the majority provide a supportive and caring service for birthing mothers. Childbirth is a natural process and our survival as a species would suggest we are particularly successful in this, despite the relatively late involvement of obstetricians (remembering that RCOG only gained its charter in the 1930s in the UK). It seems unwise to reject exactly that component of maternity care that we are now seeking to replace, notably the constant presence of a supportive carer, particularly given the value research indicates this has on labour. A sense of territorialism is gained by the frequent assertion by doctors (personally witnessed and commonly reported) that TBAs "refuse to bring mothers in" if complications develop. They infer from TBAs' reluctance to take their clients into hospitals that TBAs fear the loss of economic gain and/or power... This indicates a real lack of understanding of the situation, and perhaps even common sense, for how can a maternal death at home improve a TBA's status or position?

A more constructive path to development

It is clear that a purely clinical focus on development is unwise. Maternal and neonatal mortality and morbidity arise from incredibly complex social situations—an appreciation of which may be understood from the very poor results of the original Safe Motherhood Initiative and latterly the Millennium Goals, despite enormous resources being directed towards a variety of strategies to address the problem. I am not suggesting such initiatives are inappropriate, merely that they are sometimes initiated without an understanding of the wider situation and that the unintended consequences may prove detrimental. The routine hospitalisation of all birth is a clear example of this in countries where infection is a major risk and where resources are frequently stretched or unavailable.

Clearly, a number of clinical interventions are particularly helpful and need to be made available to all women—e.g. the use of antenatal anti-tetanus injections, or Anti-D where appropriate—but the uptake may be most successful if offered as outreach services. Another worthy aim is to have a trained skilled attendant at all births, although we need to recognise that, for a myriad of reasons, the reality of achieving this for many years is unrealistic. The continuing role of TBAs in the context of home birth therefore needs to be recognised and supported, with backup services being made available, where possible.

In addition, developing a network of referral centres, with appropriate transport facilities, is central to any maternity service for, however well trained I was as a midwife, I could achieve little when faced with a true obstetric emergency, despite all the equipment I held. Nevertheless, unnecessary hospitalisation of birth is likely to disturb the normal physiology and have an iatrogenic result with a concomitant rise in assisted delivery.

My suggestions would therefore be as follows:

- Let TBAs do the work and help them realise their full potential by giving them appropriate training and follow-up support.
- Ensure referral facilities have welcoming arms, i.e. improve clinical facilities to meet the psychological as well as physical needs of maternity 'patients'.
- Encourage TBAs to accompany the women they refer, so that they can act as a doula within the hospital environment.
- Develop maternity services with strong support and supervision offered through regular routine visits to the communities where TBAs live and work, rather than expect TBAs to attend clinics or hospitals to meet with other staff.
- Encourage communities to get involved in maternity care. Communities could retain responsibility for their mothers' own initial care and this would help to prevent a 'blame' culture from developing (with the litigation which generally ensues).
- Encourage healthcare workers to develop an awareness of traditional beliefs and practices relating to childbirth and to take these into account when giving treatment.

I would suggest we stop using the term 'developing countries' because this holds a value judgement as to what it is considered important to develop

Finally, I would suggest we stop using the term 'developing countries' because this holds a value judgement as to what it is considered important to develop. Having worked in some of the economically poorest communities, where I have experienced a wealth of riches in terms of support, care and consideration, where the new mother and baby are carefully nurtured, I wonder at just how 'developed' we have become in our industrialised societies. Our frequent management of birth with exogenous [synthetic] oxytocin impedes the flow of natural hormones which facilitate the bonding of mother and baby; postnatal care for new mother and baby has been reduced to a minimum, and in the UK it is widely recognised as a 'Cinderella' service; our previously supportive family structures have now diminished and this is to the real detriment of the new mother-baby dyad. Perhaps in our eagerness to impart new ideas to traditional societies we also have a lot to learn from them...

Trudy Stevens has been a practising midwife for 35 years, 10 of which were spent working in remote and resource-poor countries. She returned to England to read anthropology at the University of Cambridge and has subsequently been involved in both research and teaching. She has a Master's degree in social research methods and her PhD was an ethnographic study of the implementation of caseloading midwifery practice. Considering she learnt the meaning of true midwifery from the traditional birth attendants she has worked with, Trudy is passionate about the development of a more humane maternity service–which she considers would benefit midwives as much as mothers.

Reference

1 Department of Health, 1993. *Changing Childbirth. Report of the Expert Maternity Group Part 1.* London, HMSO

The 'natural caesarean' technique as inspiration for normalising practice for all types of birth

Jenny Smith

The 'natural caesarean' technique attempts to give some normality to the most abnormal birth possible: that of caesarean section. Of course, when birth takes place increasingly frequently (or even predominantly in some places) in a surgical environment the whole culture of birth changes.[1]

Some people view this negatively, but I would like to ask if greater examination of the natural caesarean technique could influence the way in which we try and improve the birthing culture for all women on mainstream labour wards.

The natural caesarean

The 'natural caesarean' is a surgical operation that encapsulates normal elements commonly only associated with natural birth (i.e. vaginal and unmedicated birth). Traditionally, during a caesarean section a drape occludes the mother's view. During the 'natural' technique the drape is removed and this allows the mother and baby to be the central focus. The parents watch the birth as the surgeon gently 'walks the baby out' by a process of gentle support, squeezing the uterus and stimulating contractions, since the uterus still contracts itself at this stage. The baby is slowly born: first the head, then one shoulder, followed by another, then the abdomen, followed by the legs. At the same time, a process of auto-resuscitation takes place with the baby breathing air as well as receiving oxygenated blood through the cord. Lung fluid is seen draining from the baby's mouth and the baby starts to cry while his body is still in the uterus. The midwife receives the baby momentarily from the surgeon and places the baby skin-to-skin, directly on the mother; babies have been known to start breastfeeding during the remainder of the surgery. This natural caesarean technique is suitable for women who have a cephalic presentation at term. (Of course, there is no space in this chapter to discuss the reasons why any one caesarean section is carried out, but reasons could vary enormously in different medical and social contexts.)

Normalising the abnormal

It may seem inconceivable to think of the most 'abnormal' birth being the solution to making birth more 'normal' on mainstream labour wards. However, could the adoption of the natural caesarean philosophy—placing the 'family' centre-stage with the 'professional family' supporting—help us to change the blueprint for mainstream labour wards so that levels of normality are increased for all women in the future, overall?

Can 'abnormal' births inspire more normality?

In fact, during the last 30 years mainstream labour wards have changed little and they have remained steeped in tradition and 'bed-conducted birth'. Perhaps this explains why some women even describe their birth as a 'dehumanising' experience.[2] Birth centres, on the other hand, offer low risk women a 'normal' active birth in a comfortable birth environment, with continuity of midwifery care. However, they only cater to a minority of women... According to data collected by BirthChoiceUK, currently around 93% of pregnant women in the UK give birth on mainstream labour wards. Some of these women will be considered high risk and may require an 'abnormal birth' for medical reasons. Since only a small minority of women (5-6%) give birth in birth centres and an even smaller number (2%) give birth at home there is inequity of birthing facilities in terms of both environment and care.[3] Perhaps this goes some way to explaining why in the UK only 62.9% of women have a spontaneous vaginal birth, 24.6% have a caesarean section and the remainder have vaginal instrumental births (12.1%)[4] —5.5% of these being forceps and 6.6% being ventouse.

In order to increase normality in a situation like this, where relatively few women have spontaneous vaginal births, a combined approach is suggested. I would like to propose that we continue offering choice of birthplace to low risk women but that we also radically refocus on improving the environment and the birthing culture of mainstream labour wards for those women who choose to give birth in a hospital.

Reconsidering what is, in fact, 'normal'

When considering definitions of 'normal' and 'abnormal' birth there no longer appears to be any clarity of definition or consensus of opinion on what the birth journey should be like. In 1997 the World Health Organization defined normal birth as follows: "Spontaneous in onset, low risk at the start of labour and remaining so throughout labour and delivery. The infant is born spontaneously in the vertex position between 37 and 42 weeks of pregnancy.[5] After birth, mother and infant are in good condition." Three definitions of 'normality' are suggested by the Royal College of Midwives, and they add the commentary that "The physiological transition from pregnancy to motherhood heralds an enormous change in each woman physically and psychologically; every system in the body is affected and the experience represents a major *rite de passage* in a woman's life".[6] Both WHO and RCM definitions mention that there is physiology at the beginning and end of the process, but they provide little detail about the actual birth journey. Abnormal birth is usually defined by birth outcome—whether forceps, ventouse or caesarean section—rather than in terms of the labour process. More recently the Maternity Care Working Party (again in the UK) has attempted to define normality of birth journey.[7] Their suggestion is a listing of what a 'normal delivery' includes and what it excludes, but this has led to heated debate amongst both women and professionals. If normal birth is defined as meaning 'without any medical intervention' (an unclear phrase in itself), by some interpretations in England only 45% of women had a normal birth in 2009 and 47% in 2010. One of the key issues of debate is why opioids are included and epidurals excluded, when considering normal birth.[8]

As there appears to be no agreement about what a normal or natural birth journey involves, perhaps the consensus could be to introduce as much normality as possible to every birth? Taking the 'natural' caesarean as my inspiration, I shall discuss its components and suggest a way forward for all births in that light.

Setting up realistic expectations and a positive approach

Women undergoing a natural caesarean section can listen to music of their choice, wear their own button-opening top, lie on their own pillow, watch the slow birth of their baby in dimmed peripheral lighting and hold their baby skin-to-skin.

Shouldn't this be the minimum standard for all women and shouldn't there be additional choices for women who also experience labour—regarding mobility, birthing positions and water in non-emergency situations?

Women who are having a planned caesarean section generally have more intense input in the antenatal period from the professional team who will be attending them during the birth, than women anticipating a non-surgical birth. The expectant mother meets a midwife, anaesthetist and obstetrician prior to the surgery and there is individualised discussion of the birth. This is not always the situation for vaginal birth and women can consequently feel unprepared for labour and birth, particularly if it is their first pregnancy.

Consultation and discussion is particularly important so that informed and realistic choices can be truly facilitated. This is because women and their babies are unique and choice is based on the woman's understanding of her own birth journey and her relationship with those providing care. it is very important that the choices offered by the hospital or birth centre are realistic and not incongruous, or choices will become the emperor's clothes. For example, if a woman expects to use a birthing pool and on arrival in labour she is told she cannot use a pool because there is no midwife who is suitably trained in water birth, the woman can become extremely disappointed and disheartened as her expectations are not met. A recently published pregnancy book highlights the dilemmas.[9] Introducing birthing pools, the text reads: "During labour, you can get in a tub of water that is large enough for you and your childbirth partner, if desired. It is not recommended to give birth in water. Many hospitals do not have a tub or pool, so be sure to check first if you are interested in this option." Later, when discussing second stage of labour it says: "Many women give birth to their babies while propped up in bed, with their legs braced against footrests. There are other birth positions you can try (lying on your side for instance) as long as your healthcare provider approves." The text is a salutary reminder that it is the midwife or obstetrician who holds the power to choose to empower women or exert their own authority, thereby limiting the possibilities for positive flexible birthing.

Should there be a minimum standard?

The birthing process

Traditionally, at caesarean section a drape occludes the mother's view. During the natural technique the drape is removed allowing the mother and baby to be the central focus.

The procedure for a caesarean section can often be as follows, as described in *Myles Textbook for Midwives* (Churchill Livingstone, 2009):[10]

"When we came to have our first baby, we didn't know what to expect (although we had been given lots of information) ...things went quickly and I was worried about having my epidural. Having my husband there helped... we brought a CD but... it was right down at the other end of the room so that we could not hear it. During the operation we were stuck under a sort of tent, so we could not see what was going on. My husband had to really strain to see our baby coming out of me, and no one asked us if we wanted to cut the cord or anything. But we did feel that everyone was kind to us and looked after us very well."

In a recent conversation a mother described her labour care as having everything in terms of environment dimmed lighting, beanbags, mats and soothing music but she felt lost and isolated because she felt no connection to the midwife, who left her for long periods of time. Her experience left her feeling unable to trust her own body or her midwife. Just as an electronic monitor cannot replace the human brain, no matter how relaxing a labour room is, it cannot replace the 'with woman' aspects of care. This is reflected in studies that have shown that a low risk woman in her first labour can be attended by 5 to 15 'masked intruders' but still left alone most of the time.[11] One-to-one care in labour has been shown to make a difference: when it was used in studies women were far more satisfied with their care and there was a lower rate of clinical intervention.[12]

Hunter recognises the difficulties. She writes: "Midwifery has a strong commitment to woman-centred care but this is frequently not achievable in practice, particularly within large institutions." However, she recognises that when midwives are able to work in a 'with woman' way, there is congruence between ideals and reality, and work is experienced as emotionally rewarding.[13]

If one-to-one care in labour really makes a difference surely our priority must be to focus on its achievement in a maternity service? The benefits have been experienced in the case of the natural caesarean, when the team works in harmony. In mainstream labour wards too, it is time for a reformation so that we can create comfortable environments and one-to-one care in labour. As discussed in *Proactive Support in Labor* (Cambridge University Press, 2009), labour room nurses are frequently given responsibilities that have "nothing to do with the birth". There should be "sufficient personnel at the bedside whose focus should be on direct, supportive care for each woman in labour."[14] In order to make this possible we need to accept that some midwives will need to change the way in which they work so that they spend more time with women in labour rooms, supporting birth, and less time managing things from their desk. It is time to 'look outside the box' and find other ways in which women can feel more supported by offering greater comforts in more complicated labours. By working in the 'greyness' of the guidelines, safety can be achieved and choices for women which are normally associated only with spontaneous birth can be integrated so as to improve the birth experience for all women.

It is useful to consider some specific examples... In the case of a woman who has a previous caesarean section scar and requires intravenous access and continuous fetal monitoring we should note that the guidelines do not prohibit the use of a birthing pool with telemetry. Likewise, a woman who is having an induction of labour with a syntocinon intravenous infusion requires continuous fetal monitoring and an infusion pump—but thanks to the use of telemetry and a battery-operated pump both can be achieved safely. Also, why can't a woman with a big baby not labour in the pool during the first stage of labour and just come out of the pool for the birth itself? Why can't a woman spend some time in a birthing pool with her baby after giving birth, even though she had an epidural in labour, as long as her motor control is now normal? Why are these creative solutions not more widely used? There are many labour ward practices that deserve a re-think. Some other potential solutions to challenges are presented in *Proactive Support of Labor,* where a "carefully orchestrated team approach aimed at a safe and rewarding normal delivery, based on the best possible evidence" is suggested.[14]

Imprints of labour ward culture also need a re-focus. For example, hospital gowns create the impression that the labouring woman is a 'patient'—someone with an illness, rather than a birthing mother. The open back causes women to struggle with back tapes so as to keep their bottoms out of view. These hospital garments should be re-designed. In a Carribean pool room[15] at Queen Charlotte's Hospital, London, many high risk women have laboured in surroundings akin to birth centres with low lights, music, beanbags, mats and birthing balls. Using the latest technology in terms of telemetry, it is also possible to normalise abnormality safely.

The birth itself

The parents watch the birth as the surgeon gently 'walks the baby out'. By a process of gentle support and squeezing to stimulate uterine contractions, the baby is slowly born, first the head then one shoulder, followed by another, then the abdomen, followed by the legs.

There has been much concern in recent years regarding medical excess in normal childbirth.[16,17] Women know what they find helpful in labour and they are clearly not getting it. In an NCT survey conducted in 2005 women highlighted the 10 most important things to them in labour. These included privacy, mobility, dimmed lighting beanbags and mats—yet many mainstream labour wards still conduct birth on a bed.[18]

The birth outcome is ultimately very important in birth but the process of birth, if not supportive, can leave women feeling emotionally traumatised. Aspects of the process which can cause emotional trauma include being left alone for long periods of time, being left lying naked after an examination or being left in bloodstained clothing.

Birth is the ultimate meeting of mother and child and it is the mother's baby and not ours as professionals. Therefore, support in labour means interacting with the woman using touch, eye contact encouragement and reassurance. Wherever possible, the mother should be given a choice. For example, she should have the opportunity to touch her own baby's head in the second stage of labour and embrace her baby skin-to-skin as soon as it is born. The mother and her partner should be invited to feel the cord pulsing and either parent can cut the cord, if this is their choice. Choices relating to third stage management also need to be discussed. Women need to know the clinical pros and cons of their labour choices. In the American College of Obstetricians and Gynecologists' text for mothers there is no discussion of physiological versus active management for placental delivery and no mention of the fact that a drug is used to expedite delivery of the placenta when active management is used. The text simply says: "This last stage is the shortest of all. It is likely to last from just a few minutes to about 20 minutes".[9]

Protection of the first hour after the birth

The midwife receives the baby momentarily from the surgeon and places the baby skin-to-skin directly with the mother. Babies have been known to commence breastfeeding during the remainder of the surgery. The baby is checked and labelled whilst still positioned on the mother's chest. The partner can do a second clamping of the cord, once a plastic clamp has been applied. The baby is weighed when surgery is completed.

Skin-to-skin contact between mother and baby is beneficial as it keeps the baby warmer, reduces baby crying at birth, improves mother-baby interaction and helps women breastfeed successfully. No negative short- or long-term effects have been recorded.[18] Despite the known benefits, it is not standard practice on mainstream labour wards for babies born by caesarean or vaginally to spend the first hour following birth skin-to-skin and this rarely occurs at the time of a caesarean section, despite the fact that it is an ideal time for the mother and baby to be together since the mother needs to be lying down while she is being sutured.

In a Cochrane Review in 2010, it was shown that delayed cord clamping improves iron status in infants up to six months after birth, although there is a possible risk of jaundice, which would require phototherapy. In vaginal birth, delaying cord clamping for two to three minutes does not increase the risk of postpartum haemorrhage.[19] Delaying cord clamping for up to 30 to 40 seconds is feasible and should be practised with both preterm and term infants born by caesarean section.[20] If evidence suggests this is good practice it would seem timely to implement delayed cord clamping for all babies. The natural caesarean technique has shown no apparent detrimental side-effects to mother and/or baby.

There may also be psychological benefits in terms of mothers' response to their babies' crying. It has been shown that mothers' brain response to their own baby-cry was significantly higher in the vaginal birth group compared to that of the caesarean birth group.[21] If mother and child bonding may be impaired with caesarean section every effort should be taken to increase the mother-child connection at any birth. Surely, it is even more important at other births if the natural caesarean technique emphasises this, so as to limit potential psychological impairment?

When trying to find solutions to increasing medical interventions and caesarean section rates it is usual to take the looking glass of normality rather than the looking glass of abnormality. I would like to suggest, by contrast, that in order to benefit all women we must look into both looking glasses at the same time as it is unlikely that there will be a significant pendulum swing away from hospital to home birthing. I would like to propose a two-pronged approach to care whereby all women can benefit from gentler birthing in the 21st century.

The turning point

Could the natural caesarean therefore herald the way forward towards normalising all births?

If we more closely examine the culture and environment of the labour ward setting, might it not be possible to achieve real choices for all women, increasing 'normality' both during women's labour journey and also during their birth? Is it not possible to balance women's expectations with the requirements of hospital policy? The 'family' needs to take centre stage and the 'professional family' needs to reclaim the art and science of midwifery and obstetrics. Midwives need to be freed up to be 'with women' and to work as partners with obstetricians, so as to develop a shared approach to birth.

By reaching this fine balance could we possibly learn from the most abnormal of births, the 'natural caesarean'? Could we not dream of reversing the trend of increasing interventions and replace it instead with a trend of decreasing intervention rates and increased birth satisfaction for all women by embracing greater 'normality' on mainstream labour wards?

Jenny Smith teaches on the mandatory training programme at Imperial College NHS Trust. She believes all women should be offered a positive birth experience. Jenny is co-author of 'The natural caesarean: a woman centred technique'[22] The 'natural caesarean' normalises caesarean section birth as far as possible. Further research is planned to examine the effects of this technique: delayed cord clamping, skin-to-skin contact and breastfeeding. Her own book *Your Body, Your Baby, Your Birth* was published in 2009 by Rodale. Jenny lectures internationally. She is the mother of four children.

References

1 Smith J, Plaat F, Fisk NM, 2008. The natural caesarean: a woman-centred technique. *BJOG* 2008; 115(8): 1037-1042.

2 Wagner M, 2007. *Born in the USA: How a Broken Maternity System Must be Fixed to Put Women and Children First*. Berkeley, CA: University of California Press.

3 http://www.BirthchoiceUK.com

4 http://www.hesonline.nhs.uk

5 World Health Organization. *Care in Normal Birth: a practical guide.* Department of Reproductive Health and Research, WHO reference number:WHO/FRH/MSM/96.24, 1996.

6 http://www.rcmnormalbirth.org.uk

7 http://www.nct.org.uk/about-us/what-we-do/maternity-services-user-involvement/making-normal-birth-a-reality

8 Hospitals try to stop women having 'abnormal' epidurals http://www.telegraph.co.uk/health/healthnews/4902795/Hospital-try-to-stop-women-having-abnormal-epidurals.html [accessed 1 March 2009]

9 American College of Obstetricians and Gynaecologists Your Pregnancy and Childbirth Month to Month (5th edition). 2010 P 158,192

10 Fraser DM, Cooper MA, 2009. *Myles Textbook for Midwives* (15th edition). Churchill Livingstone. Assisted Births 32:616 Box 32.1. Wendy and Martin's story

11 Enkin M, Keirse MJNC, Neilson J, *et al*, 2000. Hospital Practices. In: *A Guide to Effective Care in Pregnancy and Childbirth*, 3rd edition. Oxford University Press.

12 Hodnett E, Gates S, Hofmeyr GJ, Salaka C, 2003. Continuous support for women during childbirth. Cochrane database Syst Rev 2003;(3):CD003766.

13 Hunter B, 2004. Conflicting ideologies as a source of emotional work in midwifery. *Midwifery* 20:261-272, 2004.

14 Reuwer P,Bruinse H,Franx A, 2009. *Proactive Support of Labor: The Challenge of Normal Childbirth*. Cambridge University Press, 2009, 4:31.

15 Carribean Room, jentlechildbirth.org.uk

16 Wagner M, 2001. Fish Can't See Water: The Need to Humanize Birth. *International Journal of Gynaecology and Obstetrics*, 2001; 75:S 25-37.

17 Villar J, Valladares E, *et al*, 2006. Caesarean Delivery Rates and Pregnancy Outcomes: The 2005 WHO Global Survey on Maternal and Perinatal Health in Latin America. *Lancet,* 2006;367:1819-29.

18 Newburn M. Singh D, 2005. Are Women Getting the Birth Environment They Need? Report of a national survey of women's experiences, NCT, 2005.

19 Moore ER, Anderson GC, Bergman N, 2007. Early skin-to-skin contact for mothers and their healthy newborn infants. Cochrane Database of Systematic Reviews 2007, Issue 3. Art. No: CD003519. DOI: 10.1002/14651858.CD003519.pub2

20 Kakkilaya V, Pramanik AK, Ibrahim H, Hussein S, 2008. Effect of Placental Transfusion on the Blood Volume and Clinical Outcome of Infants Born by Cesarean Section. *Clin Perinatol*, 2008 Volume 35, Issue 3, Pages 561-570, Sep; (3):561-70, xi.

21 Swain JE, Tasgin E, Mayes LC, FeldmanR,Constable RT,Leckman JF, 2008. Maternal brain response to own baby-cry is affected by casarean section delivery.

Journal of Child Psychology and Psychiatry, 2008 Oct;49(10):1042-52.Epub 2008 Sep 3.

22 Smith J, Plaat F, Fisk N, 2008. The natural caesarean: a woman centred technique". *BJOG* 2008;115: 1037-1042. A film on the technique is also available on YouTube.

Promoting home birth within hospital-led cultures

Asheya Hennessey

Mothers who have given birth at home will tell you: they would never do it any other way. Many women who have given birth at home have also experienced a hospital birth, including myself, and these women know without a doubt that home is the optimal environment for supporting physiological birth, the normal unfolding of the birth process in the way that is right for that particular woman and baby. Fawn Fritzen, a mother who has given birth at the hospital and at home in Canada, says, "Having experienced both a hospital and a home birth, I know which one I would choose again in a heartbeat." Monique Barker, a mother of two from Canada who has also given birth at the hospital and at home, says, "It wouldn't be an exaggeration to say that my experience in giving birth at home was the best thing that ever happened to me."

Childbirth is a normal life process that requires caring support, and is not a disease requiring treatment. Ali, a mother who has birthed two babies at home in the United States, says, "I believe that pregnancy is not an illness, but what a woman is designed for." Home birth is the best environment for supporting physiological birth without interventions for many reasons, including the lack of medicalisation of the home environment. A hospital is designed for intervention, designed to be there as emergency support for injury or illness, and so the hospital environment, by the very fact that it is a hospital, works against the concept of birth as a normal life process. Jennifer Zimmerman, a mother of two who has given birth at the hospital and at home in the United States, says, "The birth of my son in the hospital was treated as pathological, even though it was a straightforward vaginal birth which was only six hours total of labour, only three of them spent in the hospital," and Miranda Woodall, a mother of two who has given birth at a birth centre and at home in the United States says, "I know [health care providers] want to 'help' and be proactive, but for labouring moms, a 'wait and watch' attitude would be best."

The risks of childbirth are not greater than the risks of life, particularly with good prenatal nutrition and emotional support. The purpose of the hospital in the childbirth process is the same as the rest of life: to provide emergency, and possibly surgical, care if and when it is needed. Anne Tegtmeier, who has given birth at home, addresses the issues of risk in childbirth, comparing birth to other normal, physiological functions: "People choke to death while eating, but we don't go to the hospital every time we sit down to a meal, 'just in case,' because eating is a normal bodily function that, the majority of the time, goes just fine. But to deny that choking is a possibility is dishonest." I chose to give birth at home with my second and third babies and I hired a midwife to be there both as a support for the birth process and as an expert resource in case there was a problem that posed a health risk to myself or my baby. Because birth occurs during a short window of time, it is possible to have expert help available in the safety of my own home. Monique Barker says, "It's become my opinion that hospitals are for sick people, and so long as I'm healthy, I will never choose to have a baby there."

Because of the history of midwifery, obstetrics, and birthing in much of the developed world, most of the population has trouble envisioning birth anywhere other than the hospital. There is a cultural belief, unfounded in evidence, that the hospital is a safe place to give birth. The reality is that hospital birth has risks, and in fact is riskier than home birth in terms of morbidity, interventions and complications, negative experience for both mother and baby, reduced breastfeeding rates, incidence of infection, and other outcomes, including mental health outcomes. Ali says, "I am a health care provider and I know the infectious diseases that are rampant in hospitals. We felt that our newborn would be safer at home." Most women do choose hospital birth, some of them without realising there is a choice and others because the societal belief that the hospital is safer is so pervasive that even though they are confronted with the evidence of the safety and benefits of home birth they are still not convinced.

Given the current trend to give birth only in the hospital, in order to promote normality in birth, care providers need to be more proactive in encouraging women and their families to consider home birth as a valid option. It's necessary to educate women and their families about the risks of hospital birth and the benefits of home birth. Although we mustn't ignore the risks associated with home birth, we also mustn't over-emphasise them and we must also explain how they are minimised when a midwife is in attendance.

Nevertheless, there are women who choose home birth in this predominantly hospital-birthing culture. And these women know, or discover, that home birth is birth as nature intended. Since women feel safe and comfortable in their own familiar environment, oxytocin and beta endorphins work most effectively without inhibition by adrenalin, resulting in a more effective, less painful birth process. "I would tell healthcare practitioners that the most important thing for a woman in labour is for her to feel in control and comfortable," says Miranda Woodall. Monique Barker further comments, "What if I stuck you in a bathroom full of strange doctors and told you to have a bowel movement? You might not be able to do it. If you did, it certainly wouldn't be as easy as if I'd let you go at home in your own bathroom. Our bodies have a far easier time with intimate functions if we are in a comfortable mental state, in comfortable surroundings. Creating my own environment to give birth in makes perfect sense to me." Ali says, "We felt that ... [at home] I would be able to relax. This was true and my husband and I had the best experience of our lives. I walked or stood the entire time... It was an enjoyable and loving time between us." Fawn reflects on her home birth experience: "I knew that being at home, I'd be much more likely to have the natural birth I preferred. I was able to labour and to push in the positions that were most comfortable for me. My oldest was able to come meet her little sister right away and even got into the tub with us. It was such a great bonding time for all of us."

Because home birth is usually supported by one-on-one continuous care from a midwife, the benefits of emotional and physical support from a birth professional are experienced. And because there are fewer opportunities for interventions at home (since there is no access to epidurals, morphine, IV pitocin, etc) the intense sensations and unique challenges of the birthing process are coped with using natural methods that do not interfere with the physiological, hormonal process of birth but instead support and encourage it. When I birthed at home the room was dimly lit. All was quiet and warm. I moaned, I sighed, I stood, I swayed. I groaned, I sang, I drank water, I ate grapes. I leaned on my midwife and my husband. I pushed when I felt the urge. I knelt, I squatted in the birthing tub, I let go into myself and followed my instincts and felt a rush of pure emotion, more intense than anything I had felt before—joy and relief—when I held my baby skin-to-skin on my chest for the first time and we gazed into each other's eyes.

Not only is home birth the best environment to support physiological birth, it also provides optimal preparation for the ongoing challenges of mothering and daily family life lived in the home. Rebecca Coleman, a mother who has given birth at home in Canada, says it very well: "Having a natural birth at home gave us the opportunity to grow into our family—individually, but most importantly, together. The respect and love we found, not only for each other, but also for baby Cohen, has set the tone for our lives together as a family, and has us looking forward to our next child, and also to our next birth experience. The real gift, as we see it, is that without passing control or responsibility to anyone else, and keeping birth uncomplicated, we were able to recognise how important WE are—all three of us—to our lives."

When we listen to mothers who have given birth at home, we begin to understand that home birth encourages mothers to take responsibility for their own care and choices, and that the experience of comfort , privacy, and control that a home birth supports results in a safer, healthier birth for both the mother and the baby. Mothers who have given birth at home will tell you: we did it ourselves. No one, and nothing, saved us. We, the baby and me, we did it ourselves. And that is truly normal birth.

Asheya Hennessey is the Founder and Executive Director of the Canadian consumer advocacy group, Mothers of Change for Maternity Care. She has a background in education and her passion is educating the public and health professionals about normal birth and advocating for informed choice. She also founded the Canadian lobby group Yukoners for Funded Midwifery, which is working to get midwifery integrated into the health care system of the Yukon Territory in Canada. She has three children, one born in the hospital with unnecessary medical interventions and two undisturbed births with a midwife at home.

Founding and building *Midwifery Today* to promote normal birth around the world

Jan Tritten

The story of *Midwifery Today* begins as a personal one. My mother said of me from my birth that when I came out the world said 'yes', and I said "NO." That touch of rebellion has served me well in my life's work, my calling, which is to do everything within my power to help every mother and baby to have a great birth.

When I was going to college and working in a mental hospital in California, as I was pondering my future, I remember thinking, "Doctors deliver the babies; I guess I will become a teacher." So I went to college for five years. I was educated to become a teacher and received Lifetime California Credentials, but ended up a CCM (Community Created Midwife) with no credentials. This term comes from a Mennonite midwife who I've had the privilege of meeting and interviewing. When a community needs a midwife, it basically raises her up by requesting her help with births. The concept of a CCM has become a really important one for normal birth.

In 1972 I had a 'normal' hospital birth that would change my life completely and shatter my world. I went blindly into the hospital with confidence—hadn't all mothers done this?—expecting them to help me have my natural birth. Instead, they forced a saddle block on me. Then, after having my second daughter at home, I went headlong and headstrong into an area that had all but disappeared in the United States by 1976: midwifery and home birth. It was a doctor who talked me into having a home birth! I suppose it is helpful to have had a normal (magnificent, life changing) birth to compare with an intervened and robbed hospital birth. The difference in those two births made me want to help every mother I could to experience normal birth. The power of birth cannot be underestimated; why not give every mother the best chance she can at having her life transformed for the best instead of walking around with trauma?

I spent the 12 years from 1976 to 1988 in the most miraculous homebirth practice. We had the passion and the desire to help other women. We would watch, encourage and listen to women as they became mothers. There is nothing like the transformative power of birth and I treasure that practice. It is the foundation of my work at *Midwifery Today.*

We had the passion and the desire to help other women

I started *Midwifery Today* in February 1986. I was actually writing a book about my years in homebirth practice, and as I was organising my files I heard the voice of God say, "No, don't write a book. Start a magazine for midwives." I sat down in the chair my son was born in six years before and God gave me the whole outline for the magazine in less than a half-hour. I wrote it down and phoned my mentor Marion Toepke McLean, who has written for every one of our quarterly issues, and a few other people, to help.

It took a year to get the first magazine together. It went off to the printer exactly one year after the idea was born. The mission: through networking and education, *Midwifery Today's* mission is to return midwifery care to its rightful position in the family; to make midwifery care the norm throughout the world; and redefine midwifery as a vital partnership with women.

Our name, *Midwifery Today,* is also our motto. The idea for the magazine was to change birth practices. The opening sentence in my first editorial read: "A primary reason for producing this magazine is to actively promote midwifery." *Midwifery Today* would be by the midwives and for the midwives. We would be a resource that brought the best information, ideas and ideals to practitioners, who would then change the world for the better for mothers and babies.

We put out those first issues of the magazine with the passion of a birth (and still do so today). We filled each issue with information to help midwives share their insights and ideas, all towards the goal of helping them be the absolute best midwives they could be. When we got an issue back from the printer it was like we'd had a baby! Eventually, we added information for childbirth educators and doulas. My bottom line philosophy has always been that midwifery belongs to women, not a profession. We are all midwives in a way. Professions draw lines to keep others out and midwifery cannot bear that limitation. We need to open the circle and bring everyone in. Birth is life and it belongs to all of us. It is the foundation upon which a life is based.

From the beginning, we organised each issue of the magazine around a theme and really became a place for birth practitioners to learn, share and discuss what is important to them. We also highlighted international issues and always had articles from people around the world. Eventually, we started a separate newsletter called *The International Midwife,* and one for parents called *Having a Baby Today. The Birthkit* was a newsletter that went out between issues of the magazine because people didn't want to wait three months between issues. These all had a shorter herstory than *Midwifery Today.* Our electronic newsletter *Midwifery Today Enews* was started in January 1999 and is still going strong. We have always been blessed with an excellent staff that supports our mission. One member of our staff was so excited back in 1993 about the new thing called 'the Internet' that she got a website started for us—talk about an ancient web history! She is still with us.

There was a point in 1992 when we thought we either needed to do something to make our mission viable or we would need to close the doors. There is not enough money in a small magazine to sustain the bills. I remember being at home praying and the Lord moved me again and said, "Stay humble because you do not know where I am taking you." Then He had us start doing conferences. It seemed reasonable to get the people who had written articles together with the ones who read them, like a magazine in the flesh! We started with a conference in our hometown of Eugene, Oregon, USA. Then we went to New York City and Hawaii. Then we started going all over the world—Europe, China, Japan, the Bahamas, Jamaica, Costa Rica, Mexico and Moscow, Russia.

It was, and still is, amazing grace. Each conference is different and has its own personality; and the special emotional and spiritual effects that take in people's hearts are beautiful to watch.

It was our interest in international issues that led us to start the *International Alliance of Midwives* (IAM). It began as a paper directory, then it turned into an online directory and newsletter, and it eventually became a Facebook Page. We still maintain the IAM webpage on our website.

One of our many goals has been to share the techniques we've learnt from around the world. Midwives from Denmark now use the *rebozo* (a shawl) that Mexican midwives commonly use. That tool is good for so, so many different clinical solutions, from turning posterior babies to 'closing the bones' after the birth to helping with fertility. We've had a Mexican midwife teach it at almost every conference we've done—over 50! It is quite unique to Mexico and we have helped to spread this helpful practice, along with many others, around the world.

One of the overriding issues I am concerned with is keeping good midwives practising. Midwives have told us over and over they were on the verge of quitting midwifery when the love and encouragement they received from one of our conferences rejuvenated them so much that they decided to stay and keep on working for the good of mothers and babies. The soul of a conference is really to help the registrants with whatever they are dealing with. Often it is the medicalisation of birth, which they feel stripped of any ability to influence. Mothers and babies are often the victims, but a midwife who really cares becomes a victim too. After a conference, a discouraged midwife reconnects with her ability to make a difference instead of being swamped with the negative emotions that can shoot down the best midwife working in hospital situation. Midwives often share with me how moved they were to keep working, even in medicalised hospital situations that once left them on the verge of quitting. Often they feel a surge of new and old ideas that they can apply to help women most in need of our care: those in hospitals.

At our conference in Russia in 2010 we discovered there were many midwives practising home birth around that huge country because women did not want a brutal hospital birth. Most were practising like we started in the United States when we were reviving midwifery, without credentials. They are already CCMs. The schools in many parts of the world are as brutal as the hospitals where they make students learn and then practise. How can you learn kind, loving, encouraging midwifery in those situations? It is hard, if not impossible.

While these problems exist in Russia, I also know many European countries where the schools are committing human rights violations in the way they train midwives. In response, we recently started the Global Midwifery Counsel (GMC) with the goal of redefining 'midwife', the midwife's goals and philosophy and how best to train midwives. Part of the work was already done in the IAM. This GMC is currently being developed. We're considering the best way to train midwives and possibly to certify them. Eventually, we would like to get this certification recognised by the World Health Organization, who has stated that the world needs 300,000 more midwives. The resources are right there waiting to be tapped.

There are many traditional midwives practising all over the world who maybe just need more education. This can be done in the manner of a midwives' exchange. I have friends who go out to different parts of the world to lead impromptu midwife training sessions. They find that traditional midwives are clamoring for education. No midwife wants to see a mother or baby die. I find that midwives everywhere are very open to learning when it is not top down or demeaning. The evolution of *Midwifery Today*'s mission has evolved over time, but the bottom line goal has remained the same: that every woman in the world gets a chance at a fantastic, life-changing birth experience.

We began by doing books and other projects as the need arose. Much of the copy comes from back issues of *Midwifery Today,* with some original writing to flesh out each subject. We concentrate on clinical information because that is what people seem to want from us. A few years ago we began Motherbaby Press and have published several books by other authors.

The technology used to spread our message and achieve that goal has undergone much change. When we did the first magazine the layout process was a nightmare. We laid it out on a computer but printed and pasted it on to boards that were snailmailed to the printer. Eventually, we were able to send the copy over the wires to the printer. The old layout light table gathers dust. I see a day in the not-so-distant future when the magazine will be delivered to midwives' iPads or other reading devices. I see our books being delivered in a similar way. Technology has moved faster in the past 25 years than at any other time in history. We have so many more ways to change the world but there are also so many more ways for medicine to invade the uterus, birth and postpartum period with more unproven offenses.

Social networking is one of the ways technology has changed how we do things. *Midwifery Today* has a Twitter page, and several Facebook pages, as well as a presence on several other sites. In my mission to help make the best midwives and birth practitioners possible, I have discovered that asking a midwife a question every day or two on Facebook generates some of the most interesting answers and insights. The diversity of thought is like having a virtual classroom or conference. The page is a fantastic way to learn what other midwives are thinking and to round out a midwifery education. The midwives are thanking us for providing the opportunity to talk to each other on that page. The information that midwives have within themselves is absolutely astonishing. The new technologies are providing very different ways of learning midwifery. The future will probably hold more challenges and opportunities, and it is up to us to discern how to use them to benefit mothers, babies and families.

Midwifery Today has been to me as much a calling as when God first called me into midwifery. I loved being a homebirth midwife and I love doing *Midwifery Today*. I believe it has spread an amazing amount of midwifery knowledge, ideas and ideals around the world in its almost 25 years of existence. I believe I will most likely continue with this work until God calls me home. There seems to be so much that is still needed.

One thing that encourages me is how many brilliant women have taken up this calling, each in her own special way. Robbie Davis-Floyd says that critical mass is 20% of the people knowing about birth issues. If we reach critical mass we will change the world. Critical mass means that those people who know will tell those who don't know yet about what birth can really be like—that it is the most powerful life-changing event in a woman's life; that she can either be changed for good or be traumatised, or just miss an amazing opportunity. People who know will tell people who don't that when a woman misses what is possible, all of society suffers; that the world needs strong, loving mothers; that they are the key to a better world. What could be more important work?

The story of *Midwifery Today* has been one of struggle to meet the bills but God, who had the idea, has kept it going. We attempt and carry out big projects with His help because we have never had money. Probably only well-off people or deep believers would attempt to do this. I know beyond a shadow of a doubt that besides my family this is what I was born for. I suppose when you live carrying out your dreams it follows that you love what you do. This is how it has been for me, anyway.

Each of the projects that *Midwifery Toda*y does is devoted to the goal of changing birth practices and helping birth be not only normal but miraculous. It is truly my desire that what damages mothers and babies in birth be replaced with evidence-based, heart-based knowledge that we learn and share. We need to keep working toward better birth...

Jan Tritten, mother of three, became a homebirth midwife in 1976 after the birth of her second baby at home. This birth taught her how good birth could be after a first unnecessarily medicalised birth. After working as a community midwife for 12 years, Jan founded the magazine, *Midwifery Today*, so as to promote optimal birth practices and help midwives help mothers have great births. She then created a new style of international midwifery conference, organising events all over the world, even in Japan and China. She also set up newsletters and a publishing company to further disseminate information. Seeing birth as a human rights issue, Jan's ultimate goal in life is that every woman has the most beautiful birth experience possible.

Useful contacts

1 Homepage—www.midwiferytoday.com for info on conferences and publications, as well as all kinds of useful articles related to midwifery

2 Twitter—twitter.com/MIdwiferyToday or twitter.com/jantritten">Jan

3 Facebook—www.facebook.com/MidwiferyToday

4 International Alliance of Midwives: www.facebook.com/IAMbirth

5 Birth is a Human Rights Issue—www.facebook.com/birthisahumanrightsissue

KEY QUOTES: REFLECTIONS

1 "... every human birth is a patchwork of countless meanings, from hormonal to cultural, including psychological, emotional, and spiritual aspects. Therefore, the birth of our babies should never be managed and controlled by the cultural factors of time, money or power..." (Ricardo Herbert Jones)

2 "... the use of randomised trials and the promotion of evidence-based midwifery come with a price. ... It is time to acknowledge that other qualitative research methods can be productive for researchers..." (Jette Aaroe Clausen)

3 "Technology, used as a resource and not as a means of controlling women, can be a precious tool in childbirth, nevertheless it should only be used in rare cases." (Verena Schmid)

4 "... caseload midwifery engenders a new form of professionalism which is founded on positions of equality." (Trudy Stevens)

5 "It is ... vital that midwives, mentors, student midwives, lecturing staff and supervisors of midwives learn to promote normality, be inspirational and embrace their role as advocates for women so as to empower each woman to take holistic control over the birth of her child." (Linda Wylie, et al)

6 "The actual problem with biomedical knowledge about pregnancy and birth is not that it is dominant... it is the fact that it is insufficient." (Céline Lemay)

7 "Perhaps there are things we can learn ... so that traditional approaches are not thrown out completely when birth becomes medicalised ... or when medicalised contexts attempt a return to more human values when considering the personal aspects of the experience of birth." (Mandy Forrester)

8 "... the aggressive promotion of technological 'solutions' does not appear to have led to an improvement in maternity and infant mortality rates." (Anshi Pan and Ngai Fen Cheung)

9 "I would suggest we stop using the term 'developing countries' because this holds a value judgement as to what it is considered important to develop." (Trudy Stevens)

10 "Is it not possible to balance women's expectations with the requirements of hospital policy? The 'family' needs to take centre stage and the 'professional family' needs to reclaim the art and science of midwifery and obstetrics." (Jenny Smith)

11 "When we listen to mothers who have given birth at home, we begin to understand that home birth encourages mothers to take responsibility for their own care and choices, and that the experience of comfort, privacy, and control that a home birth supports results in a safer, healthier birth for both the mother and the baby." (Asheya Hennessey)

12 "If we reach critical mass we will change the world. Critical mass means that those people who know will tell those who don't know yet about what birth can really be like—that it is the most powerful, life-changing event in a woman's life; that she can either be changed for good or be traumatised, or just miss an amazing opportunity." (Jan Tritten)

pause to think and talk...

1. Do you agree that there is a bridge which needs to be crossed? Are there gaps between what we know and what we practice, what we feel and what we do? Do you ever personally experience any dissonance in your own heart or mind between different types of 'knowing'?
2. Research or discuss the actual or probable history of equipment and procedures in your own practice. If you could re-invent the fields of midwifery and obstetrics what would they be like? What would be entirely different? Which key words would be the new buzz words?
3. What is your own attitude toward technology in various areas of your life? Is your attitude different in different spheres of activity—for example compare how your feelings are similar or different when you consider sex, cooking, leisure, fun, relaxation, work, education and childbirth.
4. How effective are rules and regulations in your own working environment? Which governing bodies and which people are responsible for the rules, regulations and even laws which affect the way in which you work? Are there any rules, regulations or laws you would change?
5. To what extent do you think protocols should 'behave' like regulations and to what extent should they simply be guidelines? How flexibly do you personally view guidelines and is your own approach similar to that of your colleagues? (If you have some experience behind you, has your approach changed as you've gained more experience?) To what extent are protocols influenced by evidence, finance, insurance and worries about litigation?
6. What personal experience do you have of birth and how do you see this in your life? Was your experience of birth positive or negative? Have you witnessed other people's positive and negative experiences? What impact have they had on you and the way in which you offer care to women?
7. How far is it possible to 'marry' old perceptions and wisdom about birth with 'new' perspectives and understanding? Which criteria can be applied when assessing anything which is 'old' or 'new'? When does a new idea become 'old' and accepted or—conversely—'old' and out-dated?
8. In the country where you live how can you personally be an agent for change? Which areas of the field of birth could you positively influence? What could you do on an international level? How could you link up with other people already working for positive change so as to work collaboratively? What could you contribute that is new and original?
9. What can you teach other caregivers—either colleagues or students—and what can they teach you? How can you optimise learning?
10. To what extent do you think men are affected by birth—either in their personal lives or in their professional lives? How much (if at all) do fathers care about how their partners give birth, in your experience? Does gender play a role at all in influencing how men or women behave when they are in the role of midwife, obstetrician, doula, nurse or maternity assistant? Consider your answers in the light of the following extracts from birth stories, all taken from *Optimal Birth: What, Why & How* (Fresh Heart, 2011).

a *"Whenever there was a choice I have always opted for nature's way in areas such as food, environment and general health. However, this had never extended to having a baby and I preferred to abdicate the responsibility to the medical profession, who appeared more than willing to take over.*

"I attended the NCT classes and that's when doubts began to creep in, especially as I learnt of all the medical hardware, paraphernalia and drugs that were deemed essential nowadays for giving birth. I began to realise that the medical profession was perhaps, after all, just as horrified as I at having the responsibility for the birth. However, we went ahead with the hospital birth of our firstborn as it was decided by a hospital screening process that Pauline's blood pressure was outside the norm, for which she was immediately admitted. Sean was eventually extracted in a very workmanlike manner, some two-and-a-half weeks of protestations, seven pessaries, two gas tanks, two doses of chemicals, 10 yards of graph paper, one cup of tea and 15 hours of narcotic trance later. It would be an understatement to say it was a very traumatic time for all of us and I was disappointed at not experiencing the joy one has heard about as the father in attendance at the birth of his first child. It was more a sense of overwhelming relief that the whole episode was over with and all three parties (physically) healthy and alive.

"16 months later we found we were expecting our second baby and this time we were determined from the outset that this baby would be born at home so that we could have more control and responsibility. Our GP reluctantly agreed to cover the birth but opposition grew from all quarters of the medical profession and eventually no doctor would agree to cover the birth at home. This again I would attribute to their horror at having the responsibility for the birth." Michael White (the second birth ended up as a normal birth, at home)

b *"My wife has very strong views about giving birth. She wanted everything to proceed with as little medical intervention as possible and without any painkilling drugs. I could relate to this at least; personally speaking I have always had a peculiar aversion to taking pills (not even an aspirin for a hangover). Covering my face with a mask has induced panic ever since a childhood trip to a drunken dentist and allowing anyone to stick a needle into my spinal column seems like asking for trouble. But it was not me who was going to give birth, it was not me who was going to have muscles and nerves stretched to breaking point and beyond. So when she asked me for opinions on everything from arnica and other homeopathic remedies to using a TENS machine, I felt like a complete fraud offering any advice at all. To compound the problem, there was my own ignorance. I thought a TENS machine was something to do with American bowling alleys and one sip of the foul-tasting raspberry leaf tea made me feel glad I was a man. But if my sense of helpless confusion was bad during the pregnancy, things were about to get a lot worse." Phil Anderton (father of four)*

c *"We had returned late on the Saturday night from a friend's wedding reception and climbed into bed, with me still feeling the effects of an over-indulgence of food and alcohol. Sleep came upon me with ease until I was rudely awakened by a sharp dig in the ribs by Karen, my beloved, who rather nervously announced that she thought it had started. Being a loving, sensitive and supportive partner, my immediate response was to enquire: 'Have you had a show yet? No?! Well go back to sleep and don't wake me until you have.' Could this really have been Mr Sensitive talking or was it the booze and lack of sleep taking over? (That's my excuse and I'm sticking to it!)" (Alan Low, father of two)*

d *"... my wife was petrified when her waters broke and we took our battered car to the hospital. The nurses spoke to her rather less well than a dog. (Actually a lot worse than a dog. Dogs at least cannot understand uncaring and cruel asides... "Yeah, she's just making a fuss. Look, she's not even one finger yet!") I sat, immature, scared and powerless. Having read all about fathers being welcomed, I was expecting someone might notice I was there..." David Newbound (father of two)*

reflect and share further...

... with Heba Zaphiriou-Zarifi

These questions are the result of an embodied living experience and many hours of working with women from varied cultures, social and religious backgrounds, many with wide and varied responsibilities and professions, and others bring wisdom trickled down through generations.

The questions are by no means exhaustive but they can perhaps be used as a starting point for personal insight or for open debate. Some may seem to challenge areas of confusion and uncertainty; some may affirm what you already know. I wish to offer this contribution alongside the dedicated work of all caregivers in the field in the spirit of facilitating a happy and wholesome birth for mother and child and, indeed, for the greater circle around them.

1 Some men and women feel the need to follow a set of collective beliefs or ideas, or perhaps to rely on their doctor, or on science to tell them how birth 'ought' to happen. How can we help those individuals see the value of relying on their own resources, on their innate knowledge, whilst still trusting medical science?

2 In what ways may women be enabled to connect with the feminine lineage in their families—their mothers, grandmothers and other kinswomen?

3 How might we support women not to lose sight of their natural capacities to give birth, even though we have the benefits of hospitals and birth centres?

4 How can we re-connect women with the traditions that have brought into being many generations? Is it possible to recognise the wisdom of the past alongside new interventions?

5 By what means can we help institutions be at the service of the individual? How can we help them put more emphasis on the individual rather than on systems or treatments?

6 How can we enhance women's capacity to learn, to rediscover the wisdom of the body, and to make informed decisions?

7 How are we to provide a forum for women to speak their dreams and share the images that arise from their physical, emotional, psychological transformations?

8 How can we help women cope with any fear of birth, guilt about making their own choices and mistrust of the normal birth? How can we transform these negative feelings so that women are more capable of proceeding with a normal, healthy birth (provided there are no medical problems)?

9 Science does not protect us from the so-called 'unreality' of the unconscious. Images that arise from the unconscious are real and need to be looked at, e.g. a tree growing out of a woman's body is seen in some cultures as an image for pregnancy. How can we help women to trust the images that speak to them during their months of pregnancy in preparation for birth?

10 Do you agree that many women today are estranged from their deepest feminine energies? Do you agree that they are confused and lost between the vital need for independence and leadership and being true to their own nature? Are they under pressure to sacrifice their own innate capacities, instinct and intuition? How can they be heard by the society they inhabit... or do they just have to fit in?

11 We are instinctual-spiritual creatures with instinctive propensities and psychic energy systems, which if encouraged in one way or another can create opportunities for women to break through to their true nature with a tremendous amount of energy and creativity. How can we facilitate this potential in women?

12 When instinctive propensities or psychic elements are suppressed women are at risk of being pulled deep into darkness, or into experiences such as postnatal depression. What might help women to accept this challenging yet perhaps inevitable journey? Is the unconscious 'underworld' capable of helping women to develop in any way? And how prepared are we to travel into those darker places of the unknown?

13 How can a woman 'wash' herself, in metaphorical terms, during her pregnancy... How can she come to terms with unresolved past issues that powerful contractions, if not pregnancy itself, will pull to the surface, like the tide? How can we help open pathways for her to be in touch with the material rising from the depths of her being?

14 How much space does the medical environment—and society itself—allow women to lead other women?

15 Many women feel the need to go through an experience of dying—perhaps some aspect of the ego 'dying' for new developments to take place. How prepared are we to support this necessary death, in order to surrender to the service of new life?

16 How are we able to face our envy of pregnancy and all other facets of feminine creativity? Some consider that giving birth is the utmost feminine experience from which some men, or even caregivers, feel excluded, however close or empathetic they are to the woman's feminine world. How can we deal with the unconscious envy of the womb? Is controlling women and their birth plan a way to control our own envy and do we fear their powerful nature?

17 How can we remind women of their uniqueness and help them to take ownership of their birth event?

18 How can professionals help to provide a field where women are not trapped in an over-medicalised system, a system which far too often shakes their trust in their deep knowing, as well as in their instinctual-spiritual body?

19 How is it possible to create an environment where women are reassured and encouraged to use their innate capacities?

20 Pregnancy and birth are powerful experiences. How are we to facilitate awareness of this to emerge in women and be in tune with them as they go through the unknown?

21 Is it possible to consider positive feelings while ignoring negative ones? Are we able to face the fear of death whilst facing birth? Are our decisions in any way an avoidance of facing the risks of death? Have we accepted that death is part of life?

22 How can women empty their womb of power-based values in order to feel less invaded and more capable of exploring their own standpoint?

23 How do we allow ourselves to be affected by a woman's experience of giving birth? How prepared are we for our lives to be touched and transformed by it?

24 Rather than stepping into the mode of doing, and of action, how can we stay in touch with a receptive, passive way of experiencing being present?

25 As a culture, how tolerant are we of pain? How can we make it a friend rather than a foe? For some women natural birth does not happen automatically. How can we direct women to resources which will help them?

26 How accepting are we of dirt, blood and excrement? Are we able to resist interference to allow the necessary opening of all orifices during birth, including the mouth for use of the voice, be it for moaning and groaning or for chanting? How are we to balance allowing the opening of orifices with our responsibility to ward off potentially life-threatening infections?

27 Most women work in collaboration. They have learnt through the generations that sharing their stories and narratives increases the bond between them. Neuroscience reminds us that the level of oxytocin increases as we are given time to connect, hence providing a quality of relationship that women thrive on. How prepared are we to help facilitate and be part of this process?

28 How can we stay open to the imagination? How can we remain open to change? How can we open ourselves to compassion for oneself and others?

Heba Zaphiriou-Zarifi is an analytical psychotherapist with a private practice in London. She runs a monthly authentic movement group for women and is a leader in BodySoul Rhythms, which allows her to bring together dream work and creativity through mask work, voice and movement improvisation. She dedicates much of her time to reconciliation and conflict resolution and has participated in conferences on war trauma. She is also the mother of three children, all born at home and in their own time.

commentary to contemplate...

These comments are extracts from birth stories included in the books *Birth: Countdown to Optimal* (2nd ed, Fresh Heart, 2011). Authors are indicated after each extract, with extra information, if necessary. Which issues does each comment raise? Do you take into account these issues in your own practice?

1 *"She wheeled a machine on a little trolley into the room and told me to lie down. I was uneasy and didn't like the situation at all any more, but I was also not going to stand up for myself. I had to be a good patient. I was not a troublemaker. The machine was a brand new portable scanner, which she had been 'wanting to try out'. I was instructed to look at the little screen, to see the baby, to make it 'real' for me. She didn't know anything about me, hadn't asked me anything about myself or my feelings, yet she seemed certain that I was in denial and this experience wasn't sinking in for me. Looking at the nondescript image on a small greyish-green screen, I thought that my changing body and swelling, tender uterus, my nausea and cravings, were certainly more real than anything she had shown me. I then got a lecture about nutrition, even though she didn't seem even vaguely interested in my personal diet or knowledge of the topic, and was sent on my way with an order to make my next appointment at reception on my way out. The whole thing took about 20 minutes and this was my 'long, personal, initial interview'. I was on the verge of tears all the way back to work. I was suddenly not so excited about this pregnancy and felt ashamed of myself, both for letting her use ultrasound on me and my baby for no good reason (even though I didn't know at the time that there were any risks associated with it) and for being so 'irresponsible' as to get pregnant without 'trying'. I tried to remember why I had been so cheerful on my way in." Anonymous*

2 *"I was very lucky to receive such outstanding care at the hospital. I believe that it was the positive attitude of the medical staff toward vaginal twin births and natural pain relief that enabled me to have such a wonderful natural birth experience." Jo Siebert*

3 *"Harper's birth at home was sweeter than I could have dreamt it. I laboured easily and powerfully with loving support from my husband, doula, and midwife. When Harper's bag of water popped, birth energy rushed through me and soon his little head began to emerge. There was a slight case of dystocia and a tight umbilical cord but we were safe in the skilful hands of our midwife. Then, all of a sudden, there he was—pink, alert, and beautiful. ... Harper is our second child to be born at home, but our first lotus birth. We now know that we would never have another baby without giving them a lotus birth." Ashley Marshall (mother deciding to let the umbilical detach naturally)*

4 *"I searched widely for a sympathetic midwife and was so lucky to eventually find one... My baby was born after a nine-hour labour. To my amazement... I became almost like an animal, or went into another level of consciousness beyond pain. The part I remember as the most difficult was the beginning—moments of fear—then gaining confidence—more moments of fear—reassurance from the midwife—then feeling like a fish in water being thrown about by the contractions and finally roaring as she came out, not with pain (as is so often the stereotype we see of labouring women) but with power It left me feeling so proud of my body." Rachel Urbach (primipara, who wanted to avoid pharmacological pain relief)*

5 *"We will never know what could have happened if we had stayed at home. One of the risks is cord prolapse. With their feet they kick so much that if the membranes rupture, cord prolapse can follow, although not necessarily, of course. Sometimes, it is a problem to know all this." Liliana Lammers (daughter's emergency caesarean with breech baby)*

6 *"I started to have contractions at 32 weeks, which caused problems as I was not allowed to go into labour. (This is because the cervix dilates in labour and this would mean the placenta would rip, causing a major haemorrhage.) After being monitored on the labour ward to see the strength and frequency of contractions I had an emergency caesarean under general anaesthetic." Anonymous (woman with Grade 4+ placenta praevia; IVF pregnancy after previous ectopic pregnancy; both mother and baby were fine after the caesarean)*

7 *"... in a small scanning room in a London hospital we were told some lifechanging news. At 35 years old I was pregnant with my third child. Actually, third and fourth children as I had discovered at a previous scan that it was twins. ... One consultant, Donald Gibb, was prepared to consider a vaginal delivery... on examination I was already 9cm dilated (this only one hour after my waters had broken). It was then inevitable that the babies were to be delivered there and then. I felt disbelief that this was happening to me. I was full of fear at what might happen to the babies, and indeed to me, and yet couldn't quite take the situation seriously. I found myself giggling inappropriately at Mr Gibb's wellington boots. The room filled up with people and equipment, and I felt as though I was appearing in some bad hospital TV drama. At the same time, I was terrified. Instinctively, I turned my back on the room and knelt on all fours on the bed. This was the same position in which I had delivered my other two children, and I couldn't imagine any other way. I remember Mr Gibb saying, "Do you want to deliver the first one like that?" and replying that I wanted to deliver them all like that. ... For 10 weeks they were exclusively fed with breastmilk, initially by tube and later from a bottle. Kate, Sophie and Louisa are now happy, healthy 3½-year-olds." Janet Hanton*

8 *"I was very frightened about my ability to give birth properly... The pregnancy went well in that I was fit and healthy, but my partner and I started to have problems and when I was six months pregnant he left home for a month. I felt desperately insecure and cried through most of my pregnancy. ... I was gnawing on the side of the birthing pool, thinking about the benefits of knives and drugs, half hoping that she wouldn't come out at all, would go back and stay safe inside me. But that doesn't happen, and finally I got that huge push urge, when all you can do is that colossal push and your whole body is intent on turning itself inside out. It did know after all what to do, I just had to get my doubts out of the way. ... What I hadn't expected was the sharper pains as my uterus contracted back again, but apparently this is a normal feature of a second childbirth. ... I had no tears and was perfectly fit. The day following Eowyn's birth we had a celebration barbecue, and I walked around Tesco shopping for it, feeling so proud and happy, as if everyone must be able to tell that I had just had a baby!" Maria Shanahan*

9 *"I tried getting into a warm bath, but this time the magic didn't work. I kept moving and visualising, but unfortunately, the midwife also kept talking and I didn't have the guts to ask her to keep quiet. I found it impossible to 'let go' while she chatted to me and I felt obliged to smile politely and respond between contractions. Maybe four hours passed and I still felt far too much in control, but I knew it was time for the baby to be born. I decided not to invite my friend to observe after all. Somehow, I felt too observed already." Deborah Jackson (more difficult birth after previous easy births)*

10 *"Having a caesarean was like getting burgled. Strange burglars, who ransack the house and leave behind world's most priceless gift, my baby son. But a burglary nonetheless. I was robbed of an experience that I had been anticipating my whole life. Sometimes life forces us to face our worst fears. Perhaps it was necessary for me to go through the caesarean first so that I would be able to appreciate the gift of a healthy birth at home. I can't take it for granted. Now over three years later I can say it was a valuable experience. After all, now I've been in an operating theatre and have experienced major surgery. Gee whiz. Kind of interesting. I've experienced all those hospital interventions and I know what it's like. If it's happened to you, I can relate. It is possible to do it another way the second time! From the day after my son's birth, I comforted myself by thinking about what I was going to do differently if I got a chance to try again. The day after I discovered I was pregnant a second time, I started looking for an independent midwife. I really did my homework. I still regret the terror and pain that my son must have felt being yanked out into bright light by strangers. He is happy and healthy and no one could say, "Here is a child who had a difficult birth." But these things are not visible to the naked eye. Wouldn't it have been so much better for him if I had been able to welcome him to the world in a gentler way? Is that why he cried inconsolably for 36 hours after his birth? They say some babies 'just are' more unsettled than others. How can I help wondering if the caesarean was the cause? Maybe I was the cause of his distress, because I was so upset. Maybe if I hadn't wanted a natural birth so much, I wouldn't have caused him such distress. But I can't be different from who I am. My husband and I were both overjoyed about the baby, nothing could change that. It was a more abstract feeling than after the second, natural birth. After the second one, I felt a physical joy. My whole being was happy. The first time, we were filled with love and wonder for our beautiful son. But my body felt sad." Nina Klose (who had another successful VBAC later)*

11 *"I have had two breech babies. The first, a boy, was born in 1999 by caesarean, the second, a girl, was born naturally in 2001. ... With my first baby, I had encountered a lot of opposition to having my son vaginally at the hospital where I was registered. ... Second time around I had an independent midwife, Judith, with lots of experience of breech birth and had also switched hospitals and booked with an obstetrician who was prepared to support my efforts for a vaginal birth. Both Judith and the obstetrician felt that the studies on breech birth had not given enough weight to the impact different skills and experience of midwives/doctors had in determining outcomes. However we were all clear that whilst we were trying for a breech birth, at any sign of problems we would go straight for a caesarean. Given this, and the small risk of a problem with my previous section, we felt we had to opt for a hospital birth. ... I was amazingly proud of myself. I had no pain relief, no interventions and no sutures and a breech baby!" Liz Woolley*

12 *"My reasons for doing it were fairly complicated. I had one child, and was grateful that she was bright and healthy, even though I lost full-time custody of her when my marriage broke up. My ex-husband's unwillingness to contemplate surrogacy was also now a factor in its favour. I was in a relationship I considered to be short-term, although he later revised his plans to travel the world, and stayed home with me, which I'm very glad about. If I remember right, I was being unreasonably independent—"I'm doing this, it's really nothing to do with you. If you want to dump me, go ahead," sort of thing—which makes it to his great credit that he was actually hugely supportive. I had a superstition that you pay for luck either by doing good, or by balancing bad luck. I was broody, I was emotionally insecure... I wouldn't say it was a fully thought-through, rational decision on the part of a woman who had her life sorted out, but I've always been glad I did it." Anonymous (a surrogate mother)*

13 *"For my second pregnancy and birth, I had wonderful, skilled, loving care from a homebirth midwife. Labour started naturally, I dilated quickly, and the urge to push came after just a few hours. But then I pushed... and pushed... and pushed... and pushed... The three different midwives reached in to try to turn the baby's head to facilitate delivery, to no avail. After six hours of pushing, as the sun rose, my midwife said my scar just didn't look right, and I walked down the stairs with my midwife and husband, got in the car, and we drove to the hospital in rush hour traffic! (At the time I lived in a western suburb of the nearby city.) I was having immense and powerful pushing contractions, kneeling backward in the car with my midwife helping me. I was admitted to the hospital, and we all agreed that after the now 7+ hours of pushing, that perhaps an epidural was in order so I could rest a bit. Everyone was very calm and professional. My midwife stayed with me the whole time. I and the baby were both doing fine according to the monitors. ... My recovery was much less painful and traumatic than after the first caesarean. There was one nurse who came in and lectured me as I emerged groggy from my anaesthesia. She told me I was lucky I came in when I did and said how dare I try a home birth after a 'failed' first birth. She also said the uterus was so thin when they did the surgery I was lucky it hadn't ruptured. I laughed. Did she know I had been in the hospital for over eight hours before the operation was performed? ... I am trying to accept that even when I do everything right, there are some variables that I don't have control over. There is some reason for everything. " Anon (unsuccessful VBAC)*

14 *"I didn't need to do anything specific to be able to give birth. I just did it. But it was essential to be in a calm, familiar place and to be attended by someone I knew well. On some level, certainly, I was anxious about whether I'd be able to pull it off. But deep down, I think I had great faith in my body. The body is wise. It could grow a fetus without my even thinking about it. What more complicated task could there be? I have to admit to having grave doubts when it came time to push. But pushing was so powerful a reflex, there was nothing I could do to stop it once it got going. Giving birth was the most powerful, elemental—and stupendous—event I have ever participated in." Nina Klose*

15 *"I was extremely poorly after the caesarean because I did end up having a haemorrhage, as well as some sort of reaction to the anaesthetic. My daughter spent a short time on the special baby ward before being whisked into the Neonatal Unit as she was having breathing difficulties. Mother and baby are now both fine—and the 'baby' is now three years old! In general, I would definitely be on the pro 'normal birth' side of things, wherever possible. My pregnancy was clinical and from the outset not only was it a traumatic experience, I was unable to hold my baby for nearly two weeks after she was born. I was not aware I had had a baby until four hours after the birth. Caesareans as a birth option are ridiculous. Mothers 'opting' to have an elective caesarean when it is not a necessity are totally nuts! I did not recover properly until four months after the birth. It is major abdominal surgery." Anonymous*

16 *"We eventually went into the hospital at about 8.00 the next morning. When we got there, a midwife examined me. "I'll just go and get someone else to have a look at you," she said. "I'm not sure if my fingers are long enough." The second midwife said that, yes, I was definitely 10cm dilated. She asked me why we hadn't come in sooner. "I just wanted to be at home," I said, "just wanted to be quiet." They thought they'd better get me to the delivery room and suggested I get in a wheelchair. "Oh, I'll walk!" I said. Of course, I was naked by this time and one of the midwives tried to hold a towel or something round me, but I told them not to bother. I really couldn't care less who saw me by that stage! The midwife was fantastic—very calm. It was like having Mum at the birth. She looked after me and didn't let the doctors in. It was just me, my husband and the midwife. It was a really intimate and relaxed atmosphere. At one point, the midwife offered me gas and air [Entonox] but I thought, "No, I'll just keep going and see if I can manage," remembering it would be the best thing for the baby if I could. And of course, I did. Somehow, the time just went past." Sarah Cave (elderly primigravida)*

17 *"I feel happy for those mothers who have experienced normal births but concerned that mothers who have experienced other births might feel that their experiences may be seen as somehow less honourable, less heroic. I've had two caesarean deliveries: each time I felt that this birth was an incredibly heroic act. I think all births must be. The first was performed as an emergency after an incredibly traumatic labour. When my beautiful baby, Tom, emerged he weighed in at almost 12 pounds! After having such a traumatic time, I chose to have my second baby by caesarean. ... I was aware that here I was, about to begin an entirely new phase of my life as a mother of two. I also realised that I was lying in exactly the same spot where I had been when Tom was born, exactly three years and two weeks before. Except that this time I was conscious, it wasn't an emergency and the circumstances surrounding the birth were different. ... Suddenly here he was!... It's not the easiest thing to breastfeed a baby when lying flat on your back with drips in the backs of your hands and no movement in your lower body, especially when it's a newborn baby who has never breastfed before. It was agony! ... Louis grew steadily and has been such a delightful baby. I'm proud of us both." Anonymous*

18 *"I had plenty of scans during my first two pregnancies. I'm not sure now it was such a great idea. During each pregnancy, I had a false positive for a serious defect! Not only did these false positives cause endless extra anxiety, which can only have been bad for the fetus, they also probably contributed to an unnecessary caesarean section for my son." Nina Klose*

19 *Over the hours, I was put on a syntocinon drip—the contractions were not strong enough and the baby had to be delivered within 12 hours, according to the hospital's rule, because of the risk of infection. I had the water sac broken so that a monitor could be attached to the baby's head. This was very upsetting and painful. I felt raped. So much water came out—I realised that before it was only a leak and was not as dangerous for infection as the full waters emptying. Then I was persuaded to have an epidural because they wanted to increase the syntocinon to speed things up. The baby's pulse was now dropping so low they were worried, so they phoned their top doctor who advised a caesarean. The epidural was wearing off now and I could feel the baby low down in the canal, almost ready to come out. They still went ahead with a general anaesthetic and I woke up to see my husband showing my lovely baby wrapped up tight in a shawl. She was born at 12.30am on Sunday, nine hours after I went to the hospital. I was so happy to have a lovely baby that I soon forgot about my ordeal. On Samantha's first birthday I relived the humiliating, disappointing and painful time of her birth. ... [Second labour:] The first sign of labour was a gush of amniotic fluid, as before. This was at 8.30pm. The real labour pains came at 10.30pm. Kathryn was born on my bed at 2.30am after four hours of labour. My husband and [midwife] were there but kept out of the way and didn't interfere." Christina Mansi (same onset of labour (SRM); first time admitted to hospital immediately, with pressure to meet time limits; second time birthing at home in a relaxed atmosphere)*

20 "The doctor who was attending me at the time (in the USA) was famous for his 'spinals', but women often had problems with them afterwards, headaches etc, and anyway I preferred it all the natural way. But finally, as by 11.00am nothing seemed to progress any more—I seem to remember that the baby was supposed to turn, which hadn't happened yet—the doctor decided to do a caesarean. When he told me I thought, "Oh well, in that case I'm going to turn over to my side, which would ease the pain somewhat." As I had wanted to move things along I had all the time stayed on my back, the position that gave me the stronger labour pain. Anyway, very soon after I turned over, things began to move inside and I felt the urge to push. They could hardly get me to the birthing room and Dorothea was born with such urgency that I was sure all my lower parts had been ripped out along with her." Ulrike von Moltke

21 *"Birth is a huge gift, but so painful." Nina Klose (caesarean, followed by two normal VBACs)*

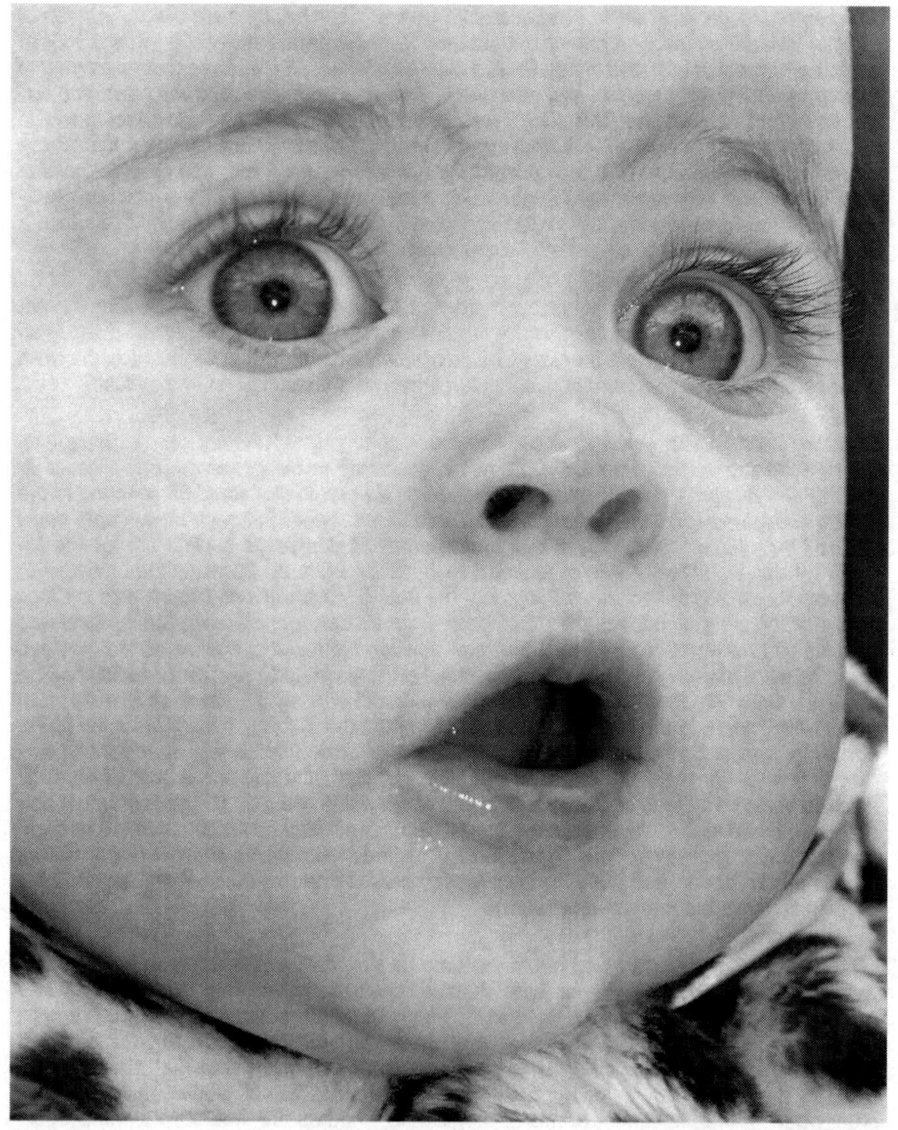

part three:

guidelines

- ways of optimising the chances...
- the way to empower women
- how to support epidural-free birth
- water birth—guided by Midwifery 2020
- the practicalities of home birth
- how to support VBAC decisions
- regulation to promote normality
- using the media successfully
- words, images and metaphors as tools
- identifying progress, gaps and ways forward

Giving normal birth the best chance

Lesley Page

Normal or straightforward birth is best for mother and baby.[1] The working definition for normal labour and birth I shall use is 'without induction, without the use of instruments, not by caesarean section and without general, spinal or epidural anaesthetic before or during delivery'.[1] The chances of having such a birth in much of the world are small. Women who intend to give birth at home are far more likely to have a normal birth, but in much of the world, even in countries where government policy supports out-of-hospital birth, having a home birth may be more difficult than choosing hospital birth. In hospitals the chance of caesarean section may be 1 in 4 in the United Kingdom and higher in other parts of the world so the chances of a woman having a normal birth in some countries become even lower.

In hospitals the chance of caesarean section may be 1 in 4 in the UK and higher in other parts of the world

Before I go any further I should acknowledge that there are parts of the world where interventions are scarce or unavailable. There are parts of the world where women give birth without professional attendance, and where maternity and perinatal mortality are very high. Each year approximately 529,000 women die during pregnancy and childbirth and over 99% of deaths occur in the developing world; approximately 11 million women suffer injury, infection or illness as a result of pregnancy or childbirth.[2] Lack of availability of medical and health care and interventions is a problem in these areas. However, this issue is outside of the scope of this chapter. I shall be focusing on giving normal birth the best chance in the developed world.

Giving normal birth the best chance involves amongst other things:

- providing genuine choice of place of birth
- giving the option for external cephalic version for breech presentation close to term
- giving the option for vaginal birth after caesarean section
- supporting women and their families adequately so that epidural use is restricted to times of genuine need
- providing one-to-one care in labour
- avoiding the use of electronic fetal monitoring
- having national and local policies in place to use evidence-based care
- fostering a philosophy of supporting normal birth within maternity services

One-to-one care helps give normality the best chance

A straightforward birth normal birth is more likely to lead to healthy outcomes for mothers and babies

In fact, given that the above factors really allow normal birth to take place, it is perverse to accept the high caesarean section rate that exists in much of the economically developed world (and also in certain sectors of many of the less economically developed parts of the world or in the emerging economies), while placing emphasis on the risks of home birth and making home birth a more difficult option. The aim is of course not only to promote normal birth but also to have outcomes which result in healthy mothers and babies, family integrity, and positive experiences of being cared for and giving birth. It is important to recognise that a straightforward normal birth is more likely to lead to these healthier outcomes because the mother does not suffer from the effect of surgery, and mother and baby have the advantage of the complex interplay of physiological processes and psychological change that is important to attachment between mother and baby, and positive support of the mother and family are important at this crucial and dramatic transition point to family life.

In general, the importance and power of human support and skilled clinical attendance has been denied and too much faith—I use the word advisedly—has been placed in the routine use of technology and medical intervention. These have their place but should be used judiciously and when indicated, not routinely.

Caesarean section as a default option

While caesarean section has become the default option, home birth is censured or frowned upon. Although in the UK it is formal government policy and joint policy of the Colleges of Midwifery and Obstetrics to give women the choice of place of birth including home birth,[3] the overall home birth rate remains low at about 3% (although there are wide variations). In some services provision of home birth is restricted on the basis of the need to staff hospitals and, meanwhile, there seems to be acceptance of the high caesarean section rate. In other parts of the world, for example the USA and Australia,[4] the Colleges of Obstetricians are against home birth, without their policies being evidence-based. In some parts of the world out-of-hospital birth has been virtually outlawed. (See, for example, Agnes Gereb's website: www.freeagnesgereb.com.)

Examination of the evidence on the outcomes of caesarean section, even when outcome measures are not confounded by medical problems, indicates increased risk to mother and baby and also to future pregnancies. The RCOG advice on consent for caesarean section gives detailed information about risks of this surgery.[5] On the other hand, an examination of the outcomes of home birth indicates that there is a lower rate of interventions for women who intend to give birth at home, and the best evidence continues to indicate that out-of-hospital birth is no less safe for the baby where pregnancy is uncomplicated.[6-10] (Although some recent studies have indicated that neonatal and perinatal mortality rates may be slightly higher for babies born out of the hospital[11-13] the methodology of these studies has been questioned.)[10 14-16]

It is inappropriate to focus on perinatal or neonatal mortality as the only indicator of safety and quality of different places of birth given the complicated combination of different risks to mother and baby associated with different places of birth. Current evidence indicates a reduction in interventions, including caesarean section, for women choosing home birth. Given the risk of these interventions to mother baby and future pregnancies, this is an important consideration when balancing risks and benefits of different places of birth.

It is inappropriate to focus on perinatal or neonatal mortality as the only indicator of safety and quality

Birth can never be risk free. As Olsen said, we can never say that birth at home is safe for all babies neither can we say that birth in the hospital is safe for all babies.[7] Even if the higher neonatal or perinatal mortality rates found in some of the studies is a valid finding, the choice of home birth is a reasonable one. Tuffnell says "the benefits of planned birth at home or in a midwifery unit mainly affect the mother. Such benefits, including a reduction in caesarean section and instrumental vaginal birth, must be considered against any assessment of risk."[11]

Balancing the risks of home and hospital birth

My focus here is not to say why undue emphasis is placed on the risk of out-of-hospital birth while the rate of caesarean section is widely accepted and justified. However it does seem strange, given that caesarean section is associated with higher maternal mortality and morbidity rates for mother and baby, increased risk of stillbirth, as well as maternal morbidity in subsequent pregnancies and reduced fertility levels.[17]

Intuitively the comparison of home birth and hospital birth seems like a stark contrast. Other options such as birth centres—either self-standing or attached to hospitals, i.e. midwifery-led units (MLUs)—and midwifery-led care within hospitals are now on offer to many women. They might seem safer because they offer a sort of 'halfway house' (in fact some are called home-from-home units). Although these forms of care are associated with advantages they are not associated with the powerful effect on the caesarean section rate of home birth.[17] It could therefore be said in this context that there is no place like home. It would be logical therefore to give higher priority to developing home birth services over others. The development of home birth services would not of course be exempt from the need to attend to quality of care. Quality of care includes safety and, as with care in any setting, attention should be paid to the factors that seem to increase the safety of home birth. Gyte and Dodwell suggest that 'women should be supported by a high quality maternity service that meets their needs, irrespective of where they give birth, including good transfer arrangements with the medical and midwifery staff receiving women at the hospital'.[10] Importantly, midwives attending home births should be well trained and competent and confident in working outside of institutions.

Giving normal birth the best chance in hospital and birth centre settings

Even if the choice of home birth is extended to and taken up by more women, many will still give birth in hospital. So, how might the normal birth rate be improved in hospital settings? Evidence arising from high quality research such as that provided through Cochrane reviews suggests that interventions should be used judiciously and these reviews also give us an idea of the kind of support that is likely to lead to normal birth. To summarise, Cochrane reviews suggest that external cephalic version should be offered for breech presentation near term; that vaginal births after caesarean sections should be offered (and perhaps encouraged); that the use of electronic fetal monitoring should be avoided; that intermittent auscultation should be used for labour when a pregnancy has been uncomplicated; that one-to-one care should be provided for women while they are in labour; and that support should be offered so as to help women avoid having an epidural. The following provides further summaries of these aspects of care in plain language, using reviews from the Cochrane Library. These notes may help provide a basis for informed discussion with women regarding these issues of choice.

External cephalic version for breech presentation at term

External cephalic version from 36 weeks reduces the chance of breech presentation at birth and caesarean section.[18]

Planned elective repeat caesarean section versus planned VBAC

When a woman has had a previous caesarean birth, there are two options for her care in a subsequent pregnancy: planned elective repeat caesarean or planned vaginal birth. Both forms of care have benefits and risks associated with them. There have been no trials to help women, their partners and their caregivers make this choice.[19]

Continuous support for women during childbirth

Continuous support in labour increases the chance of a spontaneous vaginal birth, has no identified adverse effects and results in women feeling more satisfied.[20]

Intermittent auscultation

Comparing continuous electronic monitoring of the baby's heartbeat in labour using cardiotocography (CTG, sometimes known as EFM) with intermittent monitoring (intermittent auscultation, IA), there was no difference in the incidence of cerebral palsy, although other possible long-term effects have not been fully assessed and need further study. According to the research, continuous monitoring is associated with a significant increase in caesarean section and instrumental vaginal births. Both procedures are known to carry the risks associated with a surgical procedure although specific adverse outcomes were not assessed in the studies included. [21]

Epidurals for pain relief

Epidurals are widely used for pain relief in labour. There are various types, but all involve an injection into the lower back. A review of trials showed that epidurals relieve pain better than other types of pain medication, but they can lead to more use of instruments to assist with the birth. There is no difference in caesarean delivery rates, long-term backache or effects on the baby soon after birth. However, according to this review of research, it seems that women who use epidurals are more likely to have a longer second stage labour, need their labour contractions stimulated, experience very low blood pressure, be unable to move for a period of time after the birth, have problems passing urine, and suffer from fever.[22]

Putting research into practice

Putting the knowledge from this research into practice requires reallocation of resources particularly so as to make possible the provision of one-to-one care in labour. This will mean that women are adequately supported (so as to help them cope with pain in labour) and that midwives are able to give women information (so that they can make genuinely informed choices about types of care).

One-to-one care means that women are adequately supported so as to help them cope with pain in labour

In the local National Health Service (NHS) division (currently called a 'Trust') to which I am attached (which includes a large tertiary hospital and community services, as well as small maternity hospitals or birth centres) the caesarean section rate has been successfully lowered to below the national average. This was achieved through a combination of changes:

- providing one-to-one care for the majority of women in labour
- developing a shared philosophy of care
- reducing the use of electronic fetal monitoring

The fact that the system I work within has strong community services, home birth provision, birth centres and midwifery-led care no doubt facilitated the achievement of these changes and the lowering of the caesarean rate. Two factors which may also be relevant are as follows:

- the provision of an integrated scanning and external cephalic version service for women when breech presentation is identified or suspected
- a clinic which provides advice for women who have had a previous caesarean section and who are considering type of birth in a subsequent pregnancy

It's useful to have a clinic which provides advice for women who have had a previous caesarean

We are still not providing care which is entirely in line with the guidelines implicit in the Cochrane data

In many parts of the world such services may be run by midwives or midwives and doctors working together. Dedicated clinics are helpful because the information we need to give women is based on complicated evidence and, especially in multi-ethnic, socially diverse communities, skilful communication is necessary, in which the caregiver is responsive to the woman's needs, values and feelings.

We are still not providing care which is entirely in line with the guidelines implicit in the Cochrane data. For example, the use of intermittent auscultation in labour (which the Cochrane data implicitly recommends for 'low risk' women) is still not always used routinely. Perhaps this is because this intermittent monitoring requires a culture change in the maternity services to accept this practice as well as different skills and approaches to interpretation, because the fetal heart is heard rather than seen on a paper trace. Other institutions which move to intermittent monitoring really need to provide training to staff who are used to using only EFM, and medical records need to be adapted to facilitate appropriate and frequent documentation. This is because sometimes, however good the care and the midwife-mother relationship, things may go wrong unexpectedly and good documentation may be needed in court.

The provision of one-to-one support for women to help prevent the need for an epidural and the use of intermittent auscultation both require an approach to care that involves presence (both in body and spirit) by the midwife, the ability to help find comfort in the arrangement of the house or room and furniture (chairs, beds, birthing balls, hanging ropes, birthing stools, floor mattresses, etc.), the encouragement of mobility and the appropriate use of massage and water (for example, using baths, showers and/or birthing pools).[23]

Psychological support needs to be provided in the form of words, when necessary, but also through silence. (In fact, it is becoming increasingly apparent to me that supporting women while not disturbing them is crucial to the flow of hormones and the creation of the physical and mental states that facilitate the progress of labour, the birth and the development of the relationship between mother and baby). Continuity of care necessitates flexible and effective staffing patterns, supportive relationships with women, and it may also be associated with a reduction in the caesarean section rate.[24]

Skills and attributes: the midwifery repertoire

Attendance on women in a way that gives the best chance for a normal birth requires confidence and competence. I am surprised at how many midwives I meet have never monitored the fetal heart using intermittent auscultation, or have not cared for women who do not have an epidural in situ. Learning to provide such care requires adaptation to a different culture of care and a new understanding of what 'normal' is and when the boundaries of normal have been passed.

Skills require the ability to stand back and offer support when this might be helpful, but also an understanding of when it might be helpful or necessary to be more actively involved. For example, it is important for staff to be able to assess the progress of labour in various ways, not only by carrying out vaginal examinations. (While they are sometimes helpful, many times they are not necessary at all.) Having skills to determine descent of the fetus and position of the presenting part, as well as the fetal heart rate pattern, are all important, so as to judge the health of the fetus and determine whether or not a transfer to medical care is necessary.

The ability to support women in labour so that an epidural is not required requires confidence and the use of approaches that reduce anxiety in the woman (and sometimes in other caregivers). I work with midwives who seem to exude a cloud of confidence that is contagious. Approaches such as HypnoBirthing (www.hypnobirthing.co.uk) and the use of deep relaxation, breathing and a variety of labouring and birthing positions, as well as water should be a part of every midwife's repertoire.

When transfer is required from home or MLU to the maternity ward

In the case of home births, when transfer to medical care is required the importance of clear guidelines, professional behaviour, a polite reception (on the receiving end) and mutual respect will enhance safety for both mother and baby. In other words, high standards of care and respect need to be extended to labouring women (and their caregivers) whatever their original choice of birthplace and whatever the reason for transfer, if this becomes necessary, and a collaborative, mutually respectful atmosphere between caregivers needs to prevail at all times.

My current place of practice is a small out-of-hospital birth centre in a rural location. We provide antenatal care for all women in the area, as well as a home birth and birth centre service and postnatal care. If the pregnancy is complicated we share the provision of care with local hospitals. Care is provided by midwives and midwifery support workers. All share a commitment to normal birth and help a woman choose where she is going to give birth. If there are factors in the history or pregnancy that might make out-of-hospital birth unwise we make a referral in pregnancy to medical staff that are part of the NHS Trust, who share the philosophy of promoting normal birth, where possible. This helps both the woman herself and us in making the right decision. If transfer is required in labour or after the birth we accompany the woman and/or baby in the ambulance to one of two hospitals.

What I notice in this service is the way the midwives intentionally pass on confidence to women about their ability to give birth normally from the very beginning. This is not a meaningless 'talking up' exercise because if there are likely to be problems, being some distance from the hospital, it is important to be honest about these both to ourselves and to the women we are caring for. Documentation of discussions about place of birth and the provision of literature and website addresses or other forms of communication are also important.

Resolving the paradox and recognising the perversity of current trends

Given the clear evidence on risks of caesarean section I believe we need to turn our thinking upside down. The perverse and erroneous view that home birth is too risky and that caesarean section is safe (considering the research) is a modern-day paradox. It needs to be resolved if we are to improve the start of life for babies and their mothers and give normal birth the best chance. Although it is sometimes believed and proposed that women having their first babies should give birth in a hospital 'just in case', given current evidence, I believe that women having their first babies should be told how important it is to avoid caesarean section if possible, and that out-of-hospital births are the best way of facilitating normal outcomes. No pressure must be put on women, though, because it is essential that the woman herself feels safe wherever she gives birth and that the choice of birthplace is hers alone.

A necessary priority for the future

Normal, straightforward birth should be the default pathway and the rate of caesarean section should be reduced where it is too high. This is because when caesarean section rates rise above 15% risks to reproductive health may begin to outweigh the benefits.[25] Earlier, I referred to the fact that some less economically developed countries or emerging economies, such as Brazil and China have an extremely high caesarean section rate in parts of the population, while care is restricted in other parts of the population. (The caesarean section rate given in a recent publication was 40.5% in China and 30.7% in Mexico, Brazil, the Dominican Republic and Chile and verbal reports from these parts of the world also indicate that rates are far higher in some urban hospitals.) Of course, caesarean section rates in developed countries are also rising. Countering these trends and facilitating normal birth will give families a healthier future and allow for a more equitable use of resources, simply because normal births are far less costly in terms of resources of all kinds.

The use of evidence is important in turning cultural values and practices around—but the evidence is already available and it has been available for some time. This is why we now need to do more...

- We need to develop services which demonstrate a real intention to change.
- We need to build a shared philosophy for promoting normality in birth.
- We need to set up effective governance and promote training and skills development.
- We need to give women a genuinely informed choice.
- Mostly importantly, perhaps, we need to guarantee personal support for women and their families, and guarantee that appropriate skills and knowledge are available through strong, midwifery-led services.

Normal birth should be the default—when caesarean rates rise above 15% risks may outweigh benefits

When strong midwifery leadership works in partnership with strong medical leadership the rates of both home birth and normal birth increase. We cannot be blind to the paradox of default caesarean section, given the expense this involves (in terms of both finance and public health) and the evidence on risks associated with caesarean birth. Opening our eyes and changing approaches and attitudes will require strong, collaborative leadership, but it will surely be worthwhile in terms of ensuring improved outcomes. In other words, respectful collaboration with colleagues and other medical staff is the key to turning things around, back towards normality and away from the current 'caesarean default'.

Lesley Page is visiting professor of midwifery at King's College London UK, University of Technology Sydney and University of Sydney. Her work has included clinical practice, management of large maternity services, and academic work. Professor Page has worked in the UK and Canada and has lectured in 11 countries and has many publications. She practices clinically in the NHS in Oxfordshire. She has served on three national committees in the UK including the Department of health and advisor to the House of Commons health Select Committee review of maternity services and the King's Fund.

References

1 Maternity Care Working Party. Making normal birth a reality. In: National Childbirth Trust, Royal College of Midwives, Royal College of Obstetricians and Gynaecologists, editors, 2007.

2 United Nations Population Fund. Facts about safe motherhood. In: United Nations Population Fund, editor, 2007.

3 Royal College of Midwives, Royal College of Obstetricians and Gynaecologists. Home Births, 2007.

4 Delamothe T. Throwing the baby back into the bathwater. *BMJ* 2010;341:331.

5 Royal College of Obstetricians and Gynaecologists. Caesarean Section: Consent Guidance No. 7. London: Royal College of Obstetricians and Gynaecologists, 2009.

6 Page LA. Putting science and sensitivity into practice. In: Page LA, editor. *The New Midwifery: Science and Sensitivity in Practice.* 1st ed. Edinburgh: Churchill Livingstone 2000.

7 Olsen O. Meta-analysis of the Safety of Home Birth. *BIRTH* 1997;24(1).

8 Page L. Being with Jane in Childbirth:putting science and sensitivity into practice. In: Page LA, McCandlish R, editors. *The New Midwifery: Science and Sensitivity in Practice.* Second ed. Edinburgh Churchill Livingstone, 2006.

9 Janssen PA, Saxell L, Page LA, Klein MC, Liston RM, Lee SK. Outcomes of planned home birth with registered midwife versus planned hospital birth with midwife or physician. *Canadian Medical Association Journal* 2009;181(6-7):377-383.

10 Gyte G, Dodwell M. Safety of planned home birth: an NCT review of evidence. *New Digest* 2007;40:20-29.

11 Tuffnell D. Place of delivery and adverse outcomes. Editorial. *British Medical Journal* 2010;341.

12 Evers ACC, Brouwers HAA, Hukkelhoven CWPM, Nikkels PGF, Boon J, van Egmond-Linden A. Perinatal mortality and severe morbidity in low and high risk term pregnancies in the Netherlands: prospective cohort study. *British Medical Journal* 2010;341.

13 Wax J, Lucas L, Lamont M, Pinette M, Catin A, Blackstone J. Maternal and newborn outcomes in planned home birth vs planned bospital births: a metaanalysis. *American Journal of Obstetrics and Gynecology* 2010;203:243.31-8

14 Gyte G, Newburn M, Macfarlane A. Critique of a meta-analysis by Wax and colleagues which has claimed that there is a three-times greater risk of neonatal death among babies without congenital anomalies planned to be born at home: NCT, 2010.

15 NCT. Home birth is a safe option. Press Release: NCT, 2009.

16 Newburn M. Why do medical journals get so het up about home birth? *Essentially MIDIRS* 2010;1(4):17 -22.

17 Page L, Drife J. Do we have enought evidence to judge midwife led maternity units safe? *British Medical Journal*, 2007:642-3.

18 18. Hofmeyr GJ, Kulier R. External cephalic version for breech presentation at term. *Cochrane Database of Systematic Reviews*, 1996.

19 Dodd JM, Crowther C, Huertas E, Guise J-M, Horey D. Planned elective repeat caesarean section versus planned vaginal birth for women with a previous caesarean section birth. *Cochrane Database of Systematic Reviews*, 2004.

20 Hodnett ED, Gates S, Hofmeyr GJ, Sakala C. Continuous support for women during childbirth. *Cochrane Database of Systematic Reviews*, 2007.

21 Alfirevic Z, Devane D, Gyte GML. Continuous cardiotocography (CTG) as a form of electronic fetal monitoring (EFM) for fetal assessment during labour. *Cochrane Database of Systematic Reviews*, 2006.

22 Anim-Somuah M, Smyth RMD, Howell CJ. Epidural versus non-epidural or no analgesia in labour. *Cochrane Database of Systematic Reviews*, 2005.

23 Dodwell M, Newburn M. Normal Birth as a measure of the quality of care: Evidence on safety, effectiveness and women's experience: NCT, 2010.

24 Page LA. Working With Women in Childbirth In: Sydney UoT, editor. Sydney 2004 (http://hdl.handle.net/2100/258)

25 Betran A, Merialdi M, Lauer J, Bing-Shun W, Thomas J, van Look P, et al. Rates of caesarean section: analysis of global, regional and national estimates. *Paediatric and Perinatal Epidemiology* 2007;21(2):98-113.

"I did it!"—Empowering women through maternity care best practices

Ami Goldstein

I am a midwife [a 'nurse-midwife' in the US] who functions as an attending caregiver with family medicine registrars. This is a birth that took place one night while I was on call with a registrar on one of her last nights on our maternal-child health service. We had had an extraordinarily busy day and it was just about midnight when a 16-year-old in labour with her first child walked on to Labour & Delivery. I will call her Gayle. She was in early labour and about 3-4cm. The labouring woman had requested pain medication and so was given IV morphine and promptly fell asleep. To be honest, both the registrar and I were tired so we admitted her and went to lie down while the nurse provided her care.

About 6am, I awoke and realised I had not heard from the labouring lady for quite some time. I quickly got up and went to check on her. Gayle was lying on her back in bed and looked moderately uncomfortable. Not only did she have the external fetal monitor and tocometer on but her nurse had thought it important to leave the blood pressure monitor attached to her arm, as well as a pulse oximeter attached to the opposite hand. She also had intravenous (IV) D5 Lactated Ringers fluid running. [In case you don't know, this isotonic solution with dextrose is maintenance fluid to replace oral intake. It is a mixture of sodium, chloride, lactate, potassium and calcium and is often used to bring up a woman's blood pressure after blood loss. It may also be used to stimulate urine output in a patient. The dextrose, a form of sugar, is added to supply energy. The intravenous access required for it can be used as a conduit for other medications.] While not unusual to have this occur in our hospital, it seemed odd to me that Gayle had a blood pressure cuff and pulse oximeter on. I reviewed her fetal heart tracing and vital signs. Since all seemed normal, I removed both of these items. At this point I asked Gayle if she would like to get up to go to the bathroom. When she gave me an affirmative, I assisted her up and her 16-year-old boyfriend immediately came to her side and walked with her to the bathroom.

When she returned, I suggested that she remain up and walking around. Gayle agreed and said she felt much better standing up. She began to walk back and forth. With contractions, Gayle would lean on her boyfriend for support. She had four or five women family members in the room, watching from the sofa. At this point she still had the fetal monitor on and the IV fluids running. About this time the nurses changed shift and the registrar came into the room. Our new nurse asked, "Can't she have intermittent monitoring?" I agreed this was an excellent idea and that she was in fact quite low risk. Now Gayle was moving into very active labour. She paced and moved with her contractions and made low moaning sounds. Her boyfriend was still at her side. As Gayle moved, the registrar chased behind her with her IV pole. She would walk around the bed and across the room with the registrar pushing the IV pole where she went. Again, our nurse asked, "Can't we disconnect the IV?" Again, I thought this was an excellent idea and now Gayle was truly free to move around the room, which she did continuously accompanied by her partner.

About five minutes later, as I was squatting under Gayle, who was standing, to obtain fetal heart rate with a Sonicaid, she let out a tremendous groan with a contraction and her waters broke explosively all over the floor. Quickly we attempted to clean the floor but as we were doing this, Gayle let out another groan and vomited across the floor. Again we were mopping and cleaning rapidly when Gayle roared ferociously and dropped to the floor on her hands and knees to push out her baby. Without coaching and with the support of her partner who told her how strong and wonderful she was, Gayle spontaneously pushed out her baby girl over an intact perineum. The registrar lifted the baby girl and placed her on a pillow in front of Gayle, who—crying—said: "My baby, my baby" as she lifted her and cradled her for the first time, with the help of her boyfriend.

This birth story illustrates the difference between routine hospital practices which not only interfere with normal birth and potentially cause harm and those evidence-based practices that not only support normal birth but also improve outcomes overall for women and babies. It also demonstrates that when caregivers use best maternity care women feel more in control and have improved birth experiences. Thus, the standard care package used by many hospitals and caregivers stands in contradiction to normal birth, rather than supporting it. There are a host of routine procedures which occur within the hospital setting. Many of them are used so regularly that staff may not stop to question whether or not they are even necessary. These range from continuous fetal monitoring and intravenous fluids to coached pushing with supine delivery. Individually these practices have been shown not to improve health outcomes for mothers and babies. In contrast, when childbirth care is provided based on the best available evidence, it inevitably actually supports normal birth and minimal intervention. The birth I've just described provides a view into real life when this is done.

When Gayle was admitted in labour, she was placed on the continuous fetal monitor and remained like that for many hours. Initial fetal monitoring via a non-stress test in labour fails to improve outcomes for mothers and babies. Instead, it increases the risks of caesarean section, instrumental delivery and results in no changes in Apgar scores at five minutes.[1,2] Continuous fetal monitoring throughout labour also does not contribute to healthier mothers and babies. When used and compared to intermittent fetal auscultation—using a fetoscope (Pinard) or Sonicaid—it contributes to a decrease in the rate of immediate neonatal seizure, without any long term improvements in rate of cerebral palsy.[3] There is also no significant difference in the perinatal mortality rate. While continuous fetal monitoring has minimal impact on fetal health, it has tremendous impact on maternal health with a significant increase in risk of caesarean section.

Interestingly, in research studies, continuous fetal monitoring has been compared to intermittent auscultation, with continuous monitoring considered to be the standard of care in many settings. However, intermittent monitoring has been recognised as the preferred method of fetal monitoring for women with a low risk status in the UK, the USA and Canada (by the American College of Nurse-Midwives).[4-6] When thinking about continuous fetal monitoring, it is essential to remember that most monitoring is done via wired monitors, as it was for this woman. While it is possible to maintain some mobility with continuous monitoring, it can be very challenging for the mother to feel like she can move as she would like.

Two other common interventions in the labour and delivery ward are the administration of continuous IV fluids and the restriction of food and drink taken orally. While still controversial, it is clear that oral intake during labour has minimal risks. In 2007 O'Sullivan, *et al* reviewed five randomised controlled trials and found no difference in the length of labour when mothers were allowed to eat.[7] While there was no difference in the caesarean rate, women did have fewer ketones when encouraged to eat and drink. In addition, a recent Cochrane Review concluded there were neither risks nor benefits to food and drink restrictions during labour and birth.[8] A search of the literature also reveals that there is little to no evidence that a healthy low-risk woman requires either intravenous fluids or intravenous access during a normal labour.

Furthermore, continuous IV fluids, continuous fetal monitoring, and vital sign monitoring with blood pressure cuff and pulse oximeter are medically unnecessary. These interventions do not improve outcomes for mothers and babies and they interfere with normal labour by significantly limiting the woman's ability to move. As the above patient illustrates, when wires and tubes are removed, women will feel more free to move and change position as needed during labour. Women report less pain while mobile than lying supine in bed.[9] In addition, there appears to be more uterine activity when women change from supine to lateral and upright positions than when they simply move from a supine position to a sitting position. A Cochrane review on mobility during labour has even found that labour may be shortened by approximately one hour for women who are more upright.[10]

Labour may be shortened by approximately one hour for women who are more upright

In the case I described, the labouring woman had had minimal vaginal checks after admission but clearly observable physical changes indicated she was progressing through labour. The traditional Friedman's curve was not used to assess or manage this labouring patient. The work of Philpott and Castle which has also reinforced the expectation that women should dilate 1cm per hour once active labour is achieved may not in fact be correct.[11] More recent studies suggest that labour progress occurs much more slowly, at about 0.5cm per hour.[12] A Cochrane review of labour progress charting using partograms has demonstrated that perhaps a more appropriate marker might be significant lack of labour change after four hours.[13] Evaluating Gayle's labour, she clearly did not follow a curve of 1cm per hour. Instead, she was admitted in early labour and slept for five or six hours until waking up in active labour. A recent review of the natural progress of labour from charts from 1959 to 1962 further supports the notion that this may be a common pattern. Researchers suggest that early prodromal labour [sometimes called 'false labour'] may be longer than earlier thought while active labour, once achieved, follows a more regular pattern.[14]

She clearly did not follow a curve of 1cm per hour

Usual obstetric practice requires vaginal examination to assess labour progress at regular intervals. Also useful for promoting normal outcomes, though rarely discussed outside midwifery and nursing textbooks, are other ways to assess labour progress. Changes in vocal quality, movement, nausea and vomiting as well as spontaneous rupture of membranes are all effective qualitative methods of gauging the labouring woman's progress during labour. In the case I described, caregivers observed how the woman coped with labour as well as the signs of progress such as vomiting and spontaneous rupture of membranes. Most telling of the change occurring was when Gayle changed position and her vocal quality indicated that she had begun to push and had thus entered the second stage of labour. It is possible to assess normal labour progress through this hands-off approach which minimises invasive vaginal exams. The challenge is understanding an observational and qualitative evaluation in comparison with a quantitative approach such as vaginal exams. However, meeting this challenge further supports normal labour progress without interruptive digital vaginal exams.

When Gayle moved to her hands and knees to push, she pushed spontaneously, with contractions as she felt the need to push. Her partner and the staff provided encouragement but no direction. Women who push when they have an urge to push appear different than women who are receiving coaching. On their own, women will wait until a uterine contraction intensifies prior to pushing instead of starting at the beginning of a contraction.[15] By supporting women to push as they feel they need to, rather than directing them, caregivers not only support the normal process but also decrease the risk of several potential poor outcomes, as we shall see.

This is in contrast to Valsalva pushing which is when women are directed to hold their breath and push. Valsalva pushing has been linked to adverse outcomes for both mother and baby. The continuous and increased force associated with valsalva pushing at the moment of birth is associated with worse perineal outcomes.[16,17] There is some evidence that suggests poorer perineal function long term or, perhaps, a slower return to function when valsalva technique is used during pushing.[18,19] Interestingly, when a woman holds her breath and pushes, there can be a decrease in fetal oxygen saturation accompanied by other haemodynamic changes for mother and fetus.[20,21] The impact on the fetus can be non-reassuring fetal heart tones, change in acid base balance and lower Apgar scores.

Attendants at birth may affect how a woman pushes

Attendants at birth may affect how a woman pushes. Many healthcare caregivers are trained to count during a push, to tell a woman to hold her breath and to be quiet as well as yelling the familiar "PUSH, PUSH, PUSH!" This form of routine care is not only implicated in poor fetal outcomes, it also undermines a woman's confidence in her own ability to push her baby out. This is in contrast to providing supportive care during spontaneous pushing.[22] Rather than being directive, caregivers follow the mother's lead and encourage her to follow her own body's urges. This helps the mother focus on the normality and power she has and to trust in her own instincts during second stage. In contrast to instruction, attendants provide praise and reassurance. Research has shown that mothers have increased satisfaction with spontaneous pushing.[23]

The position Gayle unconsciously chose for herself to birth in was one that would protect her perineum and provide better oxygenation for her baby during pushing. She moved to the natural hands-and-knees or modified-kneeling position. Kneeling during pushing and birth is linked with more intact perineums, less pain and greater feelings of maternal participation. The lithotomy position commonly used in the hospital setting for birth, while potentially decreasing blood loss, is associated with increased episiotomies and increased abnormal fetal heart patterns, most likely linked to increased pressure on the vena cava by the fetus.[24] More upright positions such as standing and squatting are associated with less reported maternal pain and fewer abnormal fetal heart patterns. These positions appear to be ones women assume worldwide for birth.[25]

Gayle's experience contrasts the effects of routine hospital procedures and interventions with physiological normal birth. While the individual impact of continuous fetal monitoring, remaining immobile in bed and directed pushing in the supine position is known, the combined effect of all of these compared with undisturbed birth can only be theorised. As individual interventions, many of these have been noted to result in some harm such as the increased caesarean section rate after continuous fetal monitoring. It is unknown what the additive effect of the routine obstetric care package actually is on maternal and neonatal outcomes. As a result, it is of paramount importance for caregivers to recognise that these routine interventions interfere with normal birth.

When evidence-based practices supporting normal birth are all brought together, something even more powerful becomes quite clear. All of these practices force us to conclude that women have the internal strength and ability to labour and birth their children. Simply by recognising birth as a normal process and using best practices, caregivers can provide the foundation for women to recognise their own power and accomplishment. Providing appropriate maternity care to support the evidence-based practices which effectively mean minimal intervention is not limited to any one site—i.e. it can take place in a hospital, free-standing birth centre or in women's homes.

The concept of empowerment during birth is not minor. Often the goals for birth are noted to be a "Healthy mom, healthy baby". The reality is so much more complex than that. As noted before, maternity practices that support normal birth and do not hamper labour result in improved measurable outcomes for mothers and babies. Practices which support normal birth and which do not disturb it (which are also justifiable when considering the evidence, as we have seen) also reinforce the innate power and knowledge that women have about birth instead of undermining it like many non-evidence-based obstetric interventions do. It is not enough only to provide this evidence-based care. Women also have more positive birth experiences when the midwife or obstetrician shares decision-making with them and offers appropriate balanced education of available options so that real choices can be made.[26]

There are many women who are aware of the power of labour. Many of them seek birth outside of the hospital in order to labour undisturbed and without questionable obstetric interventions. In contrast, many women who seek more traditional obstetric care may not know of the options open to them or the possibilities of labour. In some ways, it is even more powerful when a woman with minimal expectations for birth is given the opportunity through the use of evidence-based practices for normal birth, such as those outlined above, to find empowerment.

Recently I attended another first-time mother, who I'll call Rebecca, in labour with another registrar. When she was completely dilated, the mother declined to push because of the amount of pain she was experiencing. She asked to have her epidural increased. We encouraged her to try different positions but in each position she continued to experience hip and back pain. Rebecca apologised but said she just could not do this. We suggested a supported kneeling position which she was willing to attempt as a last-ditch effort. Once all the tubes and wires were rearranged, Rebecca became quiet and focused. After 15 minutes, she began to push spontaneously in this position. When asked if she wanted to move, Rebecca declined and instead began to work very hard at pushing her baby out. The room was quiet between contractions and during them only one or two voices could be heard providing encouragement, with comments such as "What a great job you're doing" or "You're so strong". Within a short period of time, the bag of waters was visible at Rebecca's introitus. Slowly, the perineum distended and more of the bag of waters with clear amniotic fluid appeared. The head descended into the bag. Quietly and incrementally, Rebecca crowned and then birthed her baby. The amniotic sac broke with the birth of the baby's shoulders. All was silent in the room except for the baby crying. The registrar passed the baby through Rebecca's legs to her saying, "Here is your baby". With triumph and joy in her voice, Rebecca lifted her baby and said to the room at large, "I did it!"

Ami Goldstein works at the School of Medicine at the University of North Carolina at Chapel Hill. She works one-to-one with house officers on labour and delivery as well as teaching evidence based maternity care. She has presented locally and nationally on best practices for mothers and babies. She has three boys who provide challenges and joys on a daily basis.

References

1 Gourounti K, Sandall J. (2007) Admission cardiotocography versus intermittent auscultation of fetal heart rate: effects on neonatal Apgar score, on the rate of caesarean sections and on the rate of instrumental delivery—a systematic review. *International Journal of Nursing Studies* 1029-35.

2 Impey L, Reynolds M, MacQuillan K, Gates S, Murphy J. and Sheil, O. (2003) Admission cardiotocography: A randomised controlled trial. *Lancet* (361):465–470.

3 Alfirevic Z, Devane D, Gyte GML. (2006) Continuous cardiotocography (CTG) as a form of electronic fetal monitoring (EFM) for fetal assessment during labour. *Cochrane Database of Systematic Reviews*, Issue 3. Art. No.: CD006066. DOI: 10.1002/14651858.CD006066.

4 Liston R, Sawchuck D and Young D, Society of Obstetrics and Gynaecologists of Canada, British Columbia Perinatal Health Program. (2007) Fetal health surveillance: Antepartum and intrapartum consensus guideline, *Journal Obstetrics Gynaecology Canada,* 29 (9 Suppl. 4):S3–56.

5 National Collaborating Centre for Women's and Children's Health Web site. (2008) Intrapartum care of healthy women and their babies during childbirth. Clinical guideline September 2007. Revised reprint 2008.

6 Intermittent Auscultation for Intrapartum Fetal Heart Rate Surveillance (replaces ACNM Clinical Bulletin #9, March 2007). American College of Nurse-Midwives.

7 O'Sullivan G, Liu B, Shennan SH, 2007. Oral intake during labor. *International Anesthesiology Clinics.* Winter;45(1):133-47.

8 Singata, M, Tranmer, J & Gyte, GML (2010). Restricting oral fluid and food intake during labour. *Cochrane Database of Systematic Reviews* (1), CD003930. doi:10.1002/14651858.CD003930.pub 2

9 Simkin P, Bolding A, 2004. Update on nonparmacologic approaches to relieve labor pain and prevent suffering. *Journal of Midwifery and Women's Health.* Nov-Dec;49(6):489-504.

10 Lawrence A, Lewis L, Hofmeyr GJ, Dowswell T, Styles C. (2009) Maternal positions and mobility during first stage labour. *Cochrane Database of Systematic Reviews*, Issue 2. Art. No.: CD003934. DOI: 10.1002/14651858.CD003934.pub2.

11 Philpott RH, Castle WM. (1972)Cervicographs in the management of labour in primigravidae, I and II. The Journal of Obstetrics and Gynaecology of the British Commonwealth,79:592– 602.

12 Albers LL, 2007. The evidence for physiologic management of the active phase of the first stage of labor. *Journal of Midwifery and Women's Health.* May-Jun;52 (3):207-15.

13 Lavender T, Hart A, Smyth RMD. (2008) Effect of partogram use on outcomes for women in spontaneous labour at term. *Cochrane Database of Systematic Reviews*, Issue 4. Art. No.: CD005461. DOI: 10.1002/14651858.CD005461.pub2.

14 Zhang J, Troendle J, Mikolajczyk R, Sundaram R, Beaver J, Fraser W. (2010) The natural history of the normal first stage of labor. *Obstetrics and Gynecology,* 115 (4): 705-710.

15 Roberts JE, Goldstein SA, Gruener JS, Maggio M, Mendez-Bauer C, 1987. A descriptive analysis of involuntary bearing-down efforts during the expulsive phase of labor. *Journal of Obstetrical Gynecology and Neonatal Nursing* 16: 48-55.

16 Beynon, CL. (1957) The normal second-stage of labour: a plea for reform in its conduct. *The Journal of obstetrics and gynaecology of the British Empire* 64: 815-820.

17 Simpson KR, James DC. (2005) Effects of immediate versus delayed pushing during second-stage labor and fetal well-being. *Nursing Research*, 54: 149-157.

18 Bloom SL, Casey BM, Schaffer JI, Mcinterie SS, Leveno KJ. (2006) A randomized trial of coached verus uncoached maternal pushing during the second stage of labor. *American Journal of Obstetrics and Gynecology*,194: 10-13.

19 Schaffer JI, Bloom SL, Casey BM, McIntire DD, Nihira MA, Leveno KJ. (2005) A randomized control trial of the effes of coached vs uncoached maternal pushing during the second stage of labor on postpartum pelvic floor structure and function. *American Journal of Obstetrics and Gynecology*,192:1692-1696.

20 Caldeyro-Barcia R, Giussi G, Storch E. (1981) The bearing down efforts and their effects of fetal heart rate, oxygenation and acid-base balance. *Journal of Perinatal Medicine*, 9:63-67.

21 Simpson KR, James DC. (2005) Effects of immediate versus delayed pushing during second-stage labor and fetal well-being. *Nursing Research*, 54: 149-157.

22 Sampselle CM, Miller JM, Luecha Y, Fischer K, Rosten L, 2005. Provider support of spontaneous pushing during the second stage of labor. *Journal of Obstetric, Gynecologic and Neonatal Nursing.* Nov-Dec;34(6):695-702.

23 Yildirim G, Kizilkaya B. (2008) Effects of pushing techniques in birth on mother and fetus: A randomized study. *Birth*, 35:25-30.

24 Gupta JK, Hofmeyr GJ, Smyth RMD. (2004) Position in the second stage of labour for women without epidural anaesthesia. *Cochrane Database of Systematic Reviews*, Issue 1. Art. No.: CD002006. DOI: 10.1002/14651858.CD002006.pub2.

25 Lefeber Y, Voohoever H. (1997) Practices and beliefs of traditional birth attendants: lessons for obstetrics in the north? *Tropical Medicine & International Health*, 2(12) 1175–1179

26 National Collaborating Centre for Women's and Children's Health. Intrapartum care care of healthy women and their babies during childbirth. 2007.

Supporting epidural-free birth: a practice of kindness, courage and skill

Alex Smith

"The midwife who was at the birth of my first daughter was quite simply sent from heaven... She read me, understood me, worked with whatever I wanted and gently encouraged me when she thought I needed it. She never criticised or questioned any of my decisions; she made me feel like it was my birth. I want every woman to experience a midwife like her. I will think about her till the day I die."

A woman is likely to remember the care she received from her midwife for the rest of her life.[1] The degree to which she realised her own power will inform how she sees herself as a person, perhaps for years to come.[2,3] It must be daunting and rather humbling for a midwife when she knows that her words and actions will form a central part of so many life stories. When a woman embarks on this journey, intending to steer her own course and to draw upon every ounce of her own power, the trusty midwife companion who offers unfailing support will always be remembered for her strength and kindness.

'Women and their families should always be treated with kindness, respect and dignity... the views, beliefs and values of the woman, her partner and her family in relation to her care and that of her baby should be sought and respected at all times.' (National Institute for Clinical Excellence, 2007)[4]

When a caring midwife holds another set of values from the mother, it invites an almost heroic act of vision, understanding and compassion on her part to fully embrace and respect the mother's view. In finding this strength and kindness the experience becomes transformative for mother and midwife alike, no matter how the birth journey unfolds. If you hold a different set of values to any mother you are attending, particularly when it comes to pain relief, it helps to hold in mind two things:

- *Epidurals are not benign*. The moment one is in place, labour and birth cease to be normal.[5] The iatrogenic sequalae resulting from epidural anaesthesia, the snowball of possible medical complications caused by this treatment, are well documented[6-11] and explained.[12,13] It is beholden upon all caregivers to be fully aware of the adverse effects of this major disturbance to the physiological processes and to practise in a way that maximises well-being rather than introduces pathology.
- *Birth is a unique opportunity for healing the past and shaping the future.* The realisation of the mother's dream birth–the one in which she kneels radiant beyond measure, her vibrant baby held safely to her warm body–is the realisation of her marathon, of her Everest, of herself.

Birth is a unique opportunity for healing the past

For a kind and caring midwife there is immense satisfaction and pride to be found in championing another woman in her efforts, and she (or he) will do everything she (or he) can to support the mother's endeavour. In order to do this successfully, a few important principles need to be respected...

Mothers benefit from complete privacy and discreet observation

There is a principle in physics which states that the observation of a phenomenon changes it

There is a principle in physics which states that the observation of a phenomenon changes it.[14] Simply by being in the presence of another person, that person's experience will be changed in one way or another. We intuitively understand this from our own experience of being watched. Even when engaged in very ordinary tasks, we sense what our observer may be thinking. (Perhaps we subconsciously glimpse a twitch of an eyebrow, or hear a subtle nuance in vocal tone, or smell the chemicals of doubt emanating from a person who is challenged by what is happening.) We feel relaxed and competent in one person's company... and quite the opposite in another's. For the woman in labour, this awareness is heightened. In the intimacy of the birthing room, the unspoken attitudes and beliefs of her midwife are transmitted to the mother and have the power to change what happens. The natural intelligence of the mother's body will ensure that her baby is born most readily into an atmosphere of privacy, peace, and philosophical harmony. The presence of a calm, supportive and respectful advocate shortens labour and increases maternal satisfaction.[15] On the other hand, in a less conducive atmosphere, the woman's cervix may start to reclose to keep her baby safely inside, an impressive ability that Gaskin refers to as Sphincter Law.[16]

The presence of a calm, supportive and respectful advocate shortens labour and increases maternal satisfaction

In order to safeguard an appropriate atmosphere, I would suggest the following:

- Ensure that only the absolute minimum number of people enter the labouring woman's room, and then always quietly and discreetly.
- Be at the same level physically as the labouring woman, or even lower. Tune into her and sense when to minimise eye and voice contact.
- Create a sense of timelessness, and quietly convey your confidence and trust in the process. Keep routine observations and other procedures to a minimum. For normal labour the benefit of these is not supported by research and they disturb the mother by stimulating her neocortex... in the same way that routine observations of vital signs and progress during love-making would disturb the average person.

Birth is a biological process—the environment is significant

The Cartesian view of the woman's body as a machine that must be measured, monitored and manipulated by others to ensure the safety of her baby is being replaced by our renewed understanding of the mind-body connection and the biological model of birth.[17] Many midwives now prefer a more humanistic and holistic approach to care, one that respects our mammalian biology and the nature of human childbirth.[18,19] A practice philosophy based on the concept of 'salutogenesis',[20] the generation of well-being, rather than on 'the assumption of pathology'[21] is most helpful for the mother. After all, the mother at term has spent nine months growing another human being within the warmth and safety of her womb. Once we appreciate the beautiful complexity and utter magnitude of this achievement it becomes easy to trust her body's ability to complete the last few hours of that process, safely and smoothly.

Perhaps the most important element of the environment is privacy. Privacy supports the process of birth because the hormones of birth, particularly oxytocin, are also those of sexual response and require the same conditions for optimal production.[22-24] Oxytocin not only produces the powerful waves of birthing energy that open the womb, it is also involved in male and female orgasm, the release of milk, and the awakening of tenderness and nurturing instincts in both men and women. It is easy to understand why, within the biological model, the mother instinctively seeks similar conditions in which to conceive, birth and feed her baby. When women in my practice are asked to visualise their ideal birthing environment, after being led into a deeper connection with their intuitive knowing and when they are given permission to set aside everything they have seen or heard about birth, they often describe a warm, dark, space, lit perhaps with firelight or candlelight, where they will be completely undisturbed. Alternatively, the mother may see herself in the seclusion of a sunlit garden. Warm water, gentle music and some token of the natural world—fruit, flowers, or the view of the sky from the window—are always in the picture. This is very similar to the setting and conditions in which another biological and physiological process, digestion, can most comfortably take place. If we were always required to eat in registered canteen-like locations with electronic gastric monitoring or other professional close monitoring—for fear of choking, food poisoning and other gastric emergencies—the close observation, monitoring and timing of our dining experience would do little to enhance it and would very likely increase the rate of indigestion. Likewise, the environment in which birth can most comfortably take place is one in which the mother has complete privacy, with the loving and unobtrusive support of her trusted midwife and other chosen companions just within reach. In such a setting the mother feels free and uninhibited. She is able to relax into an undisturbed trance-like state where the older, more primitive part of her brain, the part that regulates the hormones of birth, becomes free to orchestrate and self-monitor this natural biological process.

Perhaps the most important element of the environment is privacy—which supports the process of birth

Invite parents to bring comfort items from home

From the midwife's perspective, it helps to be aware of the way in which the 'urban structure' of the hospital channels her behaviour,[25] of how she may have become inured to the culture of the workplace, of how the institutional setting may trigger her 'inner nurse', even when this is not her intent. (With apologies to and great respect for male midwives, the use of a single pronoun makes for smoother reading.) While 'doing good by stealth' does little to legitimise attempts to promote physiological birth,[26] small acts of kindness and thoughtfulness go some way towards subverting 'assembly-line care'[27] and provide the means with which a midwife can offer the individualised, with-woman, nurturing care that supports epidural-free birth, and in fact every type of birth.

In order to create the most favourable environment, I would suggest the following:

- ♥ Offer to dim the lights. Unobtrusively screen the mother, or cocoon her with a soft shawl or a light coverlet. Build her a private nest.[28,29]
- ♥ Invite the parents to bring comfort items from home. These might include a special picture, a photo of a loved one, colourful fruit and flowers, lavender oil, some favourite music, and bedding that has been slept on for a night so that it smells reassuringly familiar. Help the parents make the room look cosy and inviting... and a little romantic. Comment on how lovely it feels to come into their room.
- ♥ Ensure that the mother and her companions have everything they need to be comfortable: enough pillows, nice chairs, a floor mattress, a birthing ball, massage oil, drinks and other nourishment, control of the lighting, fresh air, reassuring smiles... and opportunities for complete privacy.
- ♥ Encourage the use of the shower, bath or pool. If this is not possible, towels rung out in very hot water and placed on the lower back are always welcome in strong labour.

A homely setting increases the rate of epidural-free birth,[30,31] as does immersion in water.[32] Music and art (of the individual's choice) reduces the perception of pain.[33] After all, the conditions in which a woman can most easily give birth are the same in which she could most easily make love or most easily enjoy a relaxing meal.

Birth involves a psychosomatic response, so language is important

It is easy to see how the way in which the words we hear or read and the words we say to ourselves can have immediate and powerful physiological effects. Praise makes us *swell* with pride; a compliment makes us *flush* with pleasure; sweet nothings make us *melt* with desire; the mention of a particular food makes our mouths *water*; the announcement of the imminent arrival of a loved one makes us *breathe* a little faster; words of empathy *warm* our heart; good news allows us to *relax*. It is even easier to appreciate how less positive words work just as immediately and powerfully, but in reverse.

Midwives understand the importance of words and can use them as a kind of placebo in supporting the mother as she enjoys the benefits of an epidural-free labour. Placebo (Latin: 'I shall please') plays an important part in the observed effects of medical treatments,[34,35] and often demonstrates a therapeutic effect that is almost as strong as the active treatment. Both the placebo and the active treatment are significantly more effective when prescribed by a caregiver with a positive manner[36] using calming reassuring words.[37] Neuroscience is beginning to explain this phenomenon, whereby it is the attitudes, words and expectations of those involved in a 'patient's' care that are now thought to be responsible for much of any therapeutic benefit.[38,39] As a result, some researchers are suggesting that 'the placebo effect' should be renamed *the care effect.*[40]

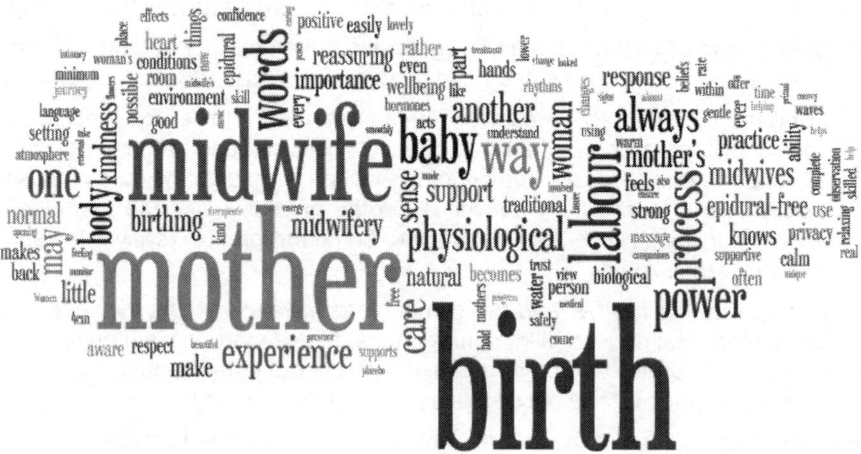

An image generated from the all the words of this chapter using www.wordle.net

"The student midwife who was at my son's birth was unbelievably kind and reassuring. She supported my husband and I in such a lovely, calm way that she enabled us to have the birth we wanted."

Mindfully structured positive messages, calmly delivered by a midwife or other caregiver who believes them to be true, will be transmitted to every cell in the woman's body creating a physiological response that will enhance and facilitate the natural process. Here are some examples of positive, progress-enhancing comments which could be used:

"Wow–3cm already!"

"You have all the time you need."

"Every minute you are coming closer to holding your baby in your arms."

"Babies always come out."

"I can see your body knows what to do."

"It's all happening beautifully."

"Simply breathe... smoothly and easily... That's perfect."

"These strong waves of labour are such a good sign."

"The power and intensity you are feeling will never be more than you can bear."

"You are as strong as a lioness."

"The hormones of pregnancy have made you stretchier than you could possibly imagine."

"This process is so good for your baby."

"Your baby is helping too... How wonderful."

"Your body is opening as naturally as a rose."

Ina May Gaskin reports a caesarean rate that has always remained under 2% over the 40 years she has been practising, even though her statistics include breech and twin births.[41] (None of her clients use epidurals.) She attributes this low rate to *an absence of fear*. Any midwife supporting epidural-free birth can share her fearlessness with the mother in her demeanour, her behaviour and in the way she speaks. As labour progresses and the mother becomes more deeply absorbed by the process, the tuned-in midwife will lower her voice and keep talking to a minimum. Respectful of the intimacy of the situation and aware of the power of her words, the skilled midwife will sense when the mother needs stillness and peace, or reassuring words. The oxytocin response requires gentle confident wooing, not brisk or anxious demand.

In order to maximise the positive effect of your communications, I would suggest the following:

- Develop rapport and empathy with the mother by listening to her with real interest and respect. Use her terminology whenever possible.
- Build the mother's confidence by using language that places the mother at the helm—no matter how her birth journey is unfolding.
- Create a relationship of trust by being 'genuine'... by being your real self. The mother will sense if you are paying 'lip service' to her beliefs. She will also sense if you are using words to steer her away from her own path. It is better to be open about your own views while remaining respectful of the mother's.
- Employ 'artful vagueness' in the way you express some ideas. This way, your positive intent can be interpreted by the mother in her own way. When you say "The baby always comes out" 'one way or another' is implied but doesn't need to be spoken. When you say "Your body knows what to do" this can imply that as well as knowing how to birth a baby, the woman's body also knows how to recover from surgery—but, again, it's not helpful for this to be spoken.
- Honour the mother as the 'doing' person, the owner of her experience, by changing the nouns of medicalised birth language back into the verbs of primal birthing. First stage, second stage and self-help techniques, are things that experts know about... Opening, breathing, moving, responding, pushing, vocalising, stretching, releasing and relaxing are things that mothers actually do.

In summary, it is helpful to remember that words elicit a very real physiological response and, like a magic spell, have the power to harm, heal or transform.

It is helpful to remember that words elicit a very real physiological response and the power to transform

Traditional midwifery skills are required

Supporting epidural-free birth calls for traditional midwifery skills rather than obstetric nursing. There is something immensely reassuring about the 'heart and hands' midwife.[42] The mother senses that here is a person who knows what they are doing—she feels in safe hands. Intermittent auscultation of the baby's heart with a Pinard stethoscope or Sonicaid is recommended in normal labour[43] and is preferred to CTG by most mothers.[44] A minimal reliance on technology normalises the experience and helps us avoid an 'atmosphere of latent anxiety'.[45] Furthermore, a low-tech approach will enhance the midwife-mother-baby connection and enable primal instinctive intuitive knowing to come back into play,[46] significantly increasing the likelihood of a lovely, straightforward birth. While technology is a valuable and very welcome resource for mothers and midwives, if required, and while a gentle and skilled vaginal examination can provide useful information before additional help is considered, respect will be restored to the mother and midwife's intuitive and perceptive ability to monitor the normal physiological process of labour by observation of external signs of progress alone.[47,48,49] Most of us are generally very practised in doing this for all other aspects of our physiological wellbeing and this ability is enhanced, for midwife and mother, in a calm, relaxing and supportive environment. Despite the legacy of Friedman and O'Driscoll (now being re-evaluated),[50,51] the skilled midwife recognises that rhythms of labour vary widely and are far too subtle to be reliably confined to a graph. The use of a partogram, even with updated curves, requires vaginal assessment of the cervix. As discussed above, the very act of observing cervical dilation, changes things. Schrödinger's cat comes to mind (if you're familiar with that)... In other words, if we had not looked, it may not have happened. This is the *observer's paradox*, a factor in the *quantum indeterminacy* of any physical state.[52] Women often talk of being 'stuck' at 4cm but later dilating very quickly. If we had not looked we may simply have noticed a magnificent woman, over time becoming more and more engrossed in her labour, her breathing and noises changing, the waves of birthing energy appearing stronger and stronger, her body sinking closer to the floor, that unique smell and gut feeling that heralds the birth, and eventually the birth itself... and we would never have known that her cervix measured 4cm until the very last hour. Yet had there been a diagnosis of 'still only 4cm', the nocebo power of finding that 'problem', the very real power of negative suggestion, would have been sufficient to make it one.[53,54] We therefore need to reinstate traditional midwifery care as the primary means of facilitating a woman's progress.

In order to ensure your practice is based on the tenets of traditional midwifery:

- ♥ Find out about the purple line and other external signs of normal progress.[47-49]
- ♥ Respect the subtle and diverse rhythms of birth and support women's natural birthing behaviours.
- ♥ Trust the research that recommends the use of intermittent monitoring of the baby's heart.[43]
- ♥ Own a beautiful Pinard stethoscope and use it a lot.
- ♥ Enjoy developing your skills in palpation and massage.[55]
- ♥ Befriend other kind and supportive midwives and learn from each other.
- ♥ Share wonderful birth stories as often as possible.
- ♥ Connect with the mother... Listen to her carefully and nurture her warmly. What this means in practice is a return to the sensitive use of heart, hands and masterly inactivity.[56]

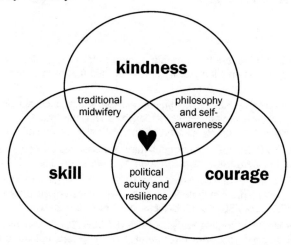

A graphic summary of challenges you might face, when offering epidural-free support

The midwifery principles I have outlined above, which support epidural-free birth are the gold standard for all midwifery practice. After all, midwives are the guardians of normal birth, and kindness, courage and skill are the basis of their work.

Nevertheless, as I write I remain very aware of the restraints that midwives experience. There is little opportunity for a hospital midwife to hold hands, stroke hair, offer mashed banana, massage feet, prepare ice-chips, mop a brow, help the mother change positions, whisper soothing affirmations, rub a sore back, convey calm confidence with the click of her knitting needles, or be mindfully still and silent. The restraints of the system sometimes appear to paralyse the very acts of traditional midwifery that best support a mother in managing the exquisite intensity of birth. It is no surprise that the temporary paralysis of the epidural may be all the midwife feels she has to offer. Yet the power of birth, embodied within the mother and her midwife, is eternally resilient. Until such time that the current maternity care crisis is resolved, small acts of kindness, courage and skill hold the power to make a difference that will be remembered forever.

Alex Smith has worked with the NCT as a childbirth educator since 1978, and as a tutor training antenatal teachers since 1982. She is also a Licensed NLP [neuro-linguistic programming] Practitioner. She continues to enjoy a deep belief in the innate ability of women to carry, birth and nurture their children, and promotes the use of language, story and metaphor as means of reawakening birthing autonomy. Alex home educated her five children and is looking forward to the birth of her tenth grandchild. She is grateful every day for having the best job in the world.

References

1 Simkin P (1992) Just another day in a woman's life? Part 11: Nature and consistency of women's long-term memory of their first birth experiences. *Birth* 19 (2):64-81

2 Peterson G (1996) Childbirth: The ordinary miracle: effects of devaluation of childbirth on women's self-esteem and family relationships. Available: http://www.birthpsychology.com/birthscene/mothers3.html [Accessed 15 September 2010]

3 Hodnett E D (2002) The impact of childbirth experiences on women's sense of self: a review of the literature. *Australian Journal of Midwifery* 15(4): 10-16

4 National Institute for Clinical Excellence. (2007) NICE Clinical Guideline 55—Intrapartum Care, p.6 Available from: http://www.nice.org.uk/nicemedia/live/11837/36280/36280.pdf [Accessed 4 November 2010]

5 The Maternity Care Working Party. NCT/RCM/RCOG (2007) Making Normal Birth a Reality. Available: http://www.rcog.org.uk/files/rcog-corp/uploaded-files/JointStatementNormalBirth2007.pdf [Accessed 6 November 2010]

6 Thorp J, Breedlove G (1996) Epidural Analgesia in Labor: An Evaluation of Risks and Benefits. *Birth* 23: 63-83

7 Enkin M, Keirse M, Renfrew M, Neilson J (2000) *A Guide to Effective Care in Pregnancy and Childbirth*. Oxford: Oxford University Press

8 Lieberman E, Davidson K, Lee-Parritz A, Shearer A (2005) Changes in fetal position during labour and their association with epidural analgesia. *Obstetrics and Gynecology* 105 (5): 974-982.

9 Anin-Somuah M, Smyth M, Howell C (2005) Epidural versus non-epidural or no analgesia for pain relief in labour (Cochrane Review) In: *Cochrane Library*, Issue 4. Chichester, UK: John Wiley and Sons Ltd.

10 Lieberman E, O'Donoghue C (2002) Unintended effects of epidural analgesia during labour: a systematic review. *American Journal of Obstetrics and Gynecology* 186(5): S31-S68

11 Lieberman E, O'Donoghue C (2002) Unintended effects of epidural analgesia during labour: a systematic review. *American Journal of Obstetrics and Gynecology* 186(5): S31-S68

12 The Maternity Care Working Party. NCT/RCM/RCOG (2007) Making Normal Birth a Reality. Available: http://www.rcog.org.uk/files/rcog-corp/uploaded-files/JointStatmentNormalBirth2007.pdf [Accessed 6 November 2010]

13 Thorp J, Breedlove G (1996) Epidural Analgesia in Labor: An Evaluation of Risks and Benefits. *Birth* 23: 63-83

14 Pritchard Lee. (No date) What is the name for a phenomenon where the presence of the observer changes the nature of the observed? Available: http://www.physlink.com/education/askexperts/ae179.cfm [Accessed 6 November 2010]

15 Hodnett ED, Gates S, Hofmeyr GJ, Sakala C. Continuous support for women during childbirth. *Cochrane Database of Systematic Reviews* 2007, Issue 3. Art. No.: CD003766. DOI: 10.1002/14651858.CD003766.pub2

16 Gaskin I.M. (2003) *Ina May's Guide to Childbirth*. New York: Bantam Dell

17 Rabuzzi KA. (1994) *Mother With Child: Transformations Through Childbirth*. Indiana, Indiana University Press

18 Davis-Floyd R. The Technocratic, Humanistic, and Holistic Paradigms of Childbirth *International Journal of Gynecology and Obstetrics*, Vol 75, Suppl No. 1, pp. S5-S23, November 2001.

19 Pylypa J (1998) *Power and Bodily Practice: Applying the Work of Foucault to Anthropology of the Body*. http://dlist.sir.arizona.edu/arizona/handle/10150/110194

20 Downe, S. (Ed.) (2004) *Normal childbirth: evidence and debate*. London: Churchill Livingstone

21 Inch, S. (1989). *Birthrights: a parent's guide to modern childbirth*. 2nd ed. London: Green Print.

22 Gaskin, I.M. (2003) *Ina May's Guide to Childbirth*. New York: Bantam Dell

23 Buckley S (2005) *Gentle Birth, Gentle Mothering: The wisdom and science of gentle choices in pregnancy, birth and parenting*. Brisbane: One Moon Press

24 Odent M. (2009) *The Functions of the Orgasms: The Highways to Transcendence*. London: Pinter & Martin

25 de Certeau, M. *The Practice of Everyday Life*, trans. Steven Rendall, University of California Press, Berkeley 1984

26 Walsh, D. (2007) Normal Birth: a Retrospective - Assessing the agenda around normal birth. Available at http://www.midirs.org/development/MIDIRSEssence.nsf/articles/68365A7CEEBAD11D802575CF003238FA [Accessed 16 October 2010]

27 Walsh, D. (2006) Subverting the assembly-line: Childbirth in a free-standing birth centre. *Social Science & Medicine* 62(6), pp.1330-1340

28 RCM (No date) Campaign for Normal Birth: Ten Top Tips. Available at http://www.rcmnormalbirth.org.uk/practice/ten-top-tips/ [Accessed 2 November 2010]

29 Walsh D. (2006) 'Nesting' and 'Matrescence' as distinctive features of a free-standing birth centre in the UK. *Midwifery* 22, 228–239

30 Hodnett ED, Downe S, Edwards N, Walsh D. Home-like versus conventional institutional settings for birth. *Cochrane Database of Systematic Reviews* 2005, Issue 1. Art. No.: CD000012.pub2. DOI: 10.1002/14651858.CD000012.pub2.

31 Lock L.R., Gibb H.J The Power of Place. *Midwifery*. 2003 Jun; 19(2): 132-9

32 Cluett ER, Burns E. Immersion in water in labour and birth. *Cochrane Database of Systematic Reviews*_2009, Issue 2. Art. No.: CD000111. DOI: 10.1002/14651858.CD000111.pub3

33 Mitchell L.A, MacDonald R.A.R, Knussen C (2008). An investigation of the effects of music and art on pain perception. *Psychology of Aesthetics, Creativity, and the Arts,* 2 (3), 162-170 DOI: 10.1037/1931-3896.2.3.162

34 Krogsbøll LT., Hróbjartsson A., Gøtzsche PC. (2009) Spontaneous improvement in randomised clinical trials: meta-analysis of three-armed trials comparing no treatment, placebo and active intervention. *BMC Medical Research Methodology* 9:1doi:10.1186/1471-2288-9-1

35 Thomson, G. (2008). *Magic in Practice. Introducing Medical NLP: The Art and Science of Language in Healing and Health.* London: Hammersmith Press Limited

36 Thomas KB. *General practice consultations: is there any point in being positive? BMJ (Clin Res Ed). 1987; 294:1200-2. [PMID: 3109581]*

37 Varelmann D., Pancaro C., Cappiello E.C., Camann W.R. Nocebo-Induced Hyperalgesia During Local Anesthetic Injection. Available at http://www.uwoanesthesia.ca/documents/Varelmann%20Nocebo%20Hyperalgesia%20AnA%202010.pdf [Accessed on 17 October 2010]

38 Seminowicz D.A. (2006) Believe in Your Placebo. *Journal of Neuroscience,* April 26 (17):4453-4454; doi:10.1523/JNEUROSCI.0789-06.2006

39 Moerman DE, Jonas WB. Deconstructing the placebo effect and finding the meaning response. *Ann Intern Med* (2002;) 136:: 471–6

40 Louhiala P., Puustinen R. (2008) Rethinking the Placebo Effect. *Med Humanities.* 34: 107-109 doi: 10.1136/jmh. 2008.000307

41 Gaskin I.M. (2003) *Ina May's Guide to Childbirth.* New York: Bantam Dell

42 Davis E. (1997) *Heart & Hands: A Midwife's Guide to Pregnancy & Birth.* Berkeley, CA: Celestial Arts

43 National Collaborating Centre for Women's and Children's Health. Intrapartum Care: care of healthy women and their babies during childbirth (for NICE). Available: http://www.nice.org.uk/nicemedia/live/11837/36275/36275.pdf [Accessed 6 November 2010]

44 Mangesi, L., Cur, B., Cur, M., Hofmeyr, G.J. (2009) Assessing the preferences of women for different methods of monitoring the fetal heart in labour. *South African Journal of Obstetrics and Gynaecology* August Vol.15.No2

45 Walsh, D. (2007) *Evidenced-based Care for Normal Labour and Birth.* Abingdon: Routledge

46 McKay, S. (1991) Shared power: the essence of humanised childbirth. *Pre and Peri-Natal Psychology,* 5(4): 283-295

47 RCM (No date) Campaign for Normal Birth: Relying on Technology. Available from http://www.rcmnormalbirth.org.uk/stories/taxi-for-north-end-road/relying-on-technology/ [Accessed 2 November 2010]

48 Walsh, D. (2007) *Evidenced-based Care for Normal Labour and Birth.* Abingdon: Routledge

49 Shepherd, A., Cheyne, H., Kennedy, S., McIntosh, C., Styles, M., Niven C. The purple line as a measure of labour progress: a longitudinal study. *BMC Pregnancy Childbirth*. 2010; 10: 54. Published online 2010 September 16. doi: 10.1186/1471-2393/10-54.

50 Lavender, T., Alfirevic, Z., Walkinshaw, S. Effect of Different Partogram Action Lines on Birth Outcomes: A Randomized Controlled Trial. *Obstetrics & Gynecology*: August 2006 - Volume 108 - Issue 2 - pp 295-302 doi: 10.1097/01.AOG.0000226862.78768.5c

51 Zhang J, Troendle JF, Yancey MK. Reassessing the labor curve in nulliparous women. *Am J Obstet Gynecol*. Oct 2002;187(4):824-8.

52 Trimmer, JD *Proceedings of the American Philosophical Society* 124, pp. 323–38 (1980), reprinted in *Quantum Theory and Measurement*, p. 152 (1983).

53 Kennedy WP. The Nocebo Reaction. *Med World* 1961;91:203-5;

54 Odent M. The Nocebo effect in prenatal care. *Primal Heath Research Newsletter* 1994; 2 (2).

55 Spenser, K.M. (2004) The primal touch of birth: Midwives Mothers and Massage. *Midwifery Today*. Issue 70. Summer 2004

56 Browne, J., Chandra, A. (2009) Slow Midwifery. *Journal of the Australian College of Midwives*. Volume 22, Issue 1, Pages 29-33 March

Water birth: a way of enhancing and promoting normality

Dianne Garland

How to enhance and promote normality?

First, let me begin with a quote:

You are a midwife…
You are helping at someone's birth.
Do good without show or fuss.
Facilitate what is happening rather than what you think ought to be happening.
If you must lead, lead so that the woman is still free and in charge.
When the baby is born the woman will rightly say: "We did this ourselves."[1]

The same words might apply to any caregiver, midwife, obstetrician, doula, doctor or other birth companion. The same concepts of facilitating and not leading are vital and sit very comfortably with the use of water.

In a more recent document, published in 2010, the Royal College of Midwives proposed their 'Campaign for Normal Birth' Top Ten Tips:[2]

- Wait and see.
- Build her a nest.
- Get her off the bed.
- Justify intervention.
- Listen to her.
- Keep a diary.
- Trust your intuition.
- Be a role model.
- Be positive.
- Promote skin-to-skin contact.

Whilst aimed at UK midwives who wish to enhance and promote normality, many of these 10 tips can be transferred to other countries. They are also relevant to the use of water during labour and birth but what are the precise implications for practice? In considering how water specifically can be used during labour and birth, I shall take a new professional document as my starting point: *Midwifery 2020: Delivering Expectations.* This report was commissioned by the Chief Nurses of the Health Departments of England, Northern Ireland, Scotland and Wales, written by the Midwifery 2020 UK Programme Board and published by the Nursing and Midwifery Council in 2010.[3]

I shall explore the six dimensions contained within the document and how they can relate to the use of water in today's maternity services. In so doing, I shall consider the use of water at home, in birth centres and in clinical hospital settings.

A report with a history and a purpose

To put this report into its historical context, it is useful to note that it is one more professional document which adds to the plethora of professional, government and consumer documents surrounding midwifery which have come out over the last few decades in the UK. These documents have had aspects of water birth included and they have either implicitly or explicitly supported water as a way to improve normality outcomes. As far back as 1992 the Winterton report and the subsequent Department of Health *Changing Childbirth* report promoted the use of water.[4,5] In fact, Winterton went so far as to write: "We recommend that all hospitals make their policy to make full provision, whenever possible, for women to choose the position that they prefer for labour and birth, with the option of a birthing pool where this is practicable." Since that date numerous other reports have been published in the UK[6-13]—but all of them appear to have failed to make 'water labour' and water birth accessible in all areas to all mothers. By the way, I shall refer to 'water labour' as well as 'water birth' because in many cases a woman may benefit from the use of water during her labour, but not wish to remain in the pool for the actual birth.

An interesting shift in perspective

Before considering the 'quality dimensions' included in the report, it is first of all interesting to note that parents' viewpoint on care is given a higher profile in this 2010 report than was previously the case. For many years practitioners and parents have written, discussed and highlighted the value they place on water labour and water birth. Meanwhile, however, it has often been only the few poor outcomes which have been reported in the press.[14-16] It seems that birth experience is finally being seen as important as a pure clinical outcome. This I deduce because *Midwifery 2020* states: "The success of maternity services should be measured in terms of actual and perceived safety, effectiveness of care and the experience of the woman and her partner... the six quality dimensions are factors to improve, increase and promote normality." It is interesting and encouraging that this report weighs perception as heavily as safety and effectiveness. After all, the quality of a woman's personal experience could arguably have an effect on bonding, as well as on longer term mental health.

It is interesting and encouraging that this report weighs perception as heavily as safety and effectiveness

The six quality dimensions

1. Person centredness

Women are entitled to choose to have a water labour and water birth, and if care is to be truly centred around the mother this option needs to discussed. The concepts of 'informed choice' and not 'informed compliance' (a contrast proposed by Mavis Kirkham at a talk in 2009)[17] highlight the issue as to whether mothers are really given all the pros and cons when using water. The benefits of using water as an analgesic are often not discussed with mothers who have a high BMI (body mass index), as these women are usually automatically excluded from using water. However, the buoyancy and mobility which water provides–it is easier to move around in water than on a bed–can really enhance a normal labour... Unfortunately, this important fact is not usually highlighted but I suggest it should be, even for women who are considered high risk. After all, it is very possible to 'risk assess' second stage options late in a woman's labour and, if it is thought to be necessary, the mother can leave the water and birth on dry land and thus use the 'normal' environment of gravity instead. There is even now some evidence supporting the use of water for mothers after a caesarean section birth[18-19] and for mothers with a Group B streptococcus infection[20]–two other groups of women who would traditionally have been excluded from using water.

Whenever women fulfil the safety criteria for a water birth, it is important that they are given the option to use a birthing pool whether they are planning to give birth in hospital, at a birth centre or at home. Currently in the UK there are many pool companies who have been working with the NHS to provide cheap options for mothers. Enlightened care providers (in the cities of Maidstone, Bradford and Sheffield,[21] for example) have started providing or hiring out pools to mothers who wish to have a home water birth.

Saving Mothers' Lives 2011–a confidential report into maternal deaths[22] states that as midwives we should act as advocates, but must establish boundaries between advocacy and collusion. This is interesting but should be placed within the nature of the report (maternal deaths)... As a midwife of 30 years, I do find it hard to understand why there are midwives who 'collude' with mothers and take actions which compromise the mothers' safety. I firmly believe that most caregivers do know boundaries for care. When difficulties arise in the UK we certainly have a robust system of support through risk management and the supervision of midwives.[23]

Water does offer challenges, though, and it is true that some mothers who seek this option are outside the 'normality criteria'. However, through my travels worldwide it has become apparent to me that while British criteria allow us to include most women in the UK, the situation is different in many other countries.

The benefits of using water are often not discussed with mothers with a high BMI... but it's easier to move around

Wherever we are based, it is certainly true that if care and water are to become person-centred, as caregivers we need to be realistic, honest and professional in the advice we offer and we need to allow the mother to make a truly informed choice for herself and her baby.

2.Safety

Several things need to be considered when offering the option of water. Whilst moving pools, handling them and infection control are important, what has all too often happened is that theses issues are placed as obstacles to using water. Often the appropriate equipment is not available due to the cost. In some centres managers have bought expensive mechanical hoists, while others have purchased lifting nets. Many consider the risks to be minimal, though, so do not purchase any supporting equipment. In fact, a robust risk assessment manager is likely to assess the risk as negligible.

Health and safety officers do need to consider how pools are placed, so as to ensure that midwives can support and facilitate each woman's labour and birth without ending up nursing a sore back afterwards, but it isn't necessary to buy a lot of expensive equipment. Risk is assessed based on the likelihood (or otherwise) of having to emergency evacuate a mother due to cardiac arrest (not fainting or haemorrhage). Assessing risk is, in fact, important because caregivers will often not offer water if they think that in an emergency they wouldn't be able to evacuate the mother. (This is why many birthing pools sit empty in hospitals.) The solution is to pre-empt any problems in the following ways:

- **In your place of work:** Review current practice. Do you already offer a low risk care pathway for VBAC mothers or are they continuously monitored, with a cannula in their hand and a less than positive attitude to outcome? What would the implications be if VBAC mothers were to use water for the first, second or third stages of labour, or for all three? Collaborate with colleagues so that all relevant personnel are involved in planning care and enhancing normality within the realms of safety and realism. In the case of all clients, review their notes before you speak to them.
- **With your clients:** Find out how your clients feel and–if they are positive about the idea of having a water labour and/or birth–find out what motivates them to use water. What has she read or heard about the pros and cons of water? If she is higher risk (e.g. if she has a high BMI) could she come and see the pool to ensure she would be able to get in and out of the pool unassisted? Does she have an ongoing condition or a problem linked to a previous labour or birth? Review medical records with the client and if she has an ongoing condition, ask her how it impacts on her daily life. What does she see as her responsibility in planning care?
- **Work with colleagues:** As soon as you have plans to introduce water birth, or have bought equipment, organise skills drills in your place of work. When I work with midwives we discuss room preparation (the importance of having the correct equipment available), as well as practical and clinical issues, e.g. how to carry out auscultation under water, how to deal with emergencies such as shoulder dystocia and postpartum haemorrhage and–if necessary–emergency evacuation.

Working with other health professionals (e.g. infection control staff, moving and handling personnel, and risk managers) you will be able to ensure that you have appropriate guidance, care pathways and professional advice to enable you to support a mother who wishes to use water. If there are issues, don't use them as an excuse not to offer water, but instead consider how you can find the resources to deal with the problem, and tap into the experience of other professionals. In this way, working through situations one by one, you will be able to further promote normality using water.

Working with other health professionals you will be able to ensure that you have appropriate guidance, care pathways and professional advice

While you are doing this, publicise any positive experiences you have. However hard we try as midwives, the media only seems to only publish negative stories about water birth. For example, in 2005 one newspaper reported a woman who'd sustained a knee injury and in 2009 there was an article which was generally unsupportive of water birth.[24,25] The positive outcomes and birth stories need to be highlighted so I would encourage you to write their stories for the local and national press and to encourage your new mothers (who have had a water labour or birth) to do the same. Surely then a more balanced impression will be made?

3. Effectiveness

Water is clearly a very effective way of promoting normality. Firstly, there is a great deal of audit surrounding the use of water to promote normality and as time has gone by more work has been published about mothers who do not fall within 'normality' criteria. Various researchers have reported shorter labours for mothers who used water.[26-28] This can be viewed from two perspectives. Firstly, there are clearly psychological benefits for mothers in having a shorter labour (although some longer labours do occur and are still within normal limits). Secondly, from a financial point of view water is certainly a relatively cheap form of pain relief. The psychological advantages can be appreciated in numerous birth stories by mothers[29] and the cost effectiveness of water as an analgesic is also emphasised in the literature.[30] For example, comparing water with epidural analgesia, although there are initial setup costs, when the equipment is available providing water is approximately eight times cheaper than drugs provided in an epidural pre-mixed bag. (Epidurals also involve associated costs, of course, such as CTG monitoring.) Clearly, water is extremely cheap when compared with an epidural. In fact, one pool manufacturer in the UK recently placed a full-page ad in the RCM *Midwives* journal which stated that while a water birth was likely to be costed at £700+, a caesarean section was likely to cost £1,370+. In the USA an uncomplicated hospital vaginal birth is said to cost around $8000 whereas an uncomplicated vaginal birth at home costs $3000—so even adding in the cost of a pool the difference in cost is apparent.[31]

A final aspect of water and effectiveness and one which many mothers use as a reason to use water is that it usually means a reduced need for pharmacological analgesics and a reduction in the number of interventions performed. In my own clinical practice of nearly 30 years (in which I have supported mothers with epidurals and all modes of intervention) I have seen that water can and does enhance physiological birth, by encouraging mobility and non-intervention. Of course, as with birth on dry land, masterly inactivity is always required on the part of the caregiver, with watchful waiting so as to assess any changes occurring during labour and the birth, and alterations in care or interventions only being used when absolutely necessary.

4. Efficiency

When considering whether or not to buy birthing pools, many caregivers wonder how many women choose to use them. Local, national and international uptake varies greatly and it is thought that it can be as low than 1% and as high as 80%. Why this huge discrepancy? My impression is that when caregivers promote the use of water rates of uptake are high, but when caregivers wait for a mother to ask for water the rates are low. It is vital that pregnant women are aware that water is available as an option, that they are aware of their caregivers' criteria for allowing their use, and also that they understand how available the pools are (taking into account the numbers of women in labour at any one time in a hospital environment). If only one pool is available it may not be realistic to expect a high uptake, so the challenge is then to obtain more pools—for use at home, in birth centres and in hospital. I challenge you to ensure that you know the water labour and water birth rates just as I suspect you are likely to know the epidural and caesarean rates. If they are low, or if your water birth facilities are not being used efficiently, I would also challenge you to consider how their use can be maximised.

5. Equity

This dimension highlights that as caregivers we need to include measures to ensure equity regardless of age, ethnicity, area of residence or socio-economic status. These issues are often emphasised, but I would like to stress how using water can promote normality for all women, even those who are otherwise often marginalised or inadequately provided for.

Consider this scenario... I meet a mother for the first time. At booking she is single, young, unemployed, has a high BMI and is non-Caucasian. She lives in one of the socio-economically deprived areas in which I work, which has a Sure Start scheme (i.e. it receives government financial support). I know this mother could be excluded from healthcare and that she may not usually interact with healthcare professionals, because it is likely she sees them as authoritarian and potentially disapproving of her lifestyle. By the way, this woman also smokes and takes recreational drugs. For her, the idea of going to hospital is daunting—hospitals are for sick people aren't they? (She tells me this at our first meeting.) She agrees to have bloods taken and a scan as she wants the best for her baby.

Then, just as she is about to leave she quietly says she would like to have a home birth. What action would we take as caregivers? Does she fall outside the 'criteria' for a home birth? How can we support her? How can we empower her to make informed decisions? The following is what I would propose:

- Individualise her care in a comfortable venue (e.g. in a small maternity unit or birth centre).
- Introduce her to some doulas so they can offer to provide her with support.
- Encourage her to attend a breastfeeding support group (e.g. one called 'Breastfeeding Buddies').
- Encourage her to attend young people's antenatal education classes with her boyfriend. (Tell her about classes which are run in her local community.)
- Ensure that all care is normalised, with home-based antenatal care, unless she needs to be referred (because of her high BMI).
- Plan her home birth with a homebirth team, using a birthing pool. (There is no cost involved if the homebirth team own the pool.)
- Explain to the woman various points about using a pool for labour and/or birth... Explain that the pool is great for pain relief and also that it'll help her move around. Explain to her that about half of labouring women leave the water for the actual birth and that this is normal. Tell her she may well benefit from gravity and from being in an upright position for the birth and that this is also perfectly normal.
- Discuss her care plan with midwifery team colleagues and explain the rationale for her choices.
- Document all actions taken and everything agreed.

I am aware that this fictional mother would be having many aspects of care that fall outside the normal care paradigm in many maternity care contexts. However, I believe that we have a duty to support this mother and in this case it means accommodating her dislike of hospitals; in a suitable environment I act as the woman's advocate and help her to voice her requests, planning a safe, realistic and professional care plan. This is in line with Centre for Maternal and Child Enquiries' (CMACE) report in 2011 which says: "Listen to the woman and act on what she tells you." It may be necessary to discuss certain possible adverse outcomes with mothers but worrying about these should not influence all care given.[32]

In summary, if we are to promote normality we need to engage with all types of parents, even those who do not fit neatly within our criteria of 'normality'. In the UK there are many caregivers who provide antenatal classes (including aquanatal, yoga-based water exercises) and there are many classes which target specific groups of mothers (e.g. teenagers, Jewish women, women who are preparing for a home birth). The caregivers who provide these classes work closely with both colleagues and consumer support groups. In the UK these are the NCT (the National Childbirth Trust), AIMS (the Association for Improvement in Maternity Services) and Doula UK. All these groups encourage mothers to obtain clear and consistent information, which does not provide an unbalanced view.

6. Timeliness

Water can assist midwives in gaining or even regaining traditional watchful skills and therefore gauging successfully how things are progressing in terms of time. Sitting and interacting, watching the nature of the labour, being a master of inactivity[33] and being positive,[34] a midwife can be intuitively aware of the subtle changes occurring in labour. Basic observations of care—temperature, pulse, respiration and blood pressure—would appear to be fundamental to good standards of care and this is recognised in CMACE 2011.[35] When caring for women who may fall outside low risk criteria (for example, women wanting a VBAC, women with a high BMI or GBS, etc) these observations are even more vital since they may indicate a change or deviation which requires immediate professional intervention. If we know what has been normal for that mother then changes—however subtle—should be apparent. The watchful, skilled caregiver will be astutely aware of change and this skill means that any caregivers who support a mother using water, particularly when outside 'normality criteria', should themselves feel educated and supported. I do not believe that we should undervalue the caregiver's perception or intuition regarding care of women and babies. Indeed, when discussing normality in terms of time factors, it would be wrong not to mention the issue of sharing and support through clinical governance. The seven pillars of clinical governance can all be utilised to ensure that we as caregivers support mothers with the choice of using water.[36] [For readers not familiar with these 'seven pillars' they are as follows: 1. clinical effectiveness and research, 2. audit, 3. risk management, 4. education and training, 5. patient and public involvement, 6. using information and IT, and 7. staffing and staff management.] The specific areas that I believe are invaluable are, multi-professional working and guidelines for care (both of which are especially important for higher risk mothers), patient/public involvement (perhaps via media coverage, amongst other methods) and auditing (i.e. keeping records and publishing results)—this last 'pillar' again being especially important when supporting higher risk mothers and ensuring that 'timely' action is taken, or not taken, as appropriate in any one woman's case.

Women's experience and satisfaction with their care

Looking at water from any and all of these six dimensions it is easy to see how using water for labour and/or birth can enhance women's experience and increase their satisfaction levels with the care they receive—and also enhance and promote normality. Given this, and the fact that many caregivers are as yet not using water as a means of improving women's experience and satisfaction with care, when successful water labours and births take place, women should be encouraged to publicise their experience, perhaps by contacting the media.[37,38]

Women should also be encouraged to inform their healthcare providers of their satisfaction or not with the service they have received. This is not about encouraging complaints but about highlighting to other caregivers what—from a woman's point of view—would really enhance care for other women in the future. Hundreds of consumer websites exist where mothers can write about experiences and ask questions,[39] but how often do we as professionals read those comments and questions? Perhaps now it's time we started doing that...

Let's find out what mothers believe enhances their labours.

With nearly 28 years of waterbirth experience, I know what I believe: promoting normality takes time but it really can be done with the right time, place, people, support and audit–and perhaps also a little water to help!

Dianne Garland has been a midwife since 1983 and has taught about water birth since 1989. Her work has taken her all over the world, from Australia to China and the United States. In the past she was involved in various government projects and on advisory panels (e.g. for RCM, RCOG and MIDIRS); she also developed an acupuncture service plan for maternity, worked closely with companies to design waterbirth equipment (e.g. the first underwater Sonicaid). Dianne now works as an expert witness, university lecturer and maintains her clinical skills on a midwife-led and consultant unit at a local hospital. In 2005 Dianne became freelance to expand these roles within her company www.midwifeexpert.com. Her newest role is as a trustee to APEC (Action on Pre-Eclampsia). She has written numerous articles and the book *Revisiting Waterbirth–an Attitude to Care* (2nd ed, Palgrave, 2010).

References

1 This is from the *Tao Te Ching* reputedly written by Lao Tzu (a contemporary of Confucius) in the 6th century BC.

2 Royal College of Midwives, Campaign for Normal Birth. Ten top tips. London RCM 2010.

3 Nursing & Midwifery Council. *Midwifery 2020: Delivering expectations*. London NMC, 2010.

4 Winterton Report. House of Commons Health Committee. Second report–*Maternity Services*. London HMSO, 1992.

5 Department of Health. *Changing Childbirth*. London HMSO, 1993.

6 Department of Health. *National Service Framework for Children, Young People and Maternity Services*. London: Department of Health, 2004.

7 Department of Health. *Maternity Matters: Choice, Access and Continuity of Care in a Safe Service*. London, Department of Health, 2007.

8 Department of Health. *High Quality Care for All*. London, Department of Health, 2008.

9 Royal College of Obstetricians and Royal College of Midwives. Immersion *in Water during Labour and Birth*. London, 2006.

10 Royal College of Midwives, Campaign for Normal Birth. Masterly inactivity. London RCM, 2006.

11 Royal College of Midwives, Royal College of Obstetricians and National Childbirth Trust. *Making Normal Birth a Reality*. London: MCWP, 2007.

12 National Institute for Health and Clinical Excellence. *Intrapartum Care*. London, 2007.

13 Healthcare Commission. *Towards Better Birth*. London, 2008.

14 Ahmed MA, Patel AD. Bilateral neuropraxia of the common peroneal nerve following water birth delivery. *Science Direct*. November 28, 2005.

15 Kassim Z, Sellars M, Greenough A. Underwater birth and neonatal respiratory distress. *British Medical Journal*, 330 pp 10-71—May 27, 2005.

16 Tuteur A. What's in the water at waterbirth? Available from: www.sciencebasedmedicine.org [accessed Nov 19, 2009].

17 Kirham M, 2009. Home birth conference, Chichester UK.

18 Sellar M. The VBAC experience in Fife. *Midwives*, Aug/Sept, pp 18-19, 2008.

19 Garland D. Is waterbirth a safe and realistic option for mothers following a previous LSCS? *MIDIRS Midwifery Digest*, 16 (2) 2006.

20 Zanetti-Dallenbach R, Lapaire A, Maertans R, Frei W, Hosli I. Waterbirth: is the water an additional reservoir for group B streptococcus? *Archives of Gynaecology and Obstetrics*, 273 pp 236-238, 2006.

21 Barnes Dresner H. The development of the Sheffield home birth pools scheme. *Essentially MIDIRS*, Vol.2 No 2, 2011 pp 47-49.

22 Centre for Maternal and Child Enquiries (CMACE). *Saving Mothers' Lives*, 2011. See http://www.cemach.org.uk/Publications-Press-Releases/Press-Releases/cmace-release-saving-mothers-lives-report.aspx [accessed 31 March 2011].

23 Nursing & Midwifery Council. Standards *for the Preparation and Practice of Supervisors*. London: NMC, 2006.

24 Ahmed MA, Patel AD. Bilateral neuropraxia of the common peroneal nerve following water birth delivery. *Science Direct*. November 28, 2005.

25 Tuteur A. What's in the water at waterbirth? Available from: ww.sciencebasedmedicine.org [accessed Nov 19, 2009].

26 Geissbuehler V, Stein S, Eberhard J. Waterbirths compared with landbirths: an observational study of nine years. *Journal of Perinatal Medicine*, 32 pp 308-14 2004.

27 Thoeni N, Zech N, Moroder L, Ploner F. Review of 1600 waterbirths: does waterbirth increase the risk of neonatal infection? *Journal of Maternal, Fetal and Neonatal Medicine*. 17 (5) May pp 357-361 2005.

28 Garland D. Is waterbirth a safe and realistic option for mothers following a previous LSCS? *MIDIRS Midwifery Digest*, 16 (2) 2006.

29 Donna S. *Birth: Countdown to Optimal* (2nd ed). Fresh Heart Publishing, 2011.

30 Garland D. Revisiting waterbirth and attitude to care. 2010, Palgrave Macmillan.

31 RCM *Midwives*. Issue 2, page 13, 2011.

32 CMACE *Saving Mothers' Lives*. 2011.

33 Royal College of Midwives, Campaign for Normal Birth. Masterly inactivity. London: RCM, 2006.

34 Tuteur A. What's in the water at waterbirth? Available from: ww.sciencebasedmedicine.org [accessed Nov 19, 2009].

35 CMACE *Saving Mothers' Lives*. 2011.

36 Scally G, Donaldson LJ. Clinical governance and the drive for quality improvement in the new HNS in England. *British Medical Journal*, 317 (7150) 4 July pp 61- 65 1998.

37 Bailey A. Enoch's home waterbirth after four c-sections. *Midwifery Today*. Spring, pp 14-5, 2009.

38 Craig R. Birth from the other side. *Midwifery Matters*, 124, Spring pp 10-12, 2010.

39 For example www.mumsnet.com or www.thebabywebsite.com.

New to using birthing pools?

Sylvie Donna

Here are some tips based on discussions I've had with various caregivers about using water in labour and/or birth. As you'll see, some are fairly self-evident, some less so... My aim is to give you some ideas for solving practical and safety issues if you are hesitant about the whole idea of water, as yet.

- ♥ If you don't already have them available in your place of work, liaise with other professionals who have set up pools and discuss how they went about it. Can two small rooms be set aside especially for the use of birthing pools?
- ♥ Explore equipment available. For example, as well as exploring pool designs, look into buying plastic birthing stools for use next to the pool, find out what birthing mats are available—and consider buying a waterproof Sonicaid for discrete auscultation during all parts of labour. Other equipment you might want to have available might include underwater torches, scoops and angled mirrors, specially designed for water births. (For general equipment see www.1cascade.com; for waterproof Sonicaids go to www.huntleigh-diagnostics.com; for emergency hoists see www.silvalealtd.co.uk and for angled mirrors see www.kentmidwiferypractice.co.uk.)
- ♥ Consider what other non-technical equipment or supplies might make the woman feel as comfortable as possible while labouring in water. For example, she may well appreciate having a big sponge, foam, pad or a folded towel to kneel on underwater, or when she gets out at any point. Also consider colours...
- ♥ Explore timings which work best physiologically. Some caregivers save water for active labour because they have observed that when women get into the water early on the effect is to slow down labour. When women get in later (after 5cm dilation), on the other hand, they've observed that water usually facilitates dilation—and is an even better appreciated form of non-pharmacological pain relief. Of course, research still needs to be done on this area.
- ♥ Ensure the temperature of the water is kept at a safe level. According to NICE clinical guidelines for intrapartum care: "the temperature of the woman and the water should be monitored hourly to ensure that the woman is comfortable and not becoming pyrexial. The temperature of the water should not be above 37.5°C."
- ♥ For information on other issues you could explore www.waterbirth.org—and the following article available online has excellent references for follow-up too: http://www.midwifery.org.uk/index.php?option=com_content&view=article&id=61:waterbirth-is-it-a-real-choice&catid=40:magazine-autumn-2009&Itemid=63.
- ♥ If a birthing pool is not available, why not encourage women to use an ordinary warm bath as a small birthing pool, if only for a few moments late on in labour? This will surely soften her perineum (just as hot compresses would), and therefore help her perineum stretch more easily for the birth itself.

pause to think and talk...

...about birthing pools

1 Do you have any experience of using water—either personally, or with clients in labour? If you do have some experience was this positive or negative? What, if anything, would you do differently next time?

2 How many different designs of birthing pool have you seen and/or tried out? How much equipment have you seen, which you have either used or would think useful?

3 Do you have any concerns about having your labouring clients use water? How do you think these might be addressed?

4 Has a pregnant woman ever asked you for a water birth? If yes, how did you respond? If no, how would you respond? How *could* you respond?

5 How do you feel about attending women who are using baths or paddling pools instead of custom-designed birthing pools? Are there any important differences and, if so, what are they?

6 What is your own view on timing of entry into warm water, whether a labouring woman is using a bath, paddling pool or custom-designed birthing pool? Have you ever witnessed a labour slowing down as a result of a woman getting into water? Have you ever seen a woman suddenly make progress soon after entering warm water? What have you observed in terms of timing? Have you done a systematic audit of what you have seen?

7 To what extent do you think women should be able to *choose* when they get into water and also when they get out? Do you differentiate between water labour and water birth—and are you happy for women to give birth in water?

8 Do you ever get into the water with a woman, or would you consider doing this? Do you encourage/allow partners and/or doulas to get in the water with the labouring/birthing woman? Why/why not?

9 What kinds of protocols do you think are important to ensure good hygiene? What do you do if/when faeces appears in the water? Should you be concerned or not, in your view?

10 How do you estimate blood loss at the moment of birth and afterwards if the woman remains in the water?

11 Do you have any concerns about women remaining in the water after they've given birth with their new baby? How do you ensure that the baby is safe and maintains his/her body heat?

12 How many birthing pools should a maternity unit ideally have, in your view?

13 Are you happy to attend women using birthing pools in their own homes?

14 What kind of preparation do you encourage?

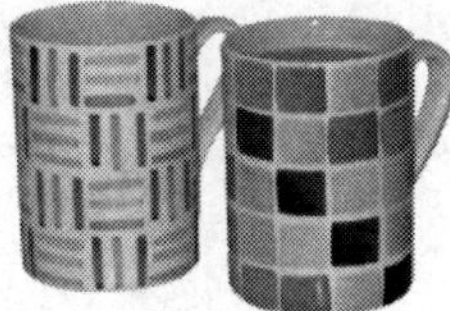

Home birth from one midwife's perspective

Valerie Bader

After nearly 13 years of practising midwifery in hospital and clinic settings, I had the opportunity to serve women who choose out-of-hospital birth. Though I fought transitioning to an out-of-hospital setting for years, I find myself completely converted to a preference for home and birth centre birth. When I began practising midwifery, I wanted to offer care for childbearing women which included medical interventions when necessary. I found that when working in the hospital setting, many of the midwives and consultants are uncomfortable allowing women to labour naturally. There is tremendous political pressure to have labour proceed quickly and have women anaesthetised. After I had the opportunity to observe an out-of-hospital birth I realised this was the setting where I belonged. I love the peacefulness of birth in an out-of-hospital setting and I enjoy being able to focus strictly on caring for the childbearing family without the political pressure to intervene unnecessarily. In the following passages I describe my homebirth practice with attention to protocols, safety, equipment, and the processes of care.

I fought transitioning to an out-of-hospital setting for years, I find myself completely converted to a preference for home and birth centre birth

Surprisingly, antenatal care proceeds similarly for women who choose out-of-hospital or hospital birth. In out-of-hospital birth, antenatal appointments last nearly twice as long (roughly an hour), and family members are included. Care begins when the woman finds she is pregnant and makes an appointment with a midwife in our practice. Factors that may exclude women from our care include: multiple gestation; substance abuse; living too far from a hospital that provides obstetric care; insulin dependent diabetes; essential hypertension; and a high likelihood that the infant would be better served being born in a hospital, usually due to a congenital abnormality. We discuss the benefits and risks of an early dating ultrasound scan, and we offer routine antenatal laboratory screening tests. Dietary habits are discussed, exercise is encouraged, and substance abuse is discouraged. We encourage antenatal vitamins, and possibly iron or calcium supplementation, depending on the client's dietary habits. Good dental hygiene is encouraged. Then, we proceed with monthly antenatal appointments until 28 weeks, bi-weekly appointments until 36 weeks, and weekly appointments after that until delivery. All in all, care is similar, although more time is spent with women at each antenatal appointment.

Surprisingly, antenatal care proceeds similarly

All of our clients are encouraged to take childbirth preparation classes, which we offer at our clinic. Classes meet six consecutive weeks, for two hours each time. One of the midwives in our practice is the instructor and the course content emphasises support and non-pharmacological pain relief in an out-of-hospital setting. During the classes participants learn about normal labour and birth, practise yoga poses to relieve stress, experience deep relaxation, and discuss risks unique to out-of-hospital birth. The final class is devoted to a discussion of breastfeeding and babycare. Not only does the content of the classes benefit participants, but the opportunity to meet like-minded families choosing out-of-hospital birth is also beneficial.

Participants learn about normal labour and birth, practise yoga poses to relieve stress, experience deep relaxation, and discuss risks unique to out-of-hospital birth

One of the non-pharmacological pain relief methods discussed at length in our childbirth classes is water birth. Our practice owns three re-usable inflatable pools and these are hired out to women who choose to use them. We discuss mechanical details such as: where to put the pool in the house, how to connect a hose to your indoor tap, how to use the air pump to inflate the pool, and how to use a water pump to get water out of the pool. We encourage women to consider water birth because of the impressive pain relief women achieve when submersed in warm water. We recommend a water temperature of 92 degrees Fahrenheit (33 degrees Centigrade) at the time of birth, so the baby doesn't get too cool. Women choosing to rent one of our inflatable pools take the pool home at about 38 weeks and we bring the pool back to the storage site when the birth has occurred.

One aspect of antenatal care that is very different for a woman choosing home birth is the 'home visit' at 36 weeks. Many women are anxious that their house will not 'measure up'. We assure them that we aren't visiting to pass judgement on their housekeeping, but merely to be sure we can find their home if it's dark when we arrive. During the visit we conduct routine antenatal surveillance and advise the woman and her partner of a strategic location for the inflatable pool. We may also determine whether the home's existing bathtub is large enough. I tell families that I need to have enough room to get in the bath with the mother, should the need arise. Finally, we determine where the washing machine and tumble dryer are so we can begin to wash the towels used during the birth before we leave the home, after the birth.

Women are anxious that their house will not 'measure up'. We assure them we aren't going to pass judgement on their housekeeping, but merely to be sure we can find their home.

We advise families that they should live no more than 30 minutes from a hospital that provides obstetric care

We advise families that they should live no more than 30 minutes from a hospital that provides obstetric care, should an emergency arise. At the 36-week home visit, we review the birth plan the woman and her partner have prepared regarding their preferences for their care during a normal birth and should unanticipated problems arise. We ask the woman which hospital she would prefer to be transferred to, should the need arise, and request that they keep that phone number readily available when in labour. Finally, we review with the woman when she should call us for signs and symptoms of labour onset. We like to know when women believe they are in early labour, although we may not go to the home immediately. Our goal is to arrive at the home when the woman is in active labour, or when contractions are five minutes apart for an hour and uncomfortable. We also request that women notify us whether or not they are in labour if they believe their membranes have ruptured.

Upon arrival at the home of a woman in active labour, I ask fairly typical assessment questions. When did labour start? Are the contractions becoming more intense? Can you feel your baby moving? When was the last time you ate, drank, and urinated? Have your membranes ruptured? I also obtain the woman's blood pressure and use a Sonicaid to check the fetal heart rate for a full minute, before, during and after a contraction. I usually wait at least an hour before evaluating cervical dilation, effacement, and fetal station. The purpose in delaying the vaginal exam is to assess how well the woman is coping with labour, estimate the phase of labour from her behaviour, and see if her contraction pattern intensifies. I often find the contractions intensify after the midwife arrives.

When I arrive at the home of a labouring woman, I bring with me a small suitcase full of equipment and an oxygen tank. In the suitcase I have standard items used in any setting for a birth: a Sonicaid, gel, measuring tape, blood pressure cuff, stethoscope, syntocinon vials and misoprostol tablets to treat postpartum haemorrhage, oral and intramuscular Vitamin K and erythromycin ointment for the ophthalmic prophylaxis. I have additional supplies for the baby: a haemostat clamp, umbilical tape and scissors. The family supplies blankets, hats, and nappies for the baby. We use the oven set at 200 degrees Fahrenheit (93.3 degrees Centigrade, less than Gas Mark ¼—i.e. only just turned on) to warm towels and blankets for the baby. I also have a self-inflating resuscitation bag for neonatal resuscitation that can be connected to the oxygen supply. Other emergency equipment I bring includes: an oxygen mask for the mother; intravenous fluids; intravenous catheters; and, blood drawing equipment. Supplies for the placenta include: a large bowl (provided by the family) and two plastic bags to put the placenta in. Finally, I bring the supplies necessary for suturing a perineal laceration: anaesthetic, syringes, suture, needle holder, and scissors.

We like to know when women believe they are in early labour, though we may not go to the home immediately

The midwife who goes to the home when the woman calls and says she is in active labour calls a second midwife to be present as the second stage approaches. The second midwife stays until the baby and placenta have delivered and the woman and baby are stable. We allow the second and third stage of labour to proceed physiologically. Women bear down to push as their body indicates. After the birth of the baby, we wait until the mother has the urge to push out her placenta. Our first choice for encouraging placental delivery and minimal postpartum bleeding is to have the mother begin to breastfeed the baby as soon as the baby indicates readiness. If bleeding is heavy after the placenta delivers, we may administer intramuscular syntocinon. Once the placenta has delivered, the baby has breastfed, and any lacerations have been sutured, we complete a thorough examination of the newborn and help the mother bathe and urinate so that she can rest. The woman who has just given birth is also encouraged to eat and drink in the postpartum period. Finally, the paperwork must be completed.

We stay at the home after a birth for at least two hours. Sleep descends on the baby and the mother just before we leave. We return to examine the mother and the newborn within 24 hours. New parents are instructed to call us with concerns about the newborn, including any respiratory or feeding difficulty. Additional home visits may be necessary prior to a clinic visit at one week depending on the status of the mother and the newborn. Our postpartum and newborn care continues until six weeks after the delivery. We see the mother and baby again at two weeks postpartum, one month postpartum, and six weeks postpartum. These visits include screening for problems, a physical exam of the mother and infant and usually counselling on how to cope with fatigue. We advise parents to have their newborn seen by a doctor at three weeks of life, to establish care. Once postpartum care has concluded, women can seek their well-woman care and family planning services from our practice, as well.

Numerous scientific papers and professional organisations support the safety of home birth

Numerous scientific papers and professional organisations support the safety of home birth. While not all women want to or should give birth at home, those who desire home birth deserve the support of caregivers. It is my sincere pleasure to work with these families who desire excellent care and who work hard to provide a peaceful birth for their child.

Valerie Bader is an instructor of clinical nursing at the University of Missouri. Her thesis for her Masters in Nursing focused on postpartum depression. She is a doctoral candidate at the University of Missouri, Kansas City, where she is studying sexuality education and unintended pregnancy. She practises midwifery in Columbia Missouri and attends home births. She attributes her satisfaction in life to her life partner, Eric Bader, her two children, inspiring nursing students, her sister midwives, and the families bearing children that she works for.

Promoting VBAC—reasons to encourage women to consider a VBAC and ways of helping them to achieve one

Hélène Vadeboncoeur

Who would have thought that in the last quarter of the 20th century having a caesarean would become commonplace for women expecting a child, in so many regions and countries of the world? It's hard to believe that so many women really need a caesarean... Could it be that at least 40% of Italian, Chinese, Mexican and Brazilian women can't give birth? Could it be that it is necessary surgery for a third of the American and Australian women who give birth each year and for 25% of British and Canadian pregnant women?[1]

How come this operation—which used to only be carried out when the life of either the mother or baby was endangered—has become another way of giving birth? It would take a whole chapter to reflect on this. Let's just say that a lot has to do with non-medical factors and that women nowadays are not necessarily less able to give birth than they have been for millennia. Happily, more and more maternal and health organisations, including some medical associations,[2] are becoming worried about the ever-increasing caesarean rates. According to recent studies carried out by the World Health Organization,[3] when caesarean rates climb beyond 15%, this operation is likely to present fewer benefits and more risks for mothers and babies. It can also lead to unnecessary maternal deaths, as implied by the rising maternal mortality rate in the USA, which has risen recently for the first time in decades.[4] Meanwhile, one large study has shown that, after more restrictive VBAC medical guidelines, diminishing VBAC rates have not lowered maternal and neonatal mortality rates.[5]

The caesarean—the surgery most commonly performed on women in the USA—has been trivialised in the last few decades. There was a time when doctors were obliged to explain why they had carried out each caesarean they performed. Not any more, though—except, perhaps, in hospital audits within studies which are carried out with the hope of exploring how to decrease caesarean rates, like the QUARISMA randomised controlled trial in Canada.[6] So why has this operation been trivialised? Not only does having a caesarean have an impact on women and babies' health, it is also more expensive than a vaginal birth. And for many women, it can be a devastating experience on an emotional level. By contrast, having a VBAC is generally better for women for many reasons, relating not only to risk and to the experience of birth itself, but also to postnatal recovery.

Having a VBAC is generally better for women...

For all these reasons, it would seem important to encourage women *not* to have a caesarean, not only the first time, but particularly when a woman has had one or more caesareans in the past, and is pregnant again. It is therefore important that you, as a midwife, doctor, obstetrician, nurse or doula, help women to consider the possibility of giving birth normally after a caesarean (of having a 'vaginal birth after caesarean'—a VBAC), and that you help them to optimise their chances of going through with it.

But first, let's take a look at your own attitudes in relation to VBAC. Your own attitudes may be important because caregivers will inevitably influence women's choices and affect their levels of success. Consider the following questions:

- How do you feel about helping women reach a decision and supporting them if they opt for a VBAC? Are you comfortable about doing this?
- Are you hesitant about supporting VBAC requests because of a difficult event you witnessed in the past—such as a uterine rupture?
- Do you have trouble with the idea of supporting a homebirth VBAC?
- Are you familiar with all the research relating to the safety of VBACs?

When considering these questions, you need to take all your feelings and experience into account. If you think that VBAC is important, in theory, but have difficulty in reality, for whatever reason, in supporting women to achieve a normal birth, it may be a good idea to refer your clients to someone who is not afraid of VBAC. Of course, another approach would be to change your perceptions and deal with your own fears... You might be able to achieve this by informing yourself about VBAC, perhaps by reading my book *Birthing Normally After A Caesarean or Two* (Fresh Heart, 2011), by talking to colleagues who are more at ease with it, or by witnessing the incredible joy that most women experience when completing a VBAC. In the end you ultimately have to respect yourself and your feelings about VBAC... However, I hope that this chapter will help you to maintain or acquire a positive outlook about this very normal way of giving birth.

Reasons to encourage women to consider a VBAC...

Reason No. 1:

A caesarean can have a devastating impact on women[7]

Many people underestimate the impact that giving birth has on women. Depending on what types of service you provide to women and what time in the childbearing year you meet clients, you may not necessarily see women again, after the baby's birth, or you may just see them for a brief medical visit. Also, it may take a while (months or years) for women who had a difficult birth experience to 'digest' it, and even to realise the emotional impact it had on them. And people around the new mother may also not always understand the sadness, anger or trauma a woman may experience after a caesarean. Family, friends, and sometimes caregivers tell new mothers: "Your baby is healthy. You're fine... Forget the birth and move on!" And the woman herself is left with emotions and feelings she can't talk to anyone about, and sometimes this may lead to depression. Or she may have signs of trauma (recurrent nightmares, obsession with what happened, avoidance of anything that has to do with the event, a tendency towards hypervigilance, etc), which can undermine the start of her relationship with her baby, make things difficult with her partner, and also, if unrecognised and untreated, lead to depression.[8]

People around the mother may not always understand

Reason No. 2:

VBAC is now supported by health authorities

Surprisingly, perhaps, after a long period of public debate in North America (dating back to the 1980s), VBAC has now been accepted by official bodies. In Europe, several decades ago VBAC was such an expected and commonplace event that there was no special name for it. In North America, by contrast, after decades of a 'no-VBAC' policy that started in the 1910s, VBAC rates starting rising at the beginning of the 1980s (while caesarean rates were diminishing), with the support of medical associations. And then, from 1997 onwards, VBAC rates started diminishing steadily. To make matters worse, the increasingly common practice of inducing labours which were planned VBACs, especially with prostaglandins to soften the cervix, led to more uterine ruptures, which gave both caregivers and pregnant women the impression that VBAC had become more dangerous.[9] Nevertheless, professional associations or health organisations are now again supporting VBAC to various degrees: RCOG and NICE in the UK, ACOG, AAFP and ACNM in the USA, SOGC in Canada, and midwives associations such as the Quebec College of Midwives, in Canada, who recently adopted progressive guidelines on VBAC.[10]

Reason No. 3:

The risk of uterine rupture is low

The fact is, that since the first studies on VBAC, the risk of uterine rupture—in a spontaneous (uninduced) VBAC—has not changed much. Some studies[11] mention that the risk ranges from 0.2% to 0.6% (i.e. 2 to 6 women per 1,000); the first consensus conference on VBAC (held in 2010 by the National Institutes of Health in the USA) evaluated it at being between 0.3% and 0.7%.[12] Of the few women who do experience uterine rupture, 5% or 6% of the babies involved in the event are seriously affected. This does not amount to a higher risk of death than for any baby during any other first pregnancy (according to the NIH).[13]

The risk of uterine rupture is low

While the risk of rupture has not changed, the knowledge about what increases that risk has now grown enormously, compared to 20 to 30 years ago, and we have a much better understanding about what lowers the risk and on what influences a woman's chances of completing a VBAC, or not. Therefore, as caregivers, you are better equipped today to help women decide, to advise them and to help them prepare for a VBAC that ever before, if only you have the necessary information at your fingertips.

Reason No. 4:

Some women have trouble organising a VBAC

It's a sad fact that not all women have easy access to VBAC. In certain countries, with some doctors, or midwives, or in some birth centres and hospitals, it may not be easy for women who want a VBAC to get permission to attempt one. For instance, in the USA, after ACOG modified its guidelines in a more restrictive way in 1999 and again in 2004, 300 hospitals had banned VBAC by 2005. So maybe the hospital your client is considering did that and has not yet revised its policies, or adjusted completely to the new ACOG and NIH guidelines, based on research. Therefore, if you can help women get the VBAC they want, you may make the difference between a woman *being able* to have a VBAC and *not being able* to have one.

Ways of supporting women

Note: For this section and the next one, you will find more information in Chapters 5 and 6 of my book Birthing Normally After A Caesarean or Two (Fresh Heart Publishing, 2011). You will also find more references in those chapters.

If a woman is having difficulty getting support, you can help a woman find another hospital (or birth centre), or a supportive caregiver, either within the institution where you work or nearby. If you are qualified to do so, you could of course offer to be her caregiver yourself. Alternatively, if your client has been refused a VBAC because of a doctor's preference, you could help her to get a second opinion on this, or even help her request a change in her hospital's VBAC policy, or register a formal complaint.

In a case where caregivers are offering a woman the opportunity of a VBAC and the woman herself is refusing, you may also be able to help. You need to be aware that a woman's refusal may be caused by various reasons, including the fact that, in our society, we live in increasing fear of labour and birth[14] and the fact that there is a lack of information about the risks of a caesarean. The evidence-based organisation Childbirth Connection has reacted by publishing *What Every Woman Should Know About Cesarean Section* (see www.childbirth connection.org/article.asp?ck=10210). A woman who previously had a very difficult birth may be too afraid of the risk (in her view) of having another one. She may have heard horrific stories around birth. Although it is perfectly legitimate for a woman like this to refuse a VBAC, when offered one, she might later retrospectively appreciate it if you explore with her why she is refusing to attempt a VBAC and, if appropriate, offer her some form of assistance. In the end, though, of course you need to remember that it is your client's choice and that having an elective caesarean may be the best option for some women.

You can also offer support in a case where a VBAC ends up being another caesarean, which will sometimes happen. This occurs usually because labour stops, or because forceps does not work, or because the baby's heartbeat becomes worrying. It is rarely due to a uterine rupture... In cases like this you will find that, often, it is the first time this client has experienced labour and she is happy to have tried and to know what labour feels like. Other clients may be more difficult to support because, for them, a lot of meaning has become attached to giving birth and when they don't achieve their goal, it is hard to bear. You can be helpful in listening to them, by expressing empathy, by directing them to needed resources, etc, and, eventually, if appropriate, informing them that a VBAC after two caesareans is indeed a possibility.

Women's families, caregivers and the institutions in which they work are influenced by our society's attitude

Mostly, you are likely to need to provide help and support during the antenatal period, i.e. offering information to clients considering a VBAC and doing everything else that entails. By this, I mean that since we live in a technologically-oriented society, where birth is medicalised, not only 'patients' (pregnant women), but also their families, their caregivers and the institutions where women give birth are influenced. The consequence of this is that helping a woman to consider having a VBAC will not just be a matter of providing information, but also of providing emotional support. Women who have had one or more caesareans need to understand what happened; they need to express how they felt during their previous births and how they have been feeling since; they need to have an accurate picture of what a VBAC *and* another caesarean would entail, in terms of both risks and advantages at the time of the birth and also postnatally. They need to be reassured that it's not crazy to want to give birth. They need to be able to work out where they stand as regards VBAC and how their own circumstances can influence their particular situation. You need to be help them take into account their own values and needs so as to help them reach a decision, not only about the VBAC itself, but also about where to give birth. They need to know that the caregivers that will take care of them and support them during the birth are knowledgeable about VBAC, that they will know how to recognise signs of danger and—most importantly—that, if necessary, they will react adequately. They probably also need to increase their confidence in their own capacity to give birth, and realise that if other women have done it, they can do it too.

Finally, they need to know that they have the right to decide how and where to give birth, as well as the right to give their informed consent or refusal when any interventions are proposed to them.

When women are making a decision, you need to tell them that...

- Most women can give birth after a caesarean. On average, 75% of women succeed in completing a VBAC. This percentage is higher in institutions where midwives are the primary caregivers.[15]
- There are very few contraindications to VBAC—the only one being having previously had what is called a 'classical' incision (i.e. a vertical incision in the upper part of the uterus). Most women have a low transverse incision, which allows for a VBAC. Another contraindication to VBAC may be uterine surgery, but not everyone agrees that this is a contraindication.
- Induction raises the risk of uterine rupture, particularly when prostaglandins are used to soften the woman's cervix.

You also need to tell your clients that...

- A caesarean really is surgery and, as such, it involves risks which are not lower than those associated with a VBAC. In fact, women need to understand that there are more risks associated with having a repeat caesarean. It presents an increased risk of death for the mother and it is not a risk-free procedure for the baby. Women also need to understand that the more caesareans they have, the more complications are likely in future pregnancies, which might affect not only the women themselves, but also their babies while they are in the womb.[16]

Finally, your clients need to understand that a VBAC offers several scientifically proven benefits for both mother and baby, especially regarding the baby's readiness to adapt to life outside the womb[17] and the bonding which occurs between mother and baby,[18] apart from the fact that it can change a woman's life and immensely increase her self-esteem. It may help her heal the emotional scar left by her caesarean(s). Having a VBAC will help the mother avoid the risks that any abdominal surgery presents, including a higher risk of death, it will mean blood transfusions are less likely, it means a lower risk of needing a hysterectomy and will mean the risk of fewer complications, such as infection. Having a VBAC will make the woman feel more in control of what happens and more part of the decision-making process, so is bound to be a more positive experience. A VBAC will help the woman to breastfeed successfully and it will mean that it is easier for the woman to bond with her baby. The baby will be less likely to suffer respiratory distress (because labour helps the baby's body prepare itself for life outside the womb) and the risk of death will also be lower. Finally, women considering whether or not to have a VBAC need to be aware that having a normal birth makes it easier for a new person to come into a family (because life is far easier postnatally) and also that giving birth normally can be a joyous and rewarding moment for everyone involved, particularly the woman who gives birth.

Your clients need to understand that a VBAC offers scientifically proven benefits for mother and baby

When women have decided on a VBAC and you are supporting them during their pregnancy...

- Some women may need your help coming to terms with their caesarean(s). They will need to understand what happened (so it will be helpful for you to see their medical notes) and they will need you to listen to them talking about how they feel. They will need to have their feelings validated and you may also have to refer them to other places so that they can receive further support. In short, you will need to help women heal emotionally from their previous caesarean(s).
- Women who have had one or more caesareans will need you to help them evaluate where they stand on the VBAC 'risk-scale'. Knowing the degree of risk their VBAC presents may also help women make more specific decisions accordingly (e.g. place of birth). Studies have shown, for instance, that several factors may play a role: the circumstances linked to a woman's previous caesarean(s), her present characteristics and situation, what happens during her pregnancy, and what happens during her VBAC. For instance, having an interval between a caesarean and a VBAC of more than 18-24 months reduces the risk of uterine rupture,[19] as does having a soft cervix at the beginning of labour.[20] Having had two caesareans, a single-layer uterine suture, and having conceived the baby shortly after the caesarean are additional factors of risk. On the contrary, having had one caesarean, a double-layer uterine suture and an interval of two years between the caesarean and the next due date are protective factors (i.e. these things lower the risk). Having a clearer idea of risk level can help women decide, for example, whether to give birth in hospital or in an out-of-hospital birth centre. Helping women use a VBAC decision aid has been shown to reduce women's anxieties around the issue of risk.[21] You may be able to help women consider how they are unique, with personal values and needs, and in doing this you may also be able to help them make decisions about their vaginal birth.
- You can help women see how you as a caregiver have the necessary knowledge about VBAC and, if appropriate, that you know how to react if complications should occur.

You will need to make women feel more *confident* about their capacity to give birth. This confidence is disappearing generally in pregnant women in modern society, as the Canadian family doctor and researcher Michael Klein emphasised,[22] but it may have been especially shaken in women who started labour and ended up having an emergency caesarean. It is helpful if you can direct women to resources (books, films, women who've already had a VBAC, special antenatal classes for women who want a VBAC, specialised websites, etc). You may also help women find ways to increase their confidence in their physical and emotional capacities to go through labour by, for example, explaining to them all the factors which are known to increase their chances of 'success'—as outlined in the next paragraph (overleaf).

- You will need to ensure that women in your care know what facilitates normal birth during labour (as detailed in the next section) and you will need to help them prepare for labour. If appropriate to a particular woman's medical history, you will also be able to reassure women who were healthy before they got pregnant,[23] who had a caesarean because of breech presentation[24] or fetal distress...[25] because in all these cases the chances of having a successful VBAC are higher. The chances of a VBAC are also higher if the woman is having a VBAC in a country where midwives are the main caregivers for normal births or if she is having a VBAC in a birth centre with a midwife,[26] or at home.[27] You will be able to offer words of encouragement and optimism if your client has already given birth vaginally previously (before or after the caesarean).[28] You can help women avoid having another caesarean by encouraging them to refuse a scan late on in their pregnancy so as to 'decide' whether their baby is too big to be born vaginally, by encouraging them to refuse medication to soften their cervix, and by encouraging them to refuse induction before 41 completed weeks—if there is no medical reason to induce—and to consider all types of induction with caution.

Offering women further support during labour...

There are many ways a caregiver can help a labouring woman to achieve a VBAC. When your client goes into labour, you will be able to reassure her if she has a favourable cervix or if her baby's head is engaged and has descended lower at the beginning of labour,[29] or even if an induction is arranged you can reassure her if her cervix is favourable.[30] (As you probably know, an induction using prostaglandins to soften the cervix increases the risk of uterine rupture.) Since your goal will be to avoid another caesarean and facilitate normal labour and birth, you will need to help your client avoid hospital routine and unnecessary procedures (such as EFM and amniotomy or staying in bed), which can all increase the risk of having another caesarean.[31]

You can help women further in the following ways:

- Help them move around during labour—to walk and change positions, whenever they want to.
- Encourage your clients to eat and drink, using their appetite and thirst as a guide.
- Encourage them to use birthing aids such as balls, birthing chairs, birthing pools, or horizontal bars (which they can hang on to while they are squatting), etc.
- Provide emotional support, by being continuously present .
- Be ready to challenge other caregivers in any case where they suggest medicalised ways of doing things during labour—such as giving birth in the supine position.

- Encourage women to keep their labours and births as normal as possible by labouring without pharmacological pain relief, if possible. Inform women about the secondary effects an epidural may have, especially its negative impact on a woman's labour.
- Welcome the presence of a doula to help your client during labour, if you can't be there.
- Encourage your client to be optimistic and positive about achieving her VBAC if her labour is progressing well–even if she's never experienced a vaginal birth before.[32]
- Be especially attentive during the time when the previous caesarean was carried out during any one particular woman's labour. (Of course, you will need to have found out in advance when this was–whether it was during the first stage of labour, or during the second stage.) Understandably, this can be a challenging time for women's confidence about their ability to give birth.

In summary, helping women choose and achieve a VBAC is now extremely important in this era of rising caesarean rates. Encouraging women to have a VBAC and facilitating VBAC labours are essential ways of promoting normal birth. Although some caesareans indeed save the lives of either mothers or babies–and we can be thankful when this is the case–we cannot really say that having a caesarean is equal to giving birth. There is a huge difference, which most caesarean mothers recognise. With your help, more and more woman will be able to achieve a VBAC.

Hélène Vadeboncoeur's thesis was on the humanisation of childbirth. She is particularly interested in issues of women's choice so wrote *Birthing Normally After A Caesarean or Two* (Fresh Heart, 2011). She has worked for Canadian health institutions on the implementation of birth centres. She is co-researcher in the QUARISMA RCT on lowering caesarean rates–and coordinator of innovative studies about emigrating to Canada and having a young child.

References

1 Organisation for Economic Co-operation and Development. OECD health data 2008: statistics and indicators for 30 countries. Paris, France: Organisation for Economic Co-operation and Development; 2008. Available at www.oecd.org/health/healthdata. Also see www.cdc.gov/mmwr/preview/mmwrhtml/mm5737a7.htm.

2 See the website of the Society of Obstetricians and Gynaecologists of Canada: www.sogc.org/projects/quarisma_f.asp

3 Villar J, Valladares E, Wojdyla D, *et al*, 2006. Caesarean delivery rates and pregnancy outcomes: The 2005 WHO global survey on maternal and perinatal health in Latin America. See www.thelancet.com DOI:10.1016/50140-6736(06)68704-7, www.ans.gov.br/portal/site/_hotsite_parto_2/publicacoes/Villar_et_al_Lancet_2006_AC.pdf; Bertran AP, Merialdi M, Lauer JA *et al*, 2007. Rates of caesarean section: analysis of global, regional and national estimates. *Paediatrics and Perinatal Epidemiology*, 21: 98-113.

4 Roan S, Girion L, 2010. Rising maternal mortality rate causes alarm, calls for action. *Los Angeles Times*, May 22; ACOG, 2006, Caesarean Delivery Associated with Increased Risk of Maternal Death from Blood Clots, Infection, Anesthesia, *ACOG News Release,* 31.

5 Zweifler J, Garza A, Hugues S, *et al,* 2006, Vaginal Birth After Caesarean in California - Before and After a Change in Guidelines. *Annals of Family Medicine*, 4:228-234.

6 See www.cpass2.umontreal.ca/quarisma/index.cgi?page=homeEN&ss=

7 Oblasser C, Ebner U, Wesp G, 2008. *Der Kaiserschnitt hat kein Gesicht*. Salzburg: Edition Riendenburg; Chaillet N, 2005. Exploratory study on women's satisfaction after a caesarean. Unpublished data; Baldwin R, Palmarini T, 1986, *Pregnant Feelings*. Berkely, CA: Celestial Arts;

8 See the evidence-based organization Childbirth Connection at: www.childbirthconnection.org/article.asp?ck=10166#psychological

9 Lydon-Rochelle M, Holt VL, Easterling TR, *et al,* 2001. Risk of Uterine Rupture during Labor among Women with a Prior Caesarean Delivery. *NEJM* 345(1): 3-8

10 See the website of the Ordre des Sages-Femmes du Québec (OSFQ): www.osfq.org.

11 Lieberman E, Ernst EK, Rooks JP, *et al,* 2004. Results of a National Study of Vaginal Birth After Caesarean in Birth Centers. *Obstet Gynecol,* 104(5 Part 1): 933-942

12 National Institutes of Health Consensus Development Conference - Vaginal Birth After Caesarean: New Insights, 2010, Final Statement, Bethesda, Maryland, March 8-10.

13 National Institutes of Health Consensus Development Conference - Vaginal Birth After Cesarean: New Insights, Bethesda, MD, March 8-10 2010 - http://consensus.nih.gov/2010/vbacstatement.htm

14 Jimenez V, 2004. Naissances: les intervenantes ont-elles vraiment le choix? Annual conference of the Association pour la santé publique du Québec, November 23-24, Montreal, Canada

15 Lieberman E, Ernst EK, Rooks JP, *et al,* 2004. Results of a National Study of Vaginal Birth After Caesarean in Birth Centers. *Obstet Gynecol,* 104(5 Part 1): 933-942.

16 See Childbirth Connection's document site: www.childbirthconnection.org/article.asp?ck=10166.

17 Li W, Weiyuan Z, Yanhui Z, 1999. The study of maternal and fetal plasma catecholamines levels during pregnancy and delivery. *Journal of Perinatal Medicine* 27(3): 195-198.

18 Oblasser C, Ebner U, Wasp G, 2008. *Der Kaiserschnitt hat kein Geslcht*. Salzburg: Edition Riendenburg

19 Bujold E, Mehta S, Bujold C, *et al,* 2002. Interdelivery interval and uterine rupture. *Am. J. Obstet Gyn*. 187(5):1199-1202; Shipp TD, Zelop CM, Repke JT, *et al.* Interdelivery interval and risk of symptomatic uterine rupture. 2001. *Obstet Gynec* 97(2):175=177.

20 Bujold E, Blackwell SC, Hendler I, *et al,* 2004. Modified Bishop's score and induction of labor in patients with a previous caesarean delivery. *Am J Obstet Gynecol,* 191(5): 1644-1648.

21 Montgomery AA, Emmett CL, Fahey T, *et al,* 2007. Two decision aids for mode of delivery among women with previous caesarean section: randomised controlled trial. *BMJ*. 334:1305.

22 Klein M, 2004. Personal communication with Dr. Vania Jimenez. Quoted in her presentation at the Annual conference of the Association pour la santé publique du Québec, Montreal, Canada, November 23-24 2004: Naissances: les intervenantes ont-elles vraiment le choix ?

23 National Institutes of Health Consensus Development Conference: Vaginal Birth After Caesarean – New Insights, Bethesda, Maryland, March 8-10, 2010.

24 Brill Y, Windrim R, 2003. Vaginal birth after caesarean section: review of antenatal predictors of success. J Obstet Gynaecol Can, 25$4): 275-286.

25 Rosen MC, Dickinson JC, Westhoff GL, 1991. Vaginal birth after caesarean: a metaanalysis of morbidity and mortality. Obstet Gynecol, 77:465-470.

26 Lieberman E, Ernst EK, Rooks JP, *et al*, 2004. Results of a national study on vaginal birth after caesarean in birth centers. Obstet Gynecol, 104(5 Part 1): 933-942.

27 Latendresse G, Murphy PA, Fullerton JT, 2005. A description of the management and outcomes of vaginal birth after caesarean birth in the homebirth setting. *J. Midwifery & Women's Health*, 50(5): 386-391.

28 Hender I, Bujold E, 2004. Effect of prior vaginal delivery or prior vaginal birth after caesarean delivery on obstetric outcomes in women undergoing trial of labor. *Obstetrics & Gynecology*. 104: 273-277; Mercer BM, Gilbert S, Landon MB, *et al*, 2008. Labor outcomes with increasing number of prior vaginal births after caesarean delivery. *Obstetrics & Gynecology*, 111:285-291.

29 Guise JM, Denman MA, Emeis C, *et al*, 2010. Agency for Healthcare Research and Quality – Evidence Report/Technology Assessment No 191, *Vaginal Birth After Caesarean: New Insights*, Publication no 10-E1001.

30 Guise JM, Denman MA, Emeis C, *et al*, 2010. Agency for Healthcare Research and Quality – Evidence Report/Technology Assessment No 191, *Vaginal Birth After Caesarean: New Insights*, Publication no 10-E1001.

31 Coalition for Improving Maternity Services, 2007. Evidence basis for the 10 steps of mother-friendly care. Systematic review. Journal of Perinatal Education. 16(1): Supplement. Winter 2007. Available at www.motherfriendly.org/products.php

32 Brill Y, Windrim R, 2003. Vaginal birth after caesarean section: review of antenatal predictors of success. *J. Obstet Gynaecol Can*, 25(4):275-286.

The role of the regulatory body in promoting normal birth

Susan Way

The UK's regulatory body for midwifery and nursing care

The Nursing and Midwifery Council (NMC) is the UK regulatory body for nurses and midwives. Its main aim is to safeguard the health and well-being of the public. It does this by maintaining a register of nurses and midwives, setting standards for education and practice, and giving guidance and advice to the professions. The NMC ensures that nurses and midwives on the register are fit to practise and deal swiftly and fairly with those who are not. (More details are available at www.nmc-uk.org.)

The NMC's role in promoting normal birth

You may be wondering how the regulatory body for nurses and midwives in the UK, is able to help promote normal birth, when often it is only known for the actions it takes to remove nurses and midwives from its register for misconduct. My aim in writing this chapter is to show that much of the work of the NMC is about supporting nurses and midwives in providing high quality care in practice, rather than holding fitness to practise hearings with a view to striking them off the register. As Warwick[1] argues, protecting the public can no longer simply be about protecting individuals from their practitioners who can potentially be removed from the register. It has to be about ensuring that individuals receive care of the highest quality from all practitioners. Focusing on the responsibilities of the individual midwife, and working collaboratively with organisations that influence and set policy at a strategic level will allow me to highlight the work the NMC does in promoting normality in childbirth.

So what is normal birth? This is a question that has exercised the regulatory body over a number of years, particularly the Statutory Midwifery Committee as it strives to ensure midwives are given the right tools, from a regulatory perspective, to practise safely and effectively. The remit of the committee is set in statute[2] (Nursing and Midwifery Order 2001) and has responsibility for advising Council on: any matter affecting midwifery, such as policy issues affecting midwifery practice, education and statutory supervision of midwives.

The Midwifery Committee's recommendations and subsequent Council decisions influence midwifery development in the UK, which affects the lives of individual women and their families under the care of UK midwives.

What is normal birth: This is a question that has exercised the regulatory body over a number of years

How the NMC promotes normality in practical terms

The current midwifery committee is comprised of 10 members, half of whom are lay members with an interest in ensuring optimal care for women and their families. The remaining members are practising midwives from the four countries of the UK. There is a requirement for Council and its committees to consult members of the wider profession and public appropriately[2] when developing standards and policy. Therefore, when advising Council, the Midwifery Committee asks members of the profession and the general public to give their opinion about any proposed changes.

The use of the term 'normality' is fundamental to the NMC

The use of the term, 'normality', is fundamental to a number of rules and standards set by the NMC. For example, the NMC has a responsibility to set standards for the training and education of student midwives. Organisations with an interest in maternity such as the Association for Improvements in the Maternity Services (AIMS) have campaigned in recent years to raise awareness of the fact that some student midwives complete their training without seeing a normal birth.[3] It is not difficult to conclude that if midwives are not confident about facilitating women to give birth normally, then this will restrict women's choice and may ultimately result in interventions that are not necessary and which are potentially harmful. In 2004, the wording of NMC standards for the education of midwives was ambiguous and it did not clearly state what the parameters of normal birth were, so the parameters were open to interpretation. The wording in that NMC document[4] reflected the European Union Directive at the time, 80/155/EEC Article 4, with the amended European Union Directive 89/594/EEC stating that students must have "personally carried out at least 40 deliveries; where this number cannot be reached owing to the lack of available women in labour, it may be reduced to a minimum of 30, provided that the student participates actively in 20 further deliveries". This raised concerns for the Midwifery Committee about how normal birth was being interpreted. Therefore, as part of their updating of the 2009 Standards for pre-registration midwifery education, the NMC took the opportunity to consult with members of the profession and public about what a normal birth is and how students can become competent in supporting women who are experiencing a pregnancy, labour and birth without complications.[5]

As part of this process the NMC took into account differing models of care, especially the model in which students hold a caseload of women during their training.[6,7] It was found that students who were exposed to caseload holding during their training were able to become grounded in the philosophy of woman-centred care, as well as having enhanced professional relationships with women. Caseload holding also facilitated the application of theory to practice in a meaningful way, resulting in students who were clinically confident and competent, and who also believed in themselves as practitioners.

Key NMC decisions which affect midwifery education

At its meeting of July 2006 the Midwifery Committee made the following decisions about pre-registration midwifery education:

- 'Normality' will be the main focus of pre-registration midwifery programmes.
- The midwifery committee will provide guidance on interventions that are not to be considered 'normal' childbirth.
- Competencies for caring for women in normal childbirth will be developed. They will include being able to identify deviations from the normal and being able to organise immediate management and referral.
- Guidance will be developed around the assessment of students' competence in normal labour.
- Student midwives must have a caseload during their training.

Student midwives must have a caseload during training

The impact of policy on criteria for qualification as a midwife

As a consequence the current education standards[8] have made more explicit the following requirements about a student's competence at the point of registration. These standards require that midwives will have:

- sound, evidence-based knowledge of facilitating the physiology of childbirth and the newborn, and competence in applying this in practice
- a knowledge of physiological, social, emotional and spiritual factors that may positively or adversely influence normal physiology, and competence in applying this in practice
- appropriate interpersonal skills (as identified in the essential skills cluster 'communication') to support women and their families
- skills in managing obstetric and neonatal emergencies, underpinned by appropriate knowledge
- status as autonomous practitioners and lead carers for women experiencing normal childbirth and the ability to support women throughout their pregnancy, labour, birth and postnatal period, in all settings including midwife-led units, birth centres and the home
- the ability to undertake critical decision-making to support appropriate referral of either the woman or baby to their health professionals or agencies when there is recognition of normal processes being adversely affected and compromised

NMC standards require that midwives have specific qualifications, knowledge and abilities

The NMC clarified what a woman could expect of a midwife

The NMC also took the opportunity to clarify what a woman could expect a newly registered midwife to do, by developing (in collaboration with a number of stakeholders) essential skills clusters. The skills clusters relate to areas where it was felt that further guidance was needed to ensure that students were exposed to different approaches of care, many of which supported normality in childbirth. The skills clusters included communication, the initial consultation between the woman and the midwife, normal labour and birth, initiating and continuation of breastfeeding, as well as the management of medicinal products.

Particularly in the labour and birth skills clusters there is reference to the demonstration of competence when the following wording is used:

- "working in partnership with women to facilitate a birth environment that supports their needs
- "measure, assess and facilitate the progress of normal labour ... using a variety of birthing aids, such as a birthing ball"

Through evidence it is known that these measures can improve the experience and outcome for women[9] and we can guess that using low-tech birthing aids (such as a birthing ball) is likely to facilitate normal birth.

The NMC's links with other stakeholders and their focus

Knowing that 'normal birth' is interpreted in many different ways the Midwifery Committee realised the importance of taking part in the work being undertaken by the Maternity Care Working Party (MCWP), a subgroup of the All Parliamentary Group on Maternity (www.appg-maternity.org.uk). The working party is an independent body, with a multidisciplinary membership that campaigns for improvements in maternity care. Its original focus, and therefore reason for being established, was to raise awareness of the rising caesarean section rate across the UK. The membership varies but includes representatives from the Royal College of Midwives, Royal College of Obstetricians & Gynaecologists, National Childbirth Trust, AIMS, Baby Lifeline, BirthChoice UK, Birth Crisis Network, British Association of Perinatal Medicine, Care Quality Commission, Foundation for the Study of Infant Deaths, HealthLink, Independent Midwives-UK, Iolanthe Midwifery Trust, NMC and the National Society for the Prevention of Cruelty to Children.

Since its early beginnings in 1998, the working party has aimed to highlight the health and social care needs of women and their families as well as the role that woman-centred maternity services can have in the promotion of public health. The MCWP wants to encourage a positive focus on normal birth so it issued a consensus statement,[10] *'Making normal birth a reality'*, which the NMC supports. The definition of normal birth adopted is one where labour starts spontaneously, progresses spontaneously without a spinal or epidural anaesthetic and the woman gives birth spontaneously.

The importance of this statement is that it gives a basis for consistency of data collection, making it possible to collect statistics for as many maternity services as possible across the UK. The statement gives recommendations for action with some practical ways of implementing them. For example the main recommendation is that attention should be paid to providing a comfortable and supportive environment for all women during labour. The statement goes on to say that providing a suitable environment will help women to relax and feel safe—a recommendation that is followed through into the NMC essential skills cluster for normal labour and birth. The statement also recommends using fewer medical procedures in labour where possible, without jeopardising safety. Examples of how this can be implemented include active one-to-one midwifery support for all women during established labour, with midwifery staffing levels remaining in line with the Royal College's recommendations of 1.0–1.4 whole time equivalent midwives per woman in labour, depending on case mix category.[11]

Individual responsibilities and the influence of the NMC

Providing safe and effective care is viewed by the NMC as not an option but integral to the daily practice of midwives. To support appropriate practice in the care environment the NMC publishes a variety of documents in the form of rules, standards, advice and guidance such as the NMC *Code: Standards of Conduct, Performance and Ethics for Nurses and* Midwives,[12] as well as the *Midwives' Rules and Standards.*[13] These documents and others can be downloaded from the NMC website www.nmc-uk.org.

The Midwives' Rules and Standards[13] and the Code[12] complement each other, identifying to the midwife the high quality of care that is expected from her while working and supporting women and their families in her care. The NMC views The Code as the basis for high quality midwifery practice, and a key tool in safeguarding the health and well-being of the public. The Code is about being professional, accountable, and being able to justify the decisions the midwife makes. It states (on page 1) that "the people in your care must be able to trust you with their health and wellbeing" and goes on to further outline four main areas in order to justify that trust:

- "You must make the care of people your first concern, treating them as individuals and respecting their dignity.
- "You must work with others to protect and promote the health and well-being of those in your care, their families and carers. And the wider community.
- "You must provide a high standard of practice and care at all times.
- "You must be open and honest, act with integrity and uphold the reputation of your profession."

What does this mean for the midwife in practice and how can these statements promote normality in the context of childbirth?

The following are a number of vignettes to illustrate how.

"You must make the care of people your first concern, treating them as individuals and respecting their dignity."

In this section of the Code[12] it states that "You must listen to people in your care and respond to their concerns and preferences." How does this influence real-life practice? Here is one example:

Mary was expecting her first baby and was looking forward to birthing her baby at home. She was considered to be at low risk of complications but her General Practitioner (GP) advised against this, commenting that all women should deliver in hospital, as [he felt] this was the safest option. Mary was disappointed with this reaction and decided to discuss it further with her midwife. The midwife first felt it important to understand the reasoning for Mary's choice so she could support her appropriately. As the midwife discussed options for place of birth with Mary it became apparent that Mary disliked being in hospitals due to a previous bad experience. The midwife was sensitive to this issue when explaining to Mary the advantages and risk of birth at home. Mary was now more confident about the choice she had made, but also understood the circumstances when it may be appropriate to reconsider the decision and choose to birth in hospital. This was helped by the midwife showing Mary around the local maternity unit in order for Mary to become familiar with the environment and to help reduce any anxiety if there was a need to transfer her there.

By understanding Mary's particular circumstances, the midwife was treating her as an individual, which helped the midwife support Mary appropriately in her choice. The midwife was able to explain the advantages and risks of birthing at home, in order for Mary to come to an informed decision. The midwife acted as Mary's advocate and supported her in her decision to continue to opt for a home birth.

"You must work with others to protect and promote the health and well-being of those in your care, their families and carers..."

In this section the Code[12] points out that you must inform someone in authority if you experience problems that prevent you from working within this Code or other nationally agreed standards. How does this influence real-life practice? Here is one example:

Sarah was a newly-qualified midwife who, in order to gain employment, moved to another part of the country. As part of Sarah's orientation programme to the new NHS Trust she was allocated a preceptor to support her during this transition. Sarah had learnt during her training that it was not necessary for all women attending hospital in labour to have an admission trace of the fetal heart done using a cardiotocograph machine (CTG). However, Sarah's preceptor challenged her on a number of occasions for not routinely undertaking an admission CTG. Sarah knew that this practice was not evidence-based and had the potential to cause unnecessary intervention and therefore potential harm to both the mother and her unborn baby. Using the national guidelines as evidence, Sarah tried to explain to her preceptor that routine admission CTGs were not necessary. However, the preceptor was unwilling to listen, saying that although she was aware of the evidence she felt it was more reassuring for the CTG to be done.

In this scenario Sarah was aware that her preceptor was working outside of the NHS Trust policy, which reflected the national guidelines[14] and that the practice was detrimental to the health and well-being of women and babies in her care. As the preceptor was unwilling to change her practice Sarah had a duty of care to raise this with someone in authority.

Potential difficulties the midwife may face and solutions

The NMC is aware that raising concerns within an organisation can be challenging and not always comfortable for the practitioner to do because of the potential conflicts that may arise.[15] In a case such as this the midwife can share her concerns with her named supervisor of midwives (SoM). Supervisors of midwives are experienced practising midwives who have undertaken additional education and training.[16] They act as positive role models for midwives, guiding and supporting them in developing skills and expertise. If a midwife requires additional education, training and support in practice, a supervisor can recommend a period of updating to be undertaken, which must be achieved.[17]

Supervisors of Midwives act as positive role models for midwives, guiding and supporting them

Supervisors of midwives are appointed by the Local Supervising Authority (LSA), which are organisations that hold statutory roles and responsibilities for supporting and monitoring the quality of midwifery practice through the mechanism of statutory supervision of midwives.[18] The primary responsibility of an LSA is to safeguard the health and well-being of women and their families. Each LSA must appoint a practising midwife to the role of LSA Midwifery Officer (LSAMO). The statutory requirements for this person and role are also set by the NMC.[19] The LSAMO is employed by the LSA to put its responsibilities into practice and this function cannot be delegated to another person or role. The LSAMO has a pivotal role in clinical governance by ensuring that the standards for supervision of midwives and midwifery practice meet the requirements set by the NMC. By appointing SoMs the LSA ensures that support, advice and guidance are available for midwives and women 24 hours a day, to increase public protection. Supervisors of midwives are accountable to the LSA for all their supervisory activities and their role is to protect the public by enabling and empowering midwives to practise safely and effectively. They also have a responsibility to bring to the attention of the LSA any practice or service issues that might undermine or jeopardise midwives' ability to care for women and their babies safely.[18]

The Local Supervising Authority Midwifery Officer has a pivotal role in clinical governance safeguarding standards

Supporting members of the public in receiving evidence-based care

The NMC works closely with members of the public in order to ensure that they understand what they can expect from a midwife and how to challenge poor care. To this end, publications are produced, such as, *Support for Parents: How supervision and supervisors of midwives can support you.*[20] One of the drivers behind writing this leaflet was the type of calls the NMC had been receiving from women and lay organisations about women not being able to access care of their choice, as well as being disappointed or distressed about the care they had received Although this only relates to a very small proportion of the calls received by the NMC on a daily basis, they were of significant concern to warrant some kind of action from the regulatory body.

The leaflet was developed in collaboration with a number of lay organisations such as the National Childbirth Trust (www.nct.org.uk), Association for Improvements in the Maternity Services (www.aims.org.uk) and Fathers Direct (www.fatherhoodinstitute.org). The publication strategy included working with MIDIRS (Midwives' Information and Resource Service—see www.midirs.org), whose own collaboration with the NCT meant they had access to a wide public audience.

The main aim of the leaflet is to inform women expecting a baby how supervision of midwives and a supervisor of midwives can support them, while at the same time supporting the midwife giving them care. Here is an example of how statutory supervision has worked well:

'In the North West Local Supervising Authority they employ a supervisor of midwives to support the role of the LSA Midwifery Officer. During 2007–2008 the midwife documented 91 cases of women needing support to explore their care options. Of these, she went on to facilitate the care of 28 of them by liaising with local supervisors, midwives and other professionals to negotiate and/or provide individual packages of care for women with very specific identified requirements. Unfortunately, in some instances, women's trust in professionals had broken down due to previous negative experiences of maternity care. However, access to the midwife employed by the LSA, who was viewed as an external, expert source of support was invaluable to them and restored their confidence, both in the health care system and in their own capabilities'.

(This example is included in the 2008 LSA report, published by the North West region of England, available on the NMC website.[21])

The Support for Parents[20] leaflet explains to women who their supervisor of midwives is and what her (or his) role is, as well as how she (or he) can support midwives with the care choices that some women make, for example around place of birth. Gnash,[22] a midwife, identifies how she used her supervisor of midwives in order to support the choice of birth environment a woman on her caseload had made. The place of birth was to be on a canal barge that was moored on the tidal part of the river. The boat would therefore rise and fall with the tide, meaning that access, via a narrow walkway was difficult, depending on whether it was high or low tide. The outcome was that the couple were satisfied with the care they received as they felt part of all the decisions that needed to be made.

The NMC and strategic working

The NMC is not a lobbying organisation and as such cannot exert influence on behalf of its members. However, it can work collaboratively with lay and government organisations at a strategic level to ensure the safety of the health and well-being of women, babies and their families. The NMC is represented at many strategic steering and advisory groups across the UK to ensure public protection is high on the policy agenda. Examples include Midwifery 2020, a working group set up by the four Chief Nurses of the UK to develop a vision of midwifery so that all midwives across the UK can fulfil women's health and social needs and meet their expectations. The NMC representatives attended all five of the workstream groups: The Core Role of the Midwife, Workforce and Workload, Education and Career Progression, Public Health, and Measuring Quality. It was a collaborative programme with the Royal College of Midwives, the NMC and diverse partners and stakeholders in maternity care, higher education, user organisations, employers and commissioners of service and education.[23] There are a number of recommendations to drive the vision to become a reality. Two of the recommendations identify key roles for midwives: one is that midwives are the lead professional for women with no complications, and the second is that midwives are the coordinator of care for all women. The role of the lead professional is to "plan, provide and review a woman's care, with input and agreement, from initial antenatal assessment through to the end of the postnatal period. In most circumstances, a midwife would take the role of lead professional for all healthy women with straightforward pregnancies."[24]

The above view is supported by two systematic reviews which conclude that when women with a low risk of complications receive midwife-led care this reduces admission to hospital and results in significantly less intervention during birth.[25,26]

An important regulatory body for promoting normality in birth

It is hoped that the snapshot given in this chapter of the work of a regulatory body for midwives shows the different ways in which such an organisation can work with members of the public and also with the professions in order to promote normality within the childbirth experience. However, the NMC is aware that care still falls short of the required high quality standards it sets for midwives and that at times the practice of midwives is called into question and investigated through the fitness to practise route.

Susan Way in her role as Lead Midwife for Education leads the development, delivery and management of midwifery education programmes at Bournemouth University. She took up this role in November 2009. From 2001 to 2009 Susan worked as a Midwifery Advisor at the Nursing and Midwifery Council, the regulatory body for nurses and midwives in the UK. This role led her to be a member of a number of advisory panels and steering groups across the UK with a focus on the safety of the health and well-being of women, their babies and their families. Her particular interests are regulation, statutory supervision and pain management following birth. Susan has two children, one of which was born in a midwife-led unit and the other at home.

References

1 Warwick C, 2009. Statutory supervision of midwives: adding value to the profession. *British Journal of Midwifery* 17(11): 686.

2 Department of Health, 2002. *Nursing and Midwifery Order 2001 Statutory Instrument No 253*. The Stationary Office: London.

3 Walsh D, 2008. Promoting normal birth: weighing the evidence. IN: Downe S, (ed) *Normal childbirth: evidence and debate* (2nd ed). London: Churchill Livingstone Elsevier, Chapter 10, 175-189.

4 Nursing and Midwifery Council, 2004. *Standards of proficiency for pre-registration midwifery education*. NMC: London. Page 34.

5 Nursing and Midwifery Council, 2005. *Consultation on a review of pre-registration midwifery education*. See http://www.nmc-uk.org/Documents/Consultations/NMC%20Consultation%20-%20pre-registration%20midwifery%20education%20-%20consultation%20document.pdf [accessed 9 December 2010].

6 Rawnson S, Fry J, Lewis P, 2008. Student Caseloading: Embedding the concept within education. *British Journal of Midwifery*. 16(10): 636-641.

7 Rawnson S, Brown S, Wilkins C, Leamon J, 2009. Student midwives' views of caseload holding: the bump study. *British Journal of Midwifery*. 17(8): 484-489.

8 Nursing and Midwifery Council, 2009. *Standards for pre-registration midwifery education*. NMC: London.

9 Penny P, Simkin PT, O'Hara MA, 2002. Nonpharmocological relief of pain during labor: systematic reviews of five methods. *American Journal of Obstetrics and Gynecology*. 186 (5): S131-S159.

10 National Childbirth Trust, Royal College of Midwives, Royal College of Obstetricians and Gynaecologists, 2007. *Making normal birth a reality: Consensus statement from the Maternity Care Working Party*. See http://www.nct.org.uk/about-us/what-we-do/policy/normalbirth [accessed 26 November 2010].

11 Royal College of Obstetricians and Gynaecologists, Royal College of Midwives, Royal College of Anaesthetists and the Royal College of Paediatrics and Child Health, 2007. *Safer childbirth: minimum standards for the delivery of care in labour*. London: RCOG Press.

12 Nursing and Midwifery Council, 2008. *The Code: standards of conduct, performance and ethics for nurses and midwives*. NMC: London.

13 Nursing and Midwifery Council, 2004. *Midwives rules and standards*. NMC: London.

14 National Institute for Health and Clinical Excellence, 2007. *Intrapartum Care: care of healthy women and their babies during childbirth*. RCOG: London.

15 Nursing and Midwifery Council, 2010. *Raising and escalating concerns: guidance for nurses and midwives*. NMC: London.

16 Nursing and Midwifery Council, 2006. *Standards for the preparation and practice of supervisors of midwives*. See http://www.nmc-uk.org/Educators/Standards-for-education/Standards-for-the-preparation-and-practice-for-supervision-of-midwives/ [accessed 10 December 2010]

17 Nursing and Midwifery Council, 2007. *Standards for the supervised practice of midwives*. See http://www.nmc-uk.org/Documents/Standards/mcStandardsGForSupervisedPracticeofMidwivess2007.pdf [accessed 10 December 2010]

18 Nursing and Midwifery Council, 2009. *Supervision, support and safety: analysis of the 2008-2009 local supervising authorities' annual reports to the Nursing and Midwifery Council*. NMC: London.

19 Nursing and Midwifery Council, 2007. *NMC Circular 12/2007: Guidance on selection and appointment of Local Supervising Authority Midwifery Officers*. NMC: London.

20 Nursing and Midwifery Council, 2009. *Support for parents: How supervision and supervisors of midwives can support you*. See http://www.nmc-uk.org/Documents/Midwifery-booklets/Support-for-parents-2009.pdf [accessed 3 December 2010].

21 North West Local Supervising Authority, 2008. *North West Local Supervising Authority annual report to the Nursing and Midwifery Council on the statutory supervision of midwives and midwifery practice 2007-2008*. See http://www.nmc-uk.org/Documents/Midwifery-LSA-reports/LSA%20Annual%20Report%20North%20West%202007%202008.pdf [accessed 3 December 2010]. Page 21.

22 Gnash L, 2009. Supervision issues in practice: supporting and advising midwives. *British Journal of Midwifery*. 17(11): 714-716.

23 Midwifery 2020 UK Programme, 2010. *Midwifery 2020: delivering expectations*. Edinburgh: Midwifery 2020 UK Programme.

24 Midwifery 2020 UK Programme, 2010. *Midwifery 2020: delivering expectations*. Edinburgh: Midwifery 2020 UK Programme. Page 24.

25 Hater M, Sandell J, Devane D, Soltani H, Gates S, 2008. *Midwife-led versus other models of care for childbearing women. Cochrane Database of Systematic Reviews* 2008, Issue 4. Art. No.: CD004667. DOI: 10.1002/14651858.CD004667.pub2. See http://onlinelibrary.wiley.com/o/cochrane/clsysrev/articles/CD004667/frame.html [accessed 9 December 2010].

26 Caird, J, Rees R, Kavanagh J, Sutcliffe K, Oliver K, Dickson K, Woodman J, Barnett-Page E, and Thomas J, 2010. *The socioeconomic value of nursing and midwifery: A rapid systematic review of reviewers*, EPPI Centre report no. 1801, London: EPPI Centre, Institute of Education, University of London.

Using the media to promote normal birth around the world

Naoli Vinaver

The role of the media in modern society

The world is harvesting the fruits of the seeds it has been planting ever since modern medicine divided the human body into segments and medical science into specialties. The process of birth has suffered greatly from the unhappy and unsuccessful ways in which woman and child have been physically and conceptually disconnected from their original natural unity and symbiotic perfection. Culturally speaking, humanity has been promoting this view of separation and inherent mistrust between mother and her child growing within, in all the different ways that we humans have for passing on our culture from generation to generation.

In the same way, as we become increasingly aware of our faults and mistakes over the years and the cultural phases and 'fashions' that we humans go through as a society, supposedly seeking an ever-better state of consciousness and health, we must also use all our means to reconstruct and undo our mistakes so that present and future generations will be able to enjoy a better experience of life.

We must use all our means to help others enjoy a better life

Modern human beings depend on many complex means to express ourselves, communicate our thoughts, profess our feelings, post our inquiries, share philosophies, debate political views and also demonstrate and prove discoveries. We have created and used drama, literature, dance, music, cinema and art in all its forms. As modernism advances, we have increasingly used the media such as radio, television, video productions, newspapers and magazines; and more recently we have started using digital media such as the Internet, with search engine systems and webpages; we now also use Facebook, video media systems such as YouTube, and the like. These media systems work as contact bridges between people who wish to share their differences and similarities in thought and work—both personally and professionally. These channels of communication have been increasing our possibilities for communication and making people feel more empowered.

When it comes to the topics of fertility, pregnancy, nutrition, labour, birth, postnatal care, breastfeeding, childrearing and so on, there are thousands of texts as well as newly-produced videos and home-movies openly shared by people over the Internet, or distributed amongst specific interest groups.

The drive individuals generally have in sharing their most intimate and often deeply catalyst moments of birth-giving mostly stems from individuals' need to share alternative options and non-conventional possibilities for giving birth in societies, cultures and communities where birth is otherwise tightly regulated and controlled, strictly regimented or even penalised if it takes place outside current conventional medical or cultural protocols.

The wide array of small-scale video and DVD productions available are often extremely low-budget personal or non-profit, organisational enterprises which aim to disseminate facts, scientific evidence, stories or documentaries which can be used to widen and deepen our world's vision of birth.

At the same time that new initiatives exist, there is also great resistance from people representing the mainstream. These are often medical or institutional representatives who want to keep things the same, stop consumers from asking questions which may make them need to modify their protocols, standards and even their laws relating to birth.

Money or economic interests are always at play in any societal state of affairs and the business of birth is widely known to be one of the largest, most profitable businesses within the healthcare system. Maintaining the status quo thus continues to be a high priority for those harvesting the most benefits so the opposing forces on the sides of 'change' and 'conservationism' clash and create a real challenge for the development of the humanisation of birth movements in the world. However, the 'battles' between those aiming to change the world and those aiming to keep it the same can be peaceful and are only true battles in the sense that they are intrinsically a clash of power.

The media can be seen as the battlefield where these battles take place—or perhaps, instead, we should consider it a peacefield—on which two or more different forms of consciousness (embracing different paradigms) consider their differences, take the opportunity to expose their uniqueness, and absorb the newness of certain concepts, philosophies or views. People on different sides have the amazing opportunity to transmute their consciousness and yield to the possibility of change and transformation.

In most communities the media is an arena and space with great potential for exposing and exchanging viewpoints, whether it takes the form of an urban newspaper, a more rural radio station, a physical magazine or a virtual webpage and whether it takes the form of radio communication, television broadcasting, community centre communication, private home gatherings, theatres, magazines, newspapers, dance forums, Internet blogs or websites.

In just a few minutes, television gives the public the chance to see and hear a person or a group of people presenting and discussing issues of great interest and current importance. Showing video clips which last even just a few seconds, gives viewers a sense of being exposed to 'the latest development' and people expect live television programmes to be the most up-to-date medium of communication. Seeing a combination of images with people opening up to share a personal viewpoint can be a very moving experience for the viewer.

Media you can personally use

Someone wanting to be at the forefront of the 'making of culture' should aim to appear on a television programme, either as a guest or presenter. It is not as difficult as it may seem. Most areas of the country have their own television channels and are eager to include people from their region, because they bring to life events happening in their area. There is usually great pride in presenting the community's local people who may have some very interesting as well as differing viewpoints, since this stimulates debate and keeps the community lively. Therefore, do not hesitate to look for ways of getting involved in a local programme so as to air your concerns and interests.

Don't hesitate to look for ways of getting involved

Radio broadcasting is similar to television, although even more accessible, as it is a less costly and a more popular form of the media. People listen to the radio while they are in their cars, at the office, at home, and while they are doing chores and other activities, so it can be a magnificent channel through which a birth activist can actively participate in the promotion of normal birth. Discussions, debates, arguments, facts, stories, questions and interviews can all take place on the radio and have an amazing impact on people who listen.

Most radio programmes welcome their listeners calling in with questions, enquiries, and comments, which turn the programme into a true exchange of views and ideas. A call-in programme can also be extremely stimulating to radio listeners who are passively or actively listening, as they can follow a debate, a challenge and its outcome with great interest and emotion, without necessarily stopping what they are doing. Radio can be a beautiful way for people to actually be a part of the world, while remaining anonymous and fully invested in their daily lives. At the same time, people's minds and hearts are touched and their consciousness and viewpoints change as a consequence.

Video productions–films as well as any other project that includes image and sound–are also very powerful tools for promoting change. Of course, the distribution of such media remains an important factor, as it is only through effective and wide distribution that messages can reach the public. Internet sites, blogs, online chats, YouTube videos, and other digital media creative projects can have a huge impact on the world as they are easily and readily accessible to all, as long as keywords and subjects are projected within search engine systems. In order for anything you participate in to have this kind of enormous impact, whenever you create something online make sure that the views you express can be backed up by scientific evidence in some way or other. This does not mean that you can only express objective, provable ideas, but if what you are expressing or disclosing is very different from what is socially accepted, it helps if you provide a 'bridge' to help people cross over from one view to another, without the need for too huge a leap of faith. Of course, this should be your aim if you want to be seen as a reliable, 'grounded' source of information and ideas.

Mentioning other reliable sources or organisations that offer similar reliable information is also a way of linking up with other people's attempts to promote change and this can be a good way of extending the solid ground that aims to promote normal birth around the world

It's worth getting involved and linking up with other people, however frightening the prospect may seem because the media is being used by all kinds of people around the globe nowadays. Online it's possible to find everything from reliable to completely unreliable information: many items or views available on the Internet are completely based on assumptions or false information. Try not to add to the misinformation but instead aim to produce material that is a truly useful resource.

Literary works and texts can be published both on paper and on the Internet. Target readership, distribution channels and finance are factors that will affect the decision as to whether paper or electronic texts will be most effective in fulfilling a particular objective. Texts have the advantage that they are long-lasting because they remain available and accessible to the public for longer than a television or radio programme, unless these are placed on the Internet—but of course the Internet has the advantage that it extends distribution so widely. Texts can be sent, read and re-read, shared by friends, discussed in groups and used as a basis for theatre plays and film or video scripts.

Ways of making your own promotional activities effective

Apparently, the only effective way of achieving long-lasting change is when people's consciousness is raised, which happens when their sensibilities are touched.

What have been the most powerful ways of affecting people's attitudes in human history? The arts seem to have been very effective. A song to a melancholic tune can reach the heart in a way that words alone may not. An image of a child emerging softly through her mother's vaginal lips over her intact perineum as she touches her baby's head with a tender hand can be much more powerful than any argument that speaks against the brutality of an unnecessary routine episiotomy which is still performed on mothers in most so-called 'civilised' countries within their modern medical systems.

Bringing together intellectual and conceptual arguments based on scientific evidence woven together and expressed through any form of artistic perspective can touch the senses of any spectator in such a powerful way that immediate change within the heart and the consciousness of that person can be achieved in a matter of minutes.

The media, bringing together elements that touch our senses, such as image and sound, combined with intelligent, sensitive and pertinent information, can create a most powerful means for promoting normal birth in our current contemporary human existence.

The actual process of creating a DVD, for example, that can then be offered to the public, is in itself a wonderfully powerful process for the individuals involved. Musicians help you create a piece of music to accompany the images in a video production, and other people such as a video editor, a graphic artist, the producer, the DVD mastering technician, etc will also be instrumental in helping you to achieve your goal. What's more, even by participating in a project which involves preparing something for the media, people who are actively involved may well experience a change of consciousness and become more aware of the issues you are trying to raise.

Consciousness-raising does not always require much energy and time, but it helps greatly if we aim to create a bridge between the source of the message and those who will be at the receiving end of it. In order for people to become sensitive to a new proposition and for the new concept to 'take root' or 'take hold' of their heart and soul, they need to feel that the new concept or need for change is actually accessible to them and possible. And perhaps, in order to start thinking in this way, they need to be challenged so that they start questioning their old preconceived ideas.

This is because, for change to take place, people must also first conceive of the possibility of things being different from the actual reality. Sometimes the human mind does not even conceive of this first step, and thus cannot create or invent a proposition to counter the current state of affairs. One must be able to imagine and dream of the possibility of things being different in order to even come up with creative ideas to inspire such changes to occur. Usually this means the first act of 'chaos' or 'openness' (where the narrowness of the mind gives way to make space for an 'otherness' to come in and make shifts) needs to be followed by a certain amount of refreshing turmoil. After that, reflection and thoughtfulness through having been touched and challenged to think again on a subject which many people assume has just one answer (the conventional answer) will bring on a shift in paradigms, or at least the motivation to open up the subject. When people are touched and challenged, they will put their old assumptions to one side so that they can consider new and exciting points of view, so they will begin to engage in this process involving chaos followed by a new reordering of ideas and possible solutions.

The media in our modern world cannot be undervalued. The different media are the main highways that connect individuals to great crowds. Different forms of the media are the river arteries that bring refreshing blood everywhere that is dry. Because of their great power, we must have the simple audacity to metaphorically launch our little boats right onto the river waters, so that we can get ourselves across and generously share our different views with people whose minds and hearts are eager to be expanded with feelings, thoughts, ideas, facts, varied angles and details, which they never before had the opportunity to ponder. Sharing is the key to growth and the key to stimulating the inner shift that leads to change.

Naoli Vinaver lives and works in rural Veracruz, Mexico. She has been an active admirer, defender and promoter of natural and instinctive birthing since she was a child. She hosted a state-wide weekly TV programme for over 6 years, celebrated by an enthusiastic public. As a midwife, she has organised midwifery conferences blending cultures as well as social groups of traditional and professional midwives over the years with the aim of maintaining the dignity and wisdom of traditional midwifery, while expanding the scope of practice of all midwives around the world. Naoli has three lovely children, born at home, and dedicates her life to teaching, creating artistic birth materials to educate and promote natural birth as well as assisting mothers and families in their home births. She has attended over 1,200 home births since 1990.

Words, metaphors and images as powerful tools for change

Sylvie Donna

A hidden storehouse of equipment for ensuring outcomes

It is possible that most of us use language with the assumption that it is an accurate and fairly unchangeable tool for conveying meaning. However, this is certainly not the case. Language acquires meaning as we use it; if you find this difficult to accept consider the evolution of the words *house*, *computer* and *shoes* in different cultures and socio-economic groups. Jimmy Choos are a far cry from Dad's lace-ups—and that's just within one household at one time!

To complicate things further, words are imbued not only with denotation (their meaning) but also connotation (the things we associate them with) so they are complex tools for influence or intervention in any situation where human beings are together. Compare the words *petite* and *trivial* for example. While both essentially mean the same thing (*small*), one is positive and the other negative. Most people are very happy for a woman to be petite, but if she asks a *trivial* question the atmosphere changes immediately. She is likely to be given a *brief* (i.e. *small*) explanation of why she is wasting everyone's time. Meanwhile, the *skinny* woman on the team is likely to improve her image by making a point *concisely*. In other words, we implicitly reveal our evaluation of concepts through the words we choose to refer to them.

If words used literally are imbued with meaning (depending on context) and if they have associations which are either positive or negative, think how powerful they become when they are used metaphorically, i.e. when they are used to create images in listeners' minds by associating one thing with another, not by saying that one thing is 'like' another (as in when we use a simile) but by saying it *is* something else. Caregivers do this every time they say that a woman's vaginal passageway is a 'canal'—a *birth canal*.

Think how influential words can become when we use them as a kind of shorthand (i.e. metonymy) to refer to a whole battery of associations (as happens when we use the word 'risk'). After all, a word is more than its surface definition. Lakoff (a cognitive linguist) used the term *idealised cognitive model* to explain this,[1] a term which embodied not just a state of associated meanings for a given term, but which also alluded to a larger set of attributes.[2] In the case of the word 'risk', for example, while a general 'surface' meaning might be 'the possibility of something bad happening'[3] a pregnant woman worrying about risk in her sixth month of pregnancy is likely to have a whole range of negative associations and 'what ifs' and may even visualise or dream about whole scenarios with long-term consequences.

Used alone, or bolstered with images, words are clearly extremely powerful tools for change, either positive or negative, and they become even more effective agents for change when combined in time and space within the complexity of human relationships. An awareness of what we are doing with the tools we have for communication in a caregiving context can give us more control to either effect change in the world... or, conversely, ensure that the status quo is maintained.

Words in pregnancy books

When a woman first becomes pregnant, all kinds of words could be said to influence her perceptions of the processes going on within her body and the likelihood (or otherwise) of a positive—let us call it 'normal'—outcome. Here are some examples, inspired from reading the bestselling book on pregnancy *What To Expect When You're Expecting* (Simon & Schuster, 2009),[4] which presents a fairly typical view of pregnancy and birth.

- In the first chapter a section is called 'What Kind of Patient Are You?' Of course, this implies that the processes of childbirth are always associated with pathology, as is usual when we use the word *patient* in other contexts. But is it really helpful to call pregnant women *patients* before any problems are discovered? What about the risk of inducing fear in a woman (which is associated with adrenaline and stress hormones) and preventing her from producing oxytocin—the hormone essential for labour to proceed smoothly—which cannot usually be produced in the presence of fear? In other words, what about the risk of creating a 'nocebo' (i.e. a negative mindset, with resultant problems), instead of its cousin, the 'placebo'?[5-7] If you as a caregiver expect outcomes to be normal and the word *patient* brings to mind abnormal outcomes, what should the women you care for be called?
- In Chapter 2 of the same pregnancy book, there is a section called 'Your Obstetric History Repeating Itself'. This phrasing suggests that this is what is going to happen to the pregnant reader, i.e. that if she had trouble coping with the pain of labour in the past, she won't be able to cope a second time; that if she previously had a caesarean, she will need one again, irrespective of the environment in which she labours, the care she receives (or doesn't receive) and her attitude and experience as a birthing woman. Another section of the book is called 'Tempting Fate the Second Time Around'—which similarly suggests that any 'trusting' approach is bound to meet with failure.
- The section called 'Reducing Risk in Any Pregnancy' suggests that *any* pregnancy is fraught with risk, not just ones where the woman is high risk. (Of course, this is true of the very terminology used in maternity care: 'low risk' and 'high risk'. Is it really necessary for *all* women and *all* caregivers to see pregnancies in terms of an experience involving 'risk'?) The 'risk' theme is further promoted in other headings, such as 'What It's Important to Know: Playing Baby Roulette' and 'The Best-Odds Diet'.
- A section entitled 'What to Take to the Hospital' suggests to women that they will certainly give birth in a hospital and not in a birth centre or at home. The choice of home birth is not even addressed since the only reference to it in the whole book is in a section entitled 'Emergency Home (or Office) Delivery'—which clearly implies that home birth is not a 'normal' option. A later section reinforces this impression with its heading 'On to the Hospital'. Through the use of phrasing, the authors are clearly influencing readers' decision-making. To what extent do you similarly compromise your clients' right to informed consent simply by not even *mentioning* some options, or by only mentioning certain options within a negative framework?

- Illustrations in the book which are intended to depict the baby's descent through the fleshy folds of his or her mother's body show a baby emerging *laterally*, so the implication is that the woman will be lying down during the second stage of labour. As we know from a knowledge of how physiology works, an upright position makes fetal descent far easier, because it causes the pelvic opening to increase substantially and of course gravity can help too.

Given this biased use of language and imagery, it is perhaps not surprising that we see negative framing of information and ideas throughout the book: every subsection begins with the heading 'What You May Be Concerned About'. Given that worry and fear are associated with non-progress in labour, since oxytocin (necessary for contractions) is produced in the presence of *loving feelings*, and inhibited by the production of adrenaline, is it such a good idea to have these negative emotions constantly highlighted during pregnancy and perhaps even early on in labour (when many women will still be referring to their pregnancy books)? Although the book has many qualities and apparently makes an effort to promote normal outcomes in many respects, the overall effect is to reinforce fear and worry, and to create the mindset of a *patient*. In other words, the emphasis is on things going wrong. Other pregnancy books are similarly guilty of using words to create more fear than joy.

What if everything were framed positively? The idea of salutogenesis—that the way people view their life has an influence on health—was introduced by the medical sociologist Aaron Antonovsky in 1990. (He called it 'salutogenic theory'.[8-10] The idea was later discussed in the context of maternity care by Soo Downe and Christine McCourt,[11] and also by Verena Schmid.[12] The idea that language can change our perceptions of who we are and how we view ourselves, particularly our status and our health, was noted by linguistics student Sarah Kiaer, who happened to be pregnant while she was doing her Master's. For her dissertation research she documented how the way in which language was used (in the UK) during her pregnancy and how words seemed to 'turn her into someone else'.[13] She also demonstrated how pregnancy is constructed as an illness and how power relations acted out in different genres of discourse (i.e. spoken and written language) help to perpetuate unequal power relations.

But what kind of book would result if everything were indeed framed positively in a book about pregnancy and birth? I explored this question in detail when I wrote *Birth: Countdown to Optimal* (Fresh Heart, 2008, 2nd ed, 2011).[14] It was an attempt to provide a realistic, but inspiring antidote to all the 'fearful' books. When I researched the topic I was amazed by how much negative language and pessimistic 'framing' I found in other books on pregnancy, particularly in week-by-week guides. The last thing many books seem to do is promote normal outcomes—and of course books, leaflets and webpages produced by hospitals or government agencies are often guilty of similar 'negative' framing. They not only have the strength of words to promote a message (whatever it is), but also the authority of the organisation. Are writers considering their use of words seriously enough when they write and are they sufficiently aware which model of birth they are implicitly promoting?

How would it be if everything were framed positively?

Metaphors and metonymy used for birth

We use metaphors more often than we realise. We talk about *raising issues* (who's lifting what up?), we *push things through* (e.g. a new policy), if we dare to we *put our oar in* and *stand up for what we believe in* (even if we're actually sitting typing at our computer), and we *call for action* without even opening our mouths. I remember thinking how metaphors were rather odd and irrelevant to me when I first studied them in English lessons at school. However, through my studies in linguistics I've come to realise that they are not only an extremely *common* form of language use, they are also an extremely *powerful* one. And—to be perfectly honest here—I wasn't even aware that metonymy existed, and it took me a while to get used to what it meant. Littlemore explains:[15]

> *Metaphor and metonymy constitute two cognitive processes which lie at the heart of much human thought and communication. In very basic terms, metaphor draws on relations of substitution and similarity, whereas metonymy draws on relations of contiguity. [According to the Cambridge Online Dictionary, 'contiguous' means 'next to or touching another, usually similar thing'.] In metaphor, one thing is seen in terms of another and the role of the interpreter is to identify points of similarity ...*
> *In metonymy, an entity is used to refer to something that it is actually related to.*

As an example of a metaphor, Littlemore suggests that a football commentator might describe a particularly easy victory as *a walk in the park*. In the field of birth, as I've already suggested, *the birth canal* is a metaphor for the very soft, folds of the vagina, which fan out under the influence of hormones (particularly oxytocin) allowing the release of the baby down through the woman's body, into the world. Another linguistics researcher, Randal Holme, argues that the very *presentation* of a placebo (e.g. its packaging) is a metaphor of its potential effect and that this will exert an unconscious influence over the patient.[16] Applying this idea to the field of maternity care, how could the presentation of a piece of maternity equipment affect perceptions of its effectiveness and effectively *symbolise* its value? How does the metaphorical power of equipment relating to 'normal' birth compare with the metaphorical power of equipment for highly interventionist births?

Littlemore's example of metonymy is the word *Hollywood* to refer to the whole of the American film industry. An example in childbirth would be the phrase *skin-to-skin contact*, which is used to refer not just to the literal contact the baby's skin makes with its mother's but also to the whole of process of postpartum bonding, because it often triggers the initiation of breastfeeding. In other words, *skin-to-skin contact* is a kind of shorthand for a much longer process. I would even argue that the word *contraction* is a case of metonymy—and a rather unhelpful one, in fact—because when a woman is said to be having a *contraction* so much more is going on physiologically: the woman's breathing spontaneously changes, her levels of oxytocin peak, the bands of muscle of her uterus draw in so as to push her baby down and make her cervix dilate—i.e. *expand* (not contract), and in terms of consciousness the woman is likely to sink deep into herself (metaphorically speaking!), particularly if she is in active labour, in an environment where she feels safe. Instead of focusing on the *contraction* of the uterine muscles to summarise this whole process, why do we not focus on the *expansion* of the cervix instead? By creating new forms of metonymy we can make unhelpful words positive.

Metaphors and metonymy are extremely common in English, so we really do need to take them seriously because they are bound to occur in our speech. When discussing language in connection with gender, linguist Mary Talbot writes:

> *Medical discourse is an important site of struggle ... The medical discourse on pregnancy and childbirth is not the only [discourse], but it is more powerful than any other, and more widespread. Antenatal care discourse [i.e. speech and writing] is upheld by the power behind the medical institution, power exercised by the medical profession. It is contemporary society's most influential discourse on the social phenomenon of maternity.*[17]

As Littlemore points out,[18] "different metaphorical meanings emerge in different discourse settings [areas of language use]" and she goes on to say that "[n]ot every discourse community uses metaphor in the same way, and many communities have their own metaphors ... that are related to, but different from, more mainstream usage." I would suggest that it is useful to consider how language is used in medical settings and how this is perceived by pregnant women who come into a medical setting fresh, when used to more 'mainstream' usage. Is it possible that a primagravida might be a little taken aback to hear the gentle folds of her body implicitly compared with a concrete canal? And if she doesn't register any shock consciously, should we perhaps reflect on what kinds of assumptions might be communicated to her (about what her body can do, in terms of opening up) through the use of a metaphor such as *birth canal*?

Metaphors are so incredibly powerful precisely because they are so discreet. In fact, it is only when metaphors are used in obviously inappropriate ways that we tend to notice them. In the film *Taking Chances*[19] characters in a small town constantly use metaphors in strange ways and this creates a strand of tension and humour throughout the film—as well as the impression that no one is really effectively communicating with anyone else successfully. (The viewer could perhaps guess that this explains why the town is approaching financial ruin.) At one point, for example, a private investigator says to the mayor, "If anything messes with my apples, that means no locating agreement, and that means no casino." The mayor replies: "I have your apples in my capable hands". The investigator replies, "I like the sound of that" but it's clear from the investigator's expression that he has absolutely no idea what's he's just agreed to. Here is a case of someone using someone else's metaphor and realising too late that he is taking on shadows of meaning of which he has no real understanding.

In a similar way, a pregnant woman is not in control of the language for pregnancy and birth when she first becomes pregnant so is, therefore, at the mercy of the current experts in that discourse community [field of language use]. Of course, those people are *you*, her caregivers—whether you are a midwife, obstetrician, doula nurse or GP. This means your new clients are unlikely to question your use of metaphors in speech because they will reasonably assume that the way in which you use words actually reflects the reality of what they are supposed to represent. However, I would like to argue that this is not the case... it is merely that the words you use reflect the reality of your *perception* of pregnancy and birth (and all that it represents), or the perception of people who you have spoken to before, or whose texts you have studied, who you have not yet challenged. And perceptions of birth are likely to be influenced by personal experience, prevailing attitudes towards risk (amongst other things) and current protocols, which implicitly convey attitudes about the risk inherent in birth.

Images used with pregnant women

Metaphors often lead us to conceive images (visual information) which we then use in more formal contexts to further reinforce our casual use of metaphor in communication. One example is the photo on the 2001 edition of Sheila Kitzinger's recently updated book *Rediscovering Birth* (Pinter & Martin, 2011),[20] All we see is a woman's hands, resting together over her naked navel, with thumbs crooked so that the space between the thumbs is the shape of a heart. Clearly, this image—which is used in many places—associates love (symbolised by the heart) with the growing baby, which we assume is behind the navel. Of course, most people would agree that this is an extremely positive image and one which is relatively harmless. But what about other images which a pregnant woman might encounter on her journey through pregnancy, labour and birth?

- Firstly, if she reads certain bestselling pregnancy books, a pregnant woman is likely to encounter images which reinforce the negative metaphor of the *birth canal*. As Holly Kennedy notes in her survey of pregnancy books,[21] in *The Girlfriend's Guide to Pregnancy* a woman will read: "A rudimentary understanding of simple physics will tip you off that a vagina that has never experienced anything larger than a super Tampax or a very well-endowed fellow is going to balk a bit at passing a watermelon through its dainty corridors."[22] This imagery is not only vivid, it is also depressing for a pregnant woman who is already apprehensive about vaginal birth. In her article analysing the language of pregnancy books Kennedy describes the range of imagery used and the extreme nature of some of this.
- Entering a delivery room a woman is likely to see colours, materials and shapes which she is more likely to associate with an engineering process than with the soft, womanly processes of birth. Bright lights positioned to make any privacy or intimacy impossible suggest that the processes about to take place need to do so in public; steel instruments, in sharp shapes suggest that cutting must be about to take place; hard, flat surfaces which are kept immaculately clear of any human fluids (on arrival) surely suggests they are not 'allowable' within this environment; posters on the walls which are intended to remind caregivers of protocols in emergencies are likely to suggest danger to the woman and the *probability* that things will go wrong.
- If a woman has read *The Girlfriend's Guide to Pregnancy,* her expectation of the birth itself is likely to be rather negative because of the metaphor used in the book. According to Kennedy, Iovine, the author, explains that "Childbirth is as messy as a pig slaughter."[23] Instead of images of birth and new life, the labouring woman has had an image of death imprinted on it—and not just any death, but a violent one and one of an animal, with which, presumably, she is supposed to identify.
- Imagery is also used by women to share their fears about vaginal damage and impairment to sexual functioning postpartum. Imagery usually involves the vagina being compared with something wide and lacking in elasticity, such as a hospital corridor—imagery which is hardly likely to reassure women that sex will be possible and even enjoyable postpartum. (Of course, the power of hormones to expand and later reduce the size of the male sexual organ is rarely mentioned in this context, although a comparison is surely appropriate.)

The power of words, metaphors and images in history

We don't need to dig far into the past to discover examples of words, metaphors and images which have caused great change. Consider how powerful words and imagery are in the following extracts. (The use of metaphor or metonymy is highlighted with my own italics.)

- **Emmeline Pankhurst speaking in Connecticut, USA in 1913, when the fight was on to get women the vote in the UK:** "I am not only here as *a soldier temporarily absent from the field at battle*; I am here—and that, I think, is the strangest part of my coming—I am here as a person who, according to the law courts of my country, it has been decided, is of no value to the community at all ... It is about eight years since the word *'militant'* was first used to describe what we were doing. It was not *militant* at all, except that it provoked militancy on the part of those who were opposed to it. When women asked questions in political meetings and failed to get answers, they were not doing anything *militant*. In Great Britain it is a custom, a time-honoured one, to ask questions of candidates for parliament and ask questions of members of the government. No man was ever put out of a public meeting for asking a question. The first people who were put out of a political meeting for asking questions, were women. They were brutally ill-used—they found themselves in jail before 24 hours had expired. ... *You have two babies very hungry and wanting to be fed. One baby is a patient baby and waits indefinitely until its mother is ready to feed it. The other baby is an impatient baby and cries lustily, screams and kicks and makes everybody unpleasant until it is fed. Well, we know perfectly well which baby is attended to first. That is the whole history of politics*."
- **Martin Luther King, speaking in Washington, USA in 1963 about the fight to establish rights for non-whites, as a black person himself:** "Let us not seek to satisfy *our thirst for freedom by drinking from the cup of bitterness and hatred*. We must forever conduct our struggle on the *high plane of dignity and discipline*. We must not allow our creative protest to degenerate into physical violence. Again and again we must rise to the *majestic heights of meeting physical force with soul force*. The marvelous new *militancy* which has *engulfed* the negro community must not lead us to a distrust of all white people, for many of our white *brothers*, as evidenced by their presence here today, have come to realise that their destiny is *tied up* with our destiny, and *their freedom is inextricably bound to our freedom. We cannot walk alone. ... I have a dream that one day even the state of Mississippi, a state sweltering with the heat of injustice, sweltering with the heat of oppression will be transformed into an oasis of freedom and justice. I have a dream* that my four little children will one day live in a nation where they will not be judged by the colour of their skin but by *the content* of their character. *I have a dream today."*
- **And finally, an extract from Oprah Winfrey's speech, which she gave on receiving the first Bob Hope Humanitarian (Emmy) Award in 22 September, 2002 (broadcast by NBC in the USA):** "*The greatest pain in life* is to be invisible. What I've learnt is that we all just want *to be heard*. And I thank all the people who continue to let me hear your stories, and by sharing your stories, you let other people *see themselves* and for a moment, *glimpse the power to change and the power to triumph*. Maya Angelou said, 'When you learn, teach. When you get, give.' ... I will continue to strive *to give back to the world what it has given to me...*"

The power of words in maternity contexts

Clearly, how or whether we speak about issues affects people's perceptions. This explains why it is not always a good idea to ask a long-term partner if he/she loves you. The very fact of asking may bring the relationship into question and result in its breakup. Considering the context of maternity, constantly referring to 'risk' will inevitably suggest to women not just that you are taking their pregnancies seriously, but also that you consider them inherently *risky*—i.e. that they are bound to be somewhere on the spectrum of risk (probably medium) because surely the odds for anyone being at the 'zero risk' end must be virtually nil... despite the fact that, physiologically speaking, birth really is a healthy process which—in a healthy woman—usually proceeds entirely smoothly. In other words, instead of promoting a view of health, i.e. a salutogenic approach, by using the word *risk* a caregiver is suggesting that pregnancy is intrinsically *unhealthy* and dangerous.

When we use metaphor, as well as words which communicate negative suggestions, the situation becomes even less salutogenic. For example, when a caregiver uses the phrase *pass through the birth canal* these few words, which are used metaphorically (since the woman does not have anything approximating to the Panama canal within her body), are problematic for two reasons. First, they imply that the passageway through which a baby passes is hard and unyielding, like a real concrete canal. (Is it not reasonable, when a metaphor is used, to assume that the target word—the word used metaphorically—has the same properties as the thing to which it refers?) Second, the words *pass through the birth canal* are problematic because they suggest that the as yet unborn baby will be moving *laterally* along the 'canal'. (Since the word *pass* gives no idea of direction, it would be reasonable for the listener to assume that the direction is similar to that of a ship passing through a real-life canal, which is laterally.) What we really need, in order to promote normal outcomes in birth is a phrase such as *descend through the flexible folds of the woman's vagina*, i.e. a phrase which communicates not only flexibility and softness, but also downward motion. Use of such a phrase will implicitly suggest to the pregnant woman that she will be upright when she is giving birth (so the baby can *descend*, not *go through* or *go along*) and that the 'canal' is now flexible and fluid—as in the folds of a dress. In changing the phrase it is not that we avoid using a metaphor... We use another metaphor, which is reasonable given that we are dealing with an area of unknown knowledge for the primagravida, but this time to good effect. In doing so, we would be taking account of a mental process proposed by the psychologist Gibbs called 'embodied cognition.'[24] He argues that "People's subjective, felt experiences of their bodies in action provides part of the fundamental grounding for language and thought"—meaning that a positive view of an experience should lead to positive language, and that this in turn should influence other people's thinking on the same experience—or vice versa.[25]

Words used in interactive contexts—i.e. in conversation—are particularly powerful agents for change. In linguistics, the field of 'pragmatics' looks at how language is used to influence practical outcomes. For example the illocutionary force—effect, if you prefer—of the utterance "It's eight o'clock!" will probably be to get someone to hurry up; it will not be an attempt to behave like a speaking clock.

We can use words to change perceptions and outcomes

We can use words, depending on how we group them and time their use, to change perceptions, behaviour and outcomes. For example, Kiaer notes in her research how the use of Yes/No questions by her doctor put her into the limited role of 'respondent', when she was attending an antenatal appointment, so it was difficult for her to ask any questions herself.[26] Other linguistics researchers have shown how depersonalised talk constructs the mother as a patient who is 'suffering from the pathology of pregnancy'[27] and as an 'object carrying a baby and a set of symptoms'.[28] Still other researchers have considered the politics of pregnancy and parenthood.[29-35]

If you consider your own use of words in conversation, how often do you think you personally ask open questions or encourage a relaxed reporting of feelings through the way in which you organise antenatal appointments? What proportion of your time is spent on 'risk checking' and what proportion on proactive salutogenic talk or action (whatever that might be)? Do you worry that your authority as a caregiver will be undermined if you stop emphasising your clients' need for you by underlining the potential for things to go wrong? If you are a man, do you compensate in any way for female (pregnant) clients' probable tendency to use (as researcher Lakoff proposed)[36] language which is notable for its 'uncertainty, weakness and excessive politeness'?

How much time do you spend on proactive salutogenic talk?

Marjorie Tew's commentary is interesting in this respect. A research statistician, teaching at a university in the UK, she explains why she started focusing on childbirth:

> *"... I was teaching students in the Department of Community Health in Nottingham University's young Medical School how much they could find out about various diseases from the available official statistics. As part of these epidemiological exercises, I discovered to my complete surprise that the relevant routine statistics did not appear to support the widely accepted hypothesis that the increased hospitalisation of birth had caused the decline by then achieved in the mortality of mothers and their new babies. At first it seemed hardly possible that I could be right in questioning the justification for what the medical world and everyone else apparently believed, but my further researches only served to confirm my initial discovery."*

In her book *Safer Childbirth? A Critical History of Maternity Care* (3rd ed, 1998, Free Association Books) Tew notes how important confidence is in ensuring good results. She argues that ongoing propaganda (i.e. the use of words in texts) from obstetricians was responsible for undermining women's confidence in their own ability to give birth and says it also undermined other caregivers' confidence in their abilities (especially midwives')—confidence which has perhaps only recently started returning in the UK and also in the USA.[37] Tew also notes how the use of ongoing tests antenatally has the unfortunate side-effect of causing caregivers to report results cautiously (since there is always the danger of false negatives or positives)—with the consequence that pregnant women become more apprehensive and more convinced of their need for specialist care (because of the apparent risks involved).[38]

Most importantly, perhaps, is the issue of how perceptions of risk affect informed choice (or consent). When reviewing literature available to pregnant women and how their apparent choices are presented, linguistics researcher Mary Talbot concludes: "All in all, choice may be more illusory than real. It is more a matter of medical procedure being presented *as if* there are choices."[39] However, the problem is further compounded by what Talbot calls 'ideological programming' which you have doubtless been subject to, if you have become a qualified caregiver.[40] What changes would be necessary in your own or your colleagues' use of language, or in the literature published by the institutions within which you work, or are affiliated to, in order to ensure that women really do have choices during pregnancy and childbirth? How could things be 'reprogrammed' within a salutogenic framework?

Our individual responsibility to take control

Remembering how things were going wrong in the town of Patriotville in the film *Taking Chances,* a place where communication was muddied through the overuse of metaphor, I wonder how much impact misuse of language has on the field of birth. Could it be that the way in which some caregivers are using language is actually influencing outcomes—making births either more or less 'normal', simply because of the impact caregivers' words are having on pregnant and labouring women? Are you as a caregiver a little too 'patriotic' towards the traditional language of midwifery and childbirth to dare to coin new uses of words? Isn't it time you moved to a new country of language use?

How would it feel to take up the challenge of changing the words and imagery used when explaining things to pregnant women in your care? To what extent would changes mean you were more effectively facilitating normal outcomes? Whether you are an empowered, confident midwife, a responsible, sensitive obstetrician, or another caregiver—e.g. a doula—attempting to fit within a complex system, how successfully do you think you promote a real feeing of health and positivity in the pregnant and labouring women you care for?

To consider a few examples of improvements which could be made, instead of saying to women who report they are in labour that they are just in 'false' labour, why not tell them they're just 'starting out'? Later on in the process, instead of using an emotionally loaded word like 'transition', why not simply say "You're nearly there"—or "The end's in sight"? How often do you encourage women in labour by telling them they're amazing, that their bodies know what to do—that their body's managed to grow a baby, so it will certainly also know how to birth it too? And what other encouraging and health-promoting ways can you think of in order to ensure positive outcomes?

As an individual who has sometimes been made very angry by the use of certain words when applied to me, and who has been profoundly affected by certain imagery created through words, I feel we all have a responsibility to consider the impact of whatever words we choose to use, whenever we speak. Not only must we be held accountable for our actions, but also for the words we use. Those small units of communication are far more powerful than we usually remember.

We all need to consider the words we choose to use

Sylvie Donna founded Fresh Heart Publishing in order to make a contribution to the world of birth—to make birth a better experience for mothers, babies and caregivers. Her own books on birth promote informed choice by providing informative and reassuring reading for mothers, or thought-provoking material for caregivers, e.g. *Optimal Birth: What, Why & How* (Fresh Heart, 2011).[41] Her aim is to inspire creative solutions to age-old problems by collating key information and posing important questions. She has three daughters, all of whom were born entirely normally, without any drugs or interventions, and each was breastfed for two or three years. She is interested in hearing from anybody who would like to publish material for either caregivers, medical students or mothers-to-be. Email: sylvie@freshheartpublishing.com.

References

1 Lakoff G, 1987. *Women, Fire and Dangerous Things: What Categories Reveal about the Mind.* Chicago: University of Chicago Press.

2 Holme R, 2004. *Mind, Metaphor and Language Teaching.* Basingstoke: Palgrave Macmillan, p 34.

3 Cambridge Online Dictionary definition, available from http://dictionary.cambridge.org/dictionary/british/risk_1 [accessed 19 Mar 2011]

4 Murkoff HE, Mazel S, 2009. What to Expect When You're Expecting. London: Simon & Schuster.

5 Odent M, 1994. The nocebo effect in prenatal care. *Primal Heath Research Newsletter*, 2(2)

6 Odent M, 1995. Back to the Nocebo effect. *Primal Heath Research Newsletter*, 5

7 Odent M, 2000. Antenatal scare. *Primal Heath Research Newsletter*, 7(4)

8 Strümpfer DJW, 1990. Salutogenesis: A new paradigm. *South African Journal of Psychology* [precise reference unknown]

9 Strümpfer DJW, 1995. The origins of health and strength: From 'salutogenesis' to 'fortigenesis'. *South African Journal of Psychology*, Vol 25(2), Jun, 81-89.

10 Bengt Lindstrom B, Eriksson M, 2006. Contextualizing salutogenesis and Antonovsky in public health development. *Health Promotion International.* Volume 21, Issue, 3, pp 238-244.

11 Downe S (ed), 2008. From being to becoming: reconstructing childbirth knowledges in *Normal Birth: Evidence and Debate.* 2nd ed. Elsevier, pp19-22.

12 Schmid V, 2007. *Salute e Nascita, la salutogenesi in gravidanza.* Milan: Apogeo.

13 Kiaer S, 2010. The construction of motherhood in the discourse of antenatal care. Unpublished MA dissertation, Lancaster University [available in the UK through inter-university loan], cited in Talbot, 2010 *Language and Gender.* Cambridge: Polity Press, pp 128-129

14 Donna, S. *Birth: Countdown to Optimal.* 2nd ed. Fresh Heart, 2011.

15 Littlemore J, 2009. *Applying Cognitive Linguistics to Second Language Learning and Teaching.* Basingstoke: Palgrave Macmillan, p 94.

16 Holme R, 2004. *Mind, Metaphor and Language Teaching.* Basingstoke: Palgrave Macmillan

17 Talbot M. *Language and Gender.* 2010, Cambridge: Polity Press, pp 128-129.

18 Littlemore J, 2009. *Applying Cognitive Linguistics to Second Language Learning and Teaching.* Basingstoke: Palgrave Macmillan, p 103.

19 *Taking Chances*, 2009. Starring Justin Long, Emmanuelle Chriqui and Rob Chorddry, among others. Director: Talmage Cooley.Studio: High Flyers (see www.highfliersplc.com).

20 Kitzinger, S, 2001. *Rediscovering Birth.* London: Little Brown. Recently republished under the same title by Pinter & Martin (2011).

21 Holly Powell Kennedy HP, Nardini K, McLeod-Waldo R, Ennis L, 2009. Top-Selling Childbirth Advice Books: A Discourse Analysis. *Birth* 36:4 Dec.

22 Iovine V, 2007. The Girlfriend's Guide to Pregnancy: Or Everything Your Doctor Won't Tell You. 2nd ed. New York: Pocket Books, p 70.

23 Ioveine V, 2007, p 74.

24 Gibbs RW Jr, Berg RA, Mental imagery and embodied Activity. *Journal of Mental Imagery,* Vol 26(1-2), Spr-Sum 2002, 1-30.

25 Gibbs RW Jr. Embodied experience and linguistic meaning. *Brain and Language.* Vol. 84, Issue 1. Jan 2003, pp 1-15.

26 Kiaer S, 2010. The construction of motherhood in the discourse of antenatal care. Unpublished MA dissertation, Lancaster University.

27 Oakley A, 1984. *The Captured Womb: A History of the Medical Care of Pregnant Women.* Oxford: Blackwell, pp 213.

28 Oakley, 1984, in Talbot M. *Language and Gender,* Polity Press, 2010, p129.

29 Lazar M, 2000. Gender, discourse and semiotics: the politics of parenthood representations. *Discourse & Society* 11(3):373-409.

30 Lazar, 2005. Performing state fatherhood: the remaking of hegemony, in *Feminist Critical Discourse Analysis: Gender, Power and Ideology in Discourse.* London: Palgrave Macmillan.

31 Marshall H, Woollett A, 2000. Fit to reproduce? The regulative role of pregnancy tests. *Feminism and Psychology* 10(3):351-66.

32 Page R, 2003. 'Cherie: lawyer, wife, mum': contradictory patterns of representation in media reports of Cherie Booth/Blair. *Discourse & Society* 14(5):559-79.

33 Rudolfsdottir, AG, 2000. 'I am not a patient, and I am not a child': the institutionalization and experience of pregnancy. *Feminism and Psychology* 10 (3):337-50.

34 Sunderland J, 2002. Baby entertainer, bumbling assistant and line manager: discourses of paternal identity in parentcraft texts. In Litosseliti L, Sunderland J (eds), 2002. *Gender Identity and Discourse Analysis.* Amsterdam/Philadelphia: John Benjamins.

35 Sunderland J, 2004. *Gendered Discourses.* London: Palgrave Macmillan.

36 Lakoff R, 1975. *Language and Women's Place.* New York: Harper & Row.

37 Tew M, 1990. *Safer Childbirth? A Critical History of Maternity Care.* London: Chapman and Hall, p 7.

38 Tew M, 1990. *Safer Childbirth? A Critical History of Maternity Care.* London: Chapman and Hall, p 18.

39 Talbot M, 2010. *Language and Gender.* Cambridge: Polity Press, p 133.

40 Talbot M, 2010, p 134.

41 Donna S, 2011. *Optimal Birth: What, Why & How.* Fresh Heart Publishing.

Identifying progress, gaps and possible ways forward

Soo Downe

Progress so far

As this book amply demonstrates, interest in the topic of normal childbirth has expanded exponentially over the last decade or so. This interest has generated important debates and insights that have taken the knowledge base a long way in a short time. Randomised trials have revealed the potential risks associated with certain interventions, when applied unnecessarily, and the value of other interventions that maximise positive, continuous, caring, relation-based care in pregnancy, childbirth and the postnatal period.[1] They have also, generally, shown that care that respects and supports the capacity of women to cope using their own resources is most likely to normalise birth and maximise well-being for mother and baby.[2]

Specifically, in high resource settings (where equipment, drugs and staff are available and accessible), this body of evidence highlights the value of out-of-hospital birth, midwife-led care, social support in pregnancy and labour, mobilisation in labour, alternative support for working with pain in labour, minimal intervention in childbirth, and peer support for breastfeeding and the development of the maternal role.[3] Even in low resource settings (where the focus of much research effort has been to find ways of reducing maternal and infant mortality) the provision of caring, compassionate, culturally sensitive, easily accessible basic services that pay attention to relationships and shared local knowledge, and that are provided as close to home as possible, seems to be a more powerful predictor of healthy survival for mother and/or baby than centralised highly technical provision.[4-7]

Qualitative studies and theoretical analysis have demonstrated why these findings have not, generally, been put into practice.[8,9] Since at least the 1980s, Foucauldian and feminist critiques have revealed the issues of power and control that dictate gender and hierarchy divisions between women and men in general, and pregnant and labouring women, midwives, nurses, obstetricians and other care workers in particular.[10,11] Such studies have also illustrated the blocking effect exerted by these power differentials when attempts are made to move towards normalising and humanising childbirth. Ethnographies have illustrated the cultural dynamics that block communication and collaboration between professional groups, and between layers of organisations and management.[12] Phenomenological studies explore the lived experience of individuals in depth, and they have powerfully illustrated the effect of current ways of 'doing' childbirth on childbearing women, their partners and families, and on caregivers. For example, Thomson and Downe used interpretive phenomenology in in-depth interviews with women who were deeply traumatised by childbirth. This study revealed that the trauma was most often associated with attitudes of maternity staff during childbirth, and that women in this situation tended to talk in terms of horror and abuse.[13] On the other hand, the same women who then went on to have a subsequent positive experience of childbirth used radically different language to describe their experience, such as 'elation' 'joy' and 'transformation.[14] These kinds of studies reinforce the increasing pressure to abandon the use of 'satisfaction' as a wholly inadequate measure of the extremes and depths of women's childbirth experience.

It seems that 'satisfaction' is a wholly inadequate measure

All of this work is creating a significant body of knowledge. However, many intractable issues remain, not least how to get what is known into practice. This chapter is largely framed around current gaps in research and evidence, with a primary focus on how to make change happen—or, in sociological terms 'praxis'.

Current and emerging debates

The definition of normal birth

There are still prolonged debates about what normal birth is.[15] These may seem trivial, but they are actually indicative of deep philosophical and pragmatic differences between stakeholders in maternity care. This is most complex when it concerns women's sense of themselves. Definitions that insist that only a completely spontaneous physiological birth is normal alienate some women who have interventions in labour. On the other hand, more inclusive definitions run the risk of being so relativist: 'anything the woman feels is normal is normal': that they could, feasibly, term as 'normal' a system in which 100% of births are caesarean sections.

Gender and hierarchy imbalance

The issue of gender and hierarchy imbalance, and so-called 'tribal' (disciplinary) divisions also remains important. The debates in this area are moving away from simplistic binary divisions of 'female/woman/midwife = good and oppressed' / 'male/doctor = bad and dominant', towards Foucauldian and critical feminist readings which acknowledge that power creates resistance, and that, as well as external agencies acting on their behalf, oppressed individuals and groups also need to be responsible for change in their circumstances.[16] This work is beginning to look at how collaboration and inter-connectivity might influence the complex dynamic systems that make up maternity care, and that cross into society, culture, and belief systems. Organisational and leadership theories, as well as complexity science, are being used to illuminate some of the complex (and complicated) inter-relationships that exist within and across boundaries.[17]

Debates are moving away from simplistic binary divisions

Technoscience

Technoscience studies have been emerging over the last 20 years or so.[18] As technology becomes increasingly integrated into maternity care, this has become an area of examination for researchers who are interested in normal childbirth. Ultrasound, fetal monitoring, central monitoring, remote tele-medicine, computerised decision-support tools and technological measurement of cervical dilation in labour all raise questions about the impact of separating out data about simple physical measurements from the complex experiences of people, which cannot always be conveyed in terms of clear data.

The separation of data from people operates on a range of levels. At the most obvious, data is translated from the individual to the machine. More subtly, the use of machines to measure and, in some cases, interpret human data shifts the gaze of the caregiver from (in the case of maternity care) the pregnant/labouring woman to the machine. At the extreme, the woman and midwife/obstetrician become invisible, and the machine becomes the ultimate decision-maker in terms of what is happening and what should be done about it. The 'norms' that are programmed into the machine become authoritative. However, these norms are usually expressed in simple terms, i.e. they only take into account a few signs and symptoms, and only those that can be measured easily. This is based on so-called linear thinking (as in A + B = C). Decision-support tools interpret this linear data based on population data and guidelines, and not on the norms of a particular individual, which may be affected by a range of physical, psychosocial, emotional, spiritual and contextual factors. Individuals who, for example, are experiencing a physiological labour which falls outside of population norms (so, for example, the labour may be longer than usual, shorter than usual, or it may have a different trajectory than usual) are assessed as 'abnormal' and therefore 'pathological' by the machine's algorithms; action is therefore taken, even though all is actually well for this particular woman and this particular baby.

Using norms to program machines has the added effect of reifying what is 'normal', so that future population studies will increasingly constrain normality into ever more precise boundaries. It also has the effect of separating the woman and the midwife because as midwives increasingly make decisions through machines, there is less and less need to be with the woman. If, on the other hand, midwives base their decision-making on touching and watching pregnant and labouring women, after learning the subtle, intuitive cues that such contact reveals, there is far more connection. When this is the case midwives also learn how to be with women in a way that 'nudges' them into coping, and they are more likely to facilitate the normal flow of each woman's labour. When machines take over decision-making and separate women from their midwives (or other caregivers), these cues and support skills and ways of being then drop from midwifery knowledge (and from the knowledge of other caregivers). This then further reinforces the supremacy of techno-science, and reduces the value and authority of the woman's own experiences and beliefs, and of midwifery—and, indeed, obstetric—expertise.

Technoscience and place of birth

One solution to the kind of scenario where pregnant women are separated from their caregivers (because of the focus on data) has been to provide continuity of midwifery care and to take birth out of hospital and away from what Foucauldian researchers would describe as the 'gaze' of the dominant way of 'doing birth'.[10] Research in this area has been very persuasive, demonstrating that out-of-hospital, midwife-led births in settings where there is good midwifery care and other support mechanisms are, generally, at least as safe as hospital births for the majority of childbearing women in resource-rich countries in terms of mortality, and that they are associated with lower levels of morbidity in both mother and baby.[19]

However, technoscience does provide another challenge to this positive picture because remote technology is becoming more effective and prevalent. One of the protective features of out-of-hospital birth has been its relative invisibility to data-collecting equipment. With no or few electronic monitors, recording devices or measurement tools, practice is dependent on the relationship between the woman and her caregiver/birth companions, and on holistic assessment of the normality of her labour, based on an expert and emphatic reading of the woman's reactions to the pregnancy and labour. As remote technology becomes more powerful, the temptation will be to introduce recording devices into the home or birth centre, so that they can transmit measurements of labour to a central point, for 'expert' review. Indeed, the potential for iPhones to record and transmit data on fetal heartbeat rates and patterns is already under discussion, meaning that women could, potentially, continuously send fetal heartbeat data during pregnancy and labour to a central monitor. This suggests that retreating to out-of-hospital settings would not prevent the accelerating influence of technology on pregnancy and childbirth. More fundamental changes would be required and women's freedom to choose more or less monitoring needs to be honoured by law, if individualised, physiological pregnancy and labour is seen to be a valuable phenomenon that needs to be protected, preserved, and promoted.

Praxis: getting evidence into practice

Realising that some caregivers are moving towards a technoscientific scenario in which data might be transmitted from home settings to a centralised point for evaluation, it becomes clear that a focus is necessary on one of the most important areas for normalising childbirth: praxis–i.e. knowing what we know, how can we make change happen? Change management theories offer a range of solutions, including transformational management,[20] product champions[21] and, even more 'nudge' approaches (which were endorsed by the UK government in 2010 as useful techniques for social change).[22] However, the experience of innovations such as the Productive Ward Initiative, which was undertaken by the NHS in England as a route to increasing ward efficiency, and, therefore, increasing the time available for staff to give personal care, has revealed that, after initial enthusiasm, sustainability is patchy.[23] Places where innovations are sustained tend to be those where there is a 'hearts and minds' change, and not just an intellectual sign-up. For example, the best evidence we have suggests that, at least for low-risk women and babies, out-of-hospital pregnancy and childbirth leads to decreased levels of intrapartum and postnatal morbidity, increased levels of breastfeeding with all the associated benefits for mother and baby in the short and longer-term, and lower costs to healthcare systems.[19] However, the overwhelming quantity of evidence which clearly points to these improved outcomes, does not seem to be sufficient to make maternity care systems promote out-of-hospital births, given that little action has as yet been taken by some stakeholders, even in this era of evidence-based medicine. This suggests that praxis in the area of normal childbirth (i.e. the translation of knowledge into new systems) needs dramatic new discoveries to effectively tip resistant maternity care systems from one way of thinking towards another.

We need dramatic new discoveries to tip resistant maternity care systems from one way of thinking towards another

Women's experience as a basis for praxis

The power of women, their partners, and midwives working together in respectful collaboration with obstetricians and managers and other colleagues cannot be underestimated. Very often, before the system suddenly shifts, it seems that it is completely impossible for it to change. (Readers who remember apartheid in South Africa or the Berlin Wall before it was brought down will appreciate this.) Then, in a few months, complete change happens. For example, in February 2011 in a city of 7 million people in China, the city leaders decreed that all midwives working in the city now have to work for three months in a new birth centre set up by Professor Cheung and her colleagues (see the chapter of this book by Ngai Fen Cheung and Anshi Pan for more information on the work undertaken by this team). The reason for this three-month placement is so as to enable midwives to learn how to support normal birth, so that the very high rate of caesarean section in the area can be reduced. Before the change, the caesarean section rate in the local hospital was above 50%. Now, in 2011, for the 1000+ low risk women per year who give birth in the birth centre, the normal birth rate is around 95%. This change came partly as a result of women having their babies in the birth centre, being transformed by the experience and talking to friends and family. Midwives across China also heard about these women's good experiences, and are now keen to make the same changes (clearly perceived as being improvements) elsewhere. Years of creating the initial conditions for change (training a few midwives to provide intrapartum care that is focused on normal birth, getting local permission, trying it out) and one small shift in a system on the edge of chaos (local women who were party officials or the wives of party officials experiencing positive normal childbirth) has rapidly and dramatically tipped a huge system potentially from one state of high rates of intervention to another of high rates of normal childbirth.

Other examples of the power of responding to women's experiences, and normalising and humanising childbirth and infant care in areas of high maternal and infant mortality, are given in work carried out in Brazil,[24] Ecuador,[25] India,[5] and Nepal.[4] For example, in one project in one region of Ecuador,[26] just paying attention to local cultural norms and treating women respectfully in hospital have been associated with a drop in infant mortality to 7.8 per 1,000 live births, which is less than half the national average. After making these changes to the quality of the service, there was just one (unrelated) maternal death due to complications, in contrast to eight deaths in horizontal deliveries the previous year; the caesarean rate was also reduced from 18% to 8% at the hospital. This offers evidence that normalising and humanising birth can both improve maternal and infant mortality rates and reduce intervention successfully. Although the effects of more respectful treatment remain to be demonstrated by controlled studies, the evidence so far suggests that humanising and normalising childbirth, and minimising mortality and morbidity rates, are not either/or options. In other words, it's clear that *in order* to minimise mortality and morbidity rates, the normalisation of birth is necessary.

Complexity science as praxis

From a complexity science perspective, dramatic shifts do occur, based on the concept of 'small in, large out'–i.e. small innovations can trigger large changes. This can be most powerful when a system is 'on the edge of chaos' and when the initial conditions are appropriate to foster such change. Dramatic new evidence is needed that will shift the 'normal science' view of pregnancy and childbirth from linear thinking about bits of bodies and systems (i.e. carrying out a specific intervention on one specific bit of the body will inevitably lead to a standard result for all women), towards an understanding of the interconnectivity of systems and an awareness that disrupting one element in the name of risk-aversion might have multiple and unknown adverse consequences for the system as a whole later in the process. What might this dramatic new evidence be? As Khun has noted, ways of knowing which are seen as legitimate can vary depending on the historical and cultural context.[27] The key feature of most current healthcare diagnosis is the super-valuation of reductionist science because the aim is to identify one, simple cause for what is seen to have gone wrong. It is becoming increasingly mainstream to accept that complex interactions determine health, well-being and illness,[28] and neuroscience does indeed provide hard evidence to support this view. In fact, in the field of neuroscience it is evident that there are complex and multiple interactions between the individual, his or her environment, physical sensations, psychological status and emotional state.[29] In other words, emotional well-being can regulate physical well-being. Metaphysical states of belief, trust, hope and joy can also promote physical healing.[30] Furthermore, interactions with caregivers can, of themselves, interfere with or promote health states in patients.[31] It may be that this is the area that can change conversations about what maternity care does, and what it is for.

Changing the conversation towards salutogenesis

Much of the intervention that occurs in both resource-rich and resource-poor maternity settings is carried out in the name of risk management. However, paradoxically, this approach, which focuses on extreme and very rare complications for the few individuals who are high risk, has generated higher levels of risk for the majority—i.e. risk aversion has, in itself, caused risk. In addition, intervention is associated with fear, guilt, and blame. A change to salutogenic thinking[32]—to a focus on what makes things go well in childbirth[33]—might be much more productive, and could also generate an atmosphere in birthing women and caregivers alike of optimism, self-belief, happiness and joy:

> *oooh you couldn't get that feeling with anything on earth drugs, alcohol, anything I just wanted to bottle it and keep it forever that feeling and I still get it*[14] (p107)

As governments move towards recognising the value of well-being as a positive attribute of health (and not just as being 'not ill') the route to creating a tipping point phenomenon might be emerging. Arguably, as noted above, it already seems to have been at least a contributor to the tipping point in one place in China, where the positive, happy, joyful stories of women have created the praxis for change. This phenomenon is viral—it spreads rapidly. Hearing one of the leading midwives from the birth centre in Hangzhou talk about her experiences recently, I could almost see the endorphins surging through her—she was passionate, excited, engaged and charismatic. Such salutogenic experiences can create heart and mind experiences that can, later, be seen as a 'small in' / 'large out' lever for change.

Much of the intervention that occurs in both resource-rich and resource-poor maternity settings is carried out in the name of risk management

Psychoimmunology as an illustration of salutogenesis and complexity thinking

The observation that positive organisational change seems to have physiological effects on those who are part of the change may be one of the most important drivers for promoting normality in birthing situations. Neuroscience—or even psycho-emotional-neuro-immunological science—is beginning to indicate something very important for childbirth activities and researchers with an interest in normal childbirth. Evidence is increasingly showing that there is a complex and fundamental interconnectivity between our emotions, our brains and our bodies at the micro-biological level.[34] Indeed, it has been known for a while that emotions can affect and be affected by physical illness. As Solomon points out, "...the immune system, operating via the central nervous and neuroendocrine systems, may act as a transducer between experience and disease."[35]

A surge in interest in psychoneuroimmunology has surfaced again recently, after spasmodic interest in this area since the 1930s. The suggestion is that stress can influence immune response in fascinating and unexpected ways. In fact, there are known links between chronic stress states and later onset of chronic illness.[35] People with more chronic stress in their lives are more likely later in life to develop cancer, for instance.[36] The relevance of this for maternity care is that mode of birth is being linked in the research literature to later immune mediated diseases, such as Type 1 diabetes in under-five year olds,[37] and to asthma and eczema.[38]–i.e. the relationship between mode of birth and Type 1 diabetes may be influenced by the amount of stress experienced by the baby during birth. Infants born after elective caesarean section have lower salivary cortisol levels (a measure of their stress response) than those born after a 'normal' vaginal birth, and both these groups tend to have lower levels of salivary cortisol than infants born after a forceps or ventouse birth.[39] However, as noted above, retrospective studies also indicate that infants with Type 1 diabetes are more likely to have been born by caesarean section,[38] so lower stress is clearly not the only thing which is important. In this study, which was a review of research on diabetes databases, with 20 studies included, there was low heterogeneity between the studies, meaning that they were similar enough to be meta-analysed. The research team found the adjusted odds ratio of risk of Type 1 diabetes in children born by caesarean section was 1.19, 95% CI 1.04-1.36, $p = 0.01$ and the team notes that this implies a 20% increase in the risk of childhood-onset Type 1 diabetes for children born after caesarean section. The accumulating data therefore suggests that a degree of stress (such as that generated by physiological labour and birth) might be necessary during childbirth to switch on immunological protective mechanisms in the neonate, but that too little or too much stress might be damaging.

To add complexity to this argument, a recent study from China apparently contradicts the suggestion that too little stress during birth might be damaging for the infant.[40] The researchers reported that, for their study population, children born after an elective caesarean section that was undertaken on maternal request (and where there were no other medical reasons for the operation) had less behavioural problems than those born after instrumental vaginal birth, indicating that low levels of stress at birth led to a calmer personality. Beyond this, there is also accumulating evidence from the field of epigenetics that stress at the time of birth may influence the infant HPA axis response for up to two months at least,[41] and that, for the first three to five days postnatally, infants born after elective caesarean section have higher levels of DNA mylenation in white blood cells than those born after spontaneous vaginal birth.[42] It is not yet clear what the long term implications of this might be, but, at the least, these outcomes demonstrate that the process of birth has a physiological effect on the baby at an epigenetic level.

Too little stress during birth might be damaging for the infant

Overall, this evidence suggests that there is a level of 'eustress'[43] (i.e. positive, or salutogenic stress) during childbirth that might be physiologically necessary for effective fetal adaptation to life. It is tempting to suggest that this level of eustress is most likely to be generated by normal, physiological, positive, socially supported pregnancy and childbirth. Research in this area might take us beyond professional territorial struggles and debates about what normal birth is and why caesarean section is too common in resource-rich countries and not common enough in resource-poor ones; it should take us beyond asking whether women should have routine access to epidurals or not, and whether choice in childbirth is a feminist issue. Hopefully, it may take us towards a better understanding of the toxic situation of high maternal and infant deaths in some countries and high levels of unnecessary intervention in others, and towards dramatically new ground where we can enjoy 'joined up', respectful, collegiate debate within and between professional disciplines, women's groups and the commissioners and managers of maternity services. These conditions may finally trigger change in maternity services provision worldwide.

Possible ways forward

It is easy to argue that the evidence which already exists on the benefits of social support in pregnancy, easy access to empathic, skilled, well-equipped caregiver support, culturally appropriate care, out-of-hospital birth for low risk women, continuous support in pregnancy, labour and the postpartum period by known caregivers in general, and by midwives in particular, and general support for physiological labour and birth should inspire governments, policy makers, managers, and practitioners to make changes immediately. However, experience reminds us that, despite the mantra that all practice must be evidence-based, such evidence is not enough to overcome deep-rooted concerns about risks or modern society's indifference to maternal health (in every country of the world). All the evidence we already have is not sufficient to inspire caregivers in the field of maternity care to re-evaluate the prevailing super-valuation of technical solutions to social issues and problems. The challenge of the gap is therefore one of praxis: how can we bring about change?

Complexity theory emphasises the connectivity of organisms and organisations at various levels and I would argue that one of the fundamental gaps in our understanding is how systems are interconnected. Understanding the interconnections on both the level of the organism (the woman's and baby's bodies) and also the organisation (the institution or system within which we work) can shift maternity care towards positive salutogenic thinking, which learns from what goes well, as well as from what has gone badly. For example, it seems that the physiology of microsystems in the body during pregnancy and labour, including biochemical, immunological and hormonal responses, is similar to the physiology of meso-systems, such as the emotion and mood of the mother. These then influence macrosystems, such as those involved with triggering the onset of labour and its ongoing progression. These systems are themselves influenced by the response of partners, companions and caregivers, and these responses are then mediated by social situations, such as the environment which people live and work in.

Understanding the influence of one part of a system on another takes research from just looking at distinct elements of the body or organisations towards an understanding of the interconnectivity of all elements

Understanding the influence of one part of a system on another takes maternity care and related research from just looking at distinct elements of the body or organisations towards an understanding of the essential interconnectivity of all elements. It also leads us away from simple assumptions, such as 'midwives are good' / 'doctors are bad', or 'hospital birth is good' / 'home and birth centre are bad', towards a much more nuanced and subtle approach to understanding pregnancy and birth and their longer-term consequences. As Einstein once said:

Problems cannot be solved at the level of understanding that created them.

Many of the authors who have contributed to this book have opened doors to new kinds of understanding for the future. I hope that the observations and ideas in this chapter also offer the potential for new lines of enquiry, and new types of praxis, with the ultimate aim being to achieve maximum well-being for mothers, fathers, babies, families, communities and societies in the future.

A much more nuanced, subtle approach to understanding pregnancy and birth is required if we are to achieve maximum well-being for all parties

Soo Downe spent 15 years working as a midwife in various clinical, research and project development roles at Derby City General Hospital. In 2001 she joined the University of Central Lancashire (UCLan) in England, set up the UCLan Midwifery Studies Research Unit in October 2002, and is now the Professor of Midwifery Studies. As well as leading various research groups nationally and internationally, she has been a member of a number of national midwifery committees. Her main research focus is the nature of, and culture around, normal birth. She leads on a number of current research grants and consultancies, including an RfPB grant for an RCT of the use of self-hypnosis in labour (the SHIP trial) and an EU COST grant focused on systems of maternity care in Europe that currently involves 17 countries and over 70 collaborators. She is the editor of *Normal Birth, Evidence and Debate* (Churchill Livingstone, 2004, 2008), and the founder of the International Normal Birth Research conference series.

References

1 Chalmers I, Enkin M, Keirse MJNC, 1998. *Effective Care in Pregnancy and Childbirth*. Oxford: Oxford University Press.

2 Hodnett ED, Fredericks S, 2003. Support during pregnancy for women at increased risk of low birthweight babies. Cochrane Database of Systematic Reviews Issue 3. Art. No.: CD000198. DOI: 10.1002/14651858.CD000198.

3 Cochrane database of pregnancy and childbirth. Available at: www.2.cochrane.org/reviews/en/topics/87.html [accessed 31st March 2011].

4 Manandhar DS, Osrin D, Shrestha BP, Mesko N, Morrison J, Tumbahangphe KM, Tamang S, Thapa S, Shrestha D, Thapa B, Shrestha JR, Wade A, Borghi J, Standing H, Manandhar M, Costello AM; Members of the MIRA Makwanpur trial team, 2004. Effect of a participatory intervention with women's groups on birth outcomes in Nepal: cluster-randomised controlled trial. *Lancet*. 11-17;364(9438):970-9.

5 Rath S, Nair N, Tripathy PK, Barnett S, Rath S, Mahapatra R, Gope R, Bajpai A, Sinha R, Costello A, Prost A, 2010. Explaining the impact of a women's group led community mobilisation intervention on maternal and newborn health outcomes: the Ekjut trial process evaluation. *BMC Int Health Hum Rights*. 10:25.

6 'Gravity Birth' Pulls Women to Ecuador Hospital (16/02/2009). Available at www.womensenews.org/story/health/090215/gravity-birth-pulls-women-ecuador-hospital [accessed 03/04/2011].

7 Misago C, Kendall C, Freitas P et al, 2001. From 'culture of dehumanization of childbirth' to 'childbirth as a transformative experience': changes in five municipalities in north-east Brazil. *Int J Gynecol Obstet* 75: S67–S72.

8 Belizan M, Meier A, Althabe F, Codazzi A, Colomar M, Buekens P, Belizan J, Walsh J, Campbell MK, 2007. Facilitators and barriers to adoption of evidence-based perinatal care in Latin American hospitals: a qualitative study. *Health Educ Res*. 22 (6):839-53.

9 Rogers EM, 1983. *Diffusion of Innovations*. New York: Free Press.

10 Arney W, 1982. *Power and the profession of obstetrics*. University of Chicago Press, Chicago.

11 Oakley A, 1986. *The Captured Womb*. A history of the medical care of pregnant women. Oxford: Blackwell.

12 Wikberg A, Bondas T, 2010. A patient perspective in research on intercultural caring in maternity care: A meta-ethnography. *Int J Qual Stud Health Well-being*, 8;5.

13 Thomson G, Downe S, 2008. Widening the trauma discourse: the link between childbirth and experiences of abuse. Journal *of Psychosomatic Obstetrics & Gynaecology*, 29(4), 268-273.

14 Thomson G, Downe S, 2010. Changing the future to change the past: women's experiences of a positive birth following a traumatic birth experience. *Journal of Reproductive and Infant Psychology*, 28(1), 102-112.

15 Maternity care working party (UK), 2007. Making Normal Birth a Reality. Available from: http://www.rcog.org.uk/womens-health/clinical-guidance/making-normal-birth-reality.

16 O'Connell R, Downe S, 2009. A metasynthesis of midwives' experience of hospital practice in publicly funded settings: compliance, resistance and authenticity. *Health* 13(6):589-609.

17 Lukas CV, Holmes SK, Cohen AB, Restuccia J, Cramer IE, Shwartz M, Charns MP, 2007. Transformational change in health care systems: an organizational model. *Health Care Manage Rev.* 32(4):309-20.

18 Casper MJ, Moore L, 2009. Missing Bodies: The Politics of Visibility—Biopolitics: Medicine, Technoscience and Health in the 21st Century, *New York Times.*

19 Hodnett ED, Downe S, Edwards N, Walsh D, 2005. Home-like versus conventional institutional settings for birth. Cochrane Database of Systematic Reviews Issue 1. Art. No.: CD000012. DOI: 10.1002/14651858.CD000012.pub2.

20 Bamford-Wade A, Moss C, 2010. Transformational leadership and shared governance: an action study. *J Nurs Manag,* 18(7):815-21.

21 Markham S K, Aiman-Smith L, 2001. Product Champions: Truths, Myths and Management. *Research-Technology Management*, 44 (3)44-50(7).

22 Thaler RH, Sunstein CR, 2008. *Nudge: Improving Decisions About Health, Wealth and Happiness* Caravan Books.

23 Institute for Innovation and Improvement, 2010. *Improving healthcare quality at scale and pace: Lessons from The Productive Ward.* Executive Summary. Available from: http://www.institute.nhs.uk/images//documents/Quality_and_value/Productive_Ward/PW%20scale%20and%20pace%20Executive%20Summary.pdf.

24 Misago C, Kendall C, Freitas P, Haneda K, Silveira D, Onuki D, Mori T, Sadamori T, Umenai T, 2001. From 'culture of dehumanization of childbirth' to 'childbirth as a transformative experience': changes in five municipalities in north-east Brazil. *Int J Gynaecol Obstet,* 75 Suppl 1:S67-72.

25 Women's health enews 16/02/2009. Gravity birth pulls women into Ecuador hospital. Available from: www.womensenews.org/article.cfm/dyn/aid/3920.

26 Kernick D, 2002. The demise of linearity in managing health services: a call for post normal health care. *J Health Serv Res Policy,* 7:121–124.

27 Kuhn, TS, 1962. *The Structure of Scientific Revolutions*. Chicago: University of Chicago Press.

28 Sweeney K, Griffiths F, 2002. *Complexity and healthcare, an introduction*. Oxford: Radcliffe Medical Press.

29 Sternberg EM, 2000. *The Balance Within : The Science Connecting Health and Emotions.* San Francisco: WH Freeman.

30 Arnaert A, Filteau N, Sourial R, 2006. Stroke patients in the acute care phase: role of hope in self-healing. *Holist Nurs Pract* 20(3):137-46.

31 Lee YY, Lin JL, 2010. Do patient autonomy preferences matter? Linking patient-centered care to patient-physician relationships and health outcomes. *Soc Sci Med,* 71(10):1811-8.

32 Antonovsky A, 1987. Unravelling the Mystery of Health—how people manage stress and stay well, San Francisco: Jossey Bass Pub.

33 Downe S, McCourt C, 2004. From being to becoming: reconstructing childbirth knowledges. In S Downe (ed.) *Normal Childbirth; Evidence & Debate*. London: Churchill Livingstone.

34 Soloman A, 1985. The emerging field of psychoneuroimmunology: Advances. *J Inst Adv Health,* 2: 6–19.

35 McEwen BS, 2007. Physiology and Neurobiology of Stress and Adaptation: Central Role of the Brain. *Physiol Rev,* 87: 873–904.

36 Effros RB, 2011. Telomere/telomerase dynamics within the human immune system: effect of chronic infection and stress. *Exp Gerontol.* 46(2-3):135-40.

37 Cardwell CR, Stene LC, Joner G, Cinek O, Svensson J, Goldacre MJ, Parslow RC, Pozzilli P, Brigis G Stoyanov D, Urbonaite B, Sipetic S, Schober E, Ionescu-Tirgoviste C, Devoti G, de Beaufort CE, Buschard K, Patterson CC, 2008. Caesarean section is associated with an increased risk of childhood-onset type 1 diabetes mellitus: a meta-analysis of observational studies. *Diabetologis,* 51(5):726-35.

38 Renz-Polster H, David MR, Buist AS, Vollmer WM, O'Connor EA, Frazier EA, Wall MA, 2005. Caesarean section delivery and the risk of allergic disorders in childhood. *Clin Exp Allergy,* 35(11):1466-72.

39 Gitau R, Menson E, Pickles V, Fisk N M, Glover V, MacLachlan N, 2001. Umbilical cortisol levels as an indicator of the fetal stress response to assisted vaginal delivery. *Eur J Obstet Gynecol Reprod Biol*, 98: 14–17.

40 Li HT, Ye R, Achenbach TM, Ren A, Pei L, Zheng X, Liu JM, 2011. Caesarean delivery on maternal request and childhood psychopathology: a retrospective cohort study in China. *BJOG,* 118(1):42-8.

41 Miller NM, Fisk NM, Modi N, Glover V, 2005. Mode of birth and infant HPA axis. Stress responses at birth: determinants of cord arterial cortisol and links with cortisol response in infancy. *BJOG,* 112(7):921-6.

42 Schlinzig T, Johansson S, Gunnar A, Ekström TJ, Norman M, 2009. Epigenetic modulation at birth—altered DNA-methylation in white blood cells after caesarean section. *Acta Paediatr,* 98(7):1096-9.

43 Selye H, 1975. Confusion and controversy in the stress field. *Journal of Human Stress,* 1: 37–44.

KEY QUOTES: GUIDELINES

1 "Opening our eyes and changing approaches and attitudes will require strong, collaborative leadership, but it will surely be worthwhile in terms of ensuring improved outcomes. In other words, respectful collaboration with colleagues and other medical staff is the key to turning things around, back towards normality and away from the current 'caesarean default'." (Lesley Page)

2 "In some ways, it is even more powerful when a woman with minimal expectations for birth is given the opportunity through the use of evidence-based practices for normal birth ... to find empowerment." (Ami Goldstein)

3 "The restraints of the system sometimes appear to paralyse the very acts of traditional midwifery that best support a mother in managing the exquisite intensity of birth. ... Until such time that the current maternity care crisis is resolved, small acts of kindness, courage and skill hold the power to make a difference that will be remembered forever." (Alex Smith)

4 "'Failure to progress' in labour, or dystocia, is one of the most common reasons for caesarean section." (Sarah Davies)

5 "With nearly 28 years of ... experience, I know what I believe: promoting normality takes time but it really can be done with the right time, place, people, support and audit—and perhaps also a little water to help!" (Dianne Garland)

6 "Numerous scientific papers and professional organisations support the safety of home birth. While not all women want to or should give birth at home, those who desire home birth deserve the support of caregivers." (Valerie Bader)

7 "Encouraging women to have a VBAC and facilitating VBAC labours are essential ways of promoting normal birth. Although some caesareans indeed save the lives of either mothers or babies—and we can be thankful when this is the case—we cannot really say that having a caesarean is equal to giving birth. There is a huge difference, which most caesarean mothers recognise." (Hélène Vadeboncoeur)

8 "In most circumstances, a midwife would take the role of lead professional for all healthy women with straightforward pregnancies." (Susan Way)

9 "Sharing is the key to growth and the key to stimulating the inner shift that leads to change." (Naoli Vinaver)

10 "Not only must we be held accountable for our actions, but also for the words we use. Those small units of communication are far more powerful than we usually remember." (Sylvie Donna)

11 "Understanding the interconnections on both the level of the organism (the woman's and baby's bodies) and also the organisation (the institution or system within which we work) can shift maternity care towards positive salutogenic thinking, which learns from what goes well, as well as from what has gone badly." (Soo Downe)

pause to think and talk...

...about guidelines

1. In your own personal situation, what steps can you take to give normal birth 'the best chance' of success? Is there anything that you or your colleagues are currently doing which is making it more difficult for women to have normal births—considering your approach to care antenatally, intrapartum and postpartum? How would you go about making changes?
2. Have you ever observed situations in which birthing women become empowered because of the way in which they give birth? How can you facilitate feelings of empowerment in the women you care for?
3. Which methods and approaches do you find work for women in your care, who avoid having epidurals? How do women best cope with any pain?
4. How do you ensure your clients have optimally informed choice? How do you feel informed choice differs from informed consent and what can you do to ensure that 'consent' is never pressurised or coerced?
5. Have you ever attended a water birth? Do you feel confident about providing care to women who choose to labour and/or give birth in water? In your current working situation, what practical measures do you need to take in order to ensure that all (or most) women can have a water labour or birth if they so choose? Where can you get information and equipment?
6. Have you ever attended a home birth? Have you ever given birth yourself at home? If 'yes', how was your experience (as a caregiver and/or as a mother)? If 'no', how do you feel about attending home births? What practical steps could you take in order to make it possible to offer a homebirth choice within your own practice?
7. Have you ever attended a VBAC or had one yourself? How do you feel about VBACs? Why do you think the history of VBACs is rather complicated and political? To what extent do the attitudes of women who are pregnant after a caesarean generally differ from those of their caregivers? What can you do to support VBACs yourself?
8. Have you ever engaged with the media in any way personally? If you wrote articles for websites, what would you write about? If you were to appear on radio or TV, what would you want to talk about? What can you do now?
9. Observe your own use of words over the next few days and weeks. How do you personally use metaphors and imagery? What reactions have you observed in pregnant women when you change the way you speak?
10. In your view, what progress has been made to 'normalise' birth? What still needs to be done? How can you help to push forward the normal birth agenda? What short- and long-term contribution could you make?

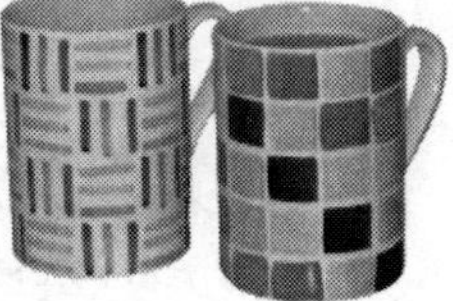

reflect and share further...

Below are extracts from the book *Optimal Birth: What, Why & How* (Sylvie Donna, Fresh Heart 2011)—authors are indicated after each extract. Questions for reflection and discussion are by Sylvie Donna, as elsewhere.

Ultrasound

Our unit policy is for regular serial scans. However, it only appears to be safe, doesn't it? Research is not conclusive so I feel it should be used as with all medical intervention and technology—when it's needed and not routinely. Following this philosophy, I chose to have two scans: an anomaly scan at 20 weeks and one further scan at 34 weeks to check presentation (they were both cephalic)—so I could then plan how to manage my labour. Growth was diagnosed clinically on palpation. **Debbie Brindley (a midwife)**

1 How well do you know the research on ultrasound? What's your conclusion?

2 When (if ever) do you think it's appropriate to use ultrasound of any kind?

Pushing

My experience illustrates that even in the case of a wonderfully skilled midwife who has a great rapport with a family and strong intentions of respecting the birthing mother's privacy and innate power, the tendency to 'help' can run so deep in caregivers that it can pop up even when the midwife's truest intention is to empower the woman.

Sandi apologised the next day for insisting on me pushing out the baby, saying that she knew, based on our antenatal conversations, that I didn't want that. She acknowledged that the baby was never in any distress and she didn't know why she had been so insistent on me pushing. I think that it came from her wanting me to be out of pain and her concept that she knew what I could do to get out of pain. I think she made a mistake in trying to 'rescue' the birthing woman by directing me, rather than pointing me back to what I could know in my own body. **Beth Dubois (a nurse who had two physiological births)**

[To protect her privacy and to respect her openness, the name 'Sandi' is not the real name of the midwife. Beth and I respect her postnatal honesty and humility. Everything else is unchanged.]

3 To what extent do you feel you need to be in 'control' of women?

4 How can you effectively and safely balance action with wise inaction?

5 How often do you 'debrief' with a woman postnatally to explore how effective or ineffective your 'care' has been from the woman's point of view? Do you reflect alone too, so as to work towards 'best' approaches?

Mode of delivery

My idea is to introduce a sort of futuristic strategy of childbirth which is partly what I have already practised. It is based on having a good understanding of physiology and of the basic needs of human beings in labour—for privacy, a sense of security, etc. If the midwife behaves in a motherly way and disturbs the woman as little as possible, either it works or a caesarean is necessary. This strategy makes it possible to avoid the two main alternatives as much as possible: drugs (which all have side effects) and difficult interventions by the vaginal route (difficult forceps and so on). If we avoid these alternatives, there are really only two possibilities: a completely undisturbed physiological labour or a caesarean section. **Michel Odent (former hospital manager/surgeon/midwife)**

6 What are the possible implications and consequences of this kind of approach—in terms of maternal choice, approach to care, the pharmaceutical industry, maternity hospital architecture, design and staffing and outcomes?

7 What is the current approach and how does it differ? What others are there?

Prematurity

Much has been written about the benefits of kangaroo mother care (KMC), which was introduced into neonatal care in response to high mortality and morbidity in resource poor countries. ... Bergman, a highly respected expert has confirmed through much of his writings on KMC that to separate mother and baby is detrimental to the baby's future. Separation causes stress in newborn infants, and continued levels of raised stress hormones are toxic to the infant's developing brain. KMC (also called 'skin-to-skin care') is one practice that will keep mother and baby together. Not only is this practice vital for term newborn babies but it's also of fundamental importance for premature infants. **Luisa Cescutti-Butler (Senior Lecturer in Midwifery).**

8 Have you ever seen or facilitated kangaroo mother care?

9 Do you agree there could be advantages?

Maternal perceptions of birth

... while I feel passionately about the value of physiological childbirth and consider individualised midwifery care and home birth the gold standard, I also think it's important for women to have the right to choose what they feel comfortable with. Who can truly say what is optimal for anyone else? And most of us who have powerful unmedicated births have a difficult time during some part of the birth, even if it turns out to be a beneficial experience overall, or perhaps it's even the difficulty we go through that makes it such a beneficial experience. I have heard it called a rite of passage and in a traditional rite of passage, there is typically adversity that is overcome. **Beth Dubois.**

10 What's your own view? *Should* birth be a rite of passage? What about choice? How is it possible to promote normality while still facilitating real choice? What is implicitly promoted in any case when you do 'nothing different'?

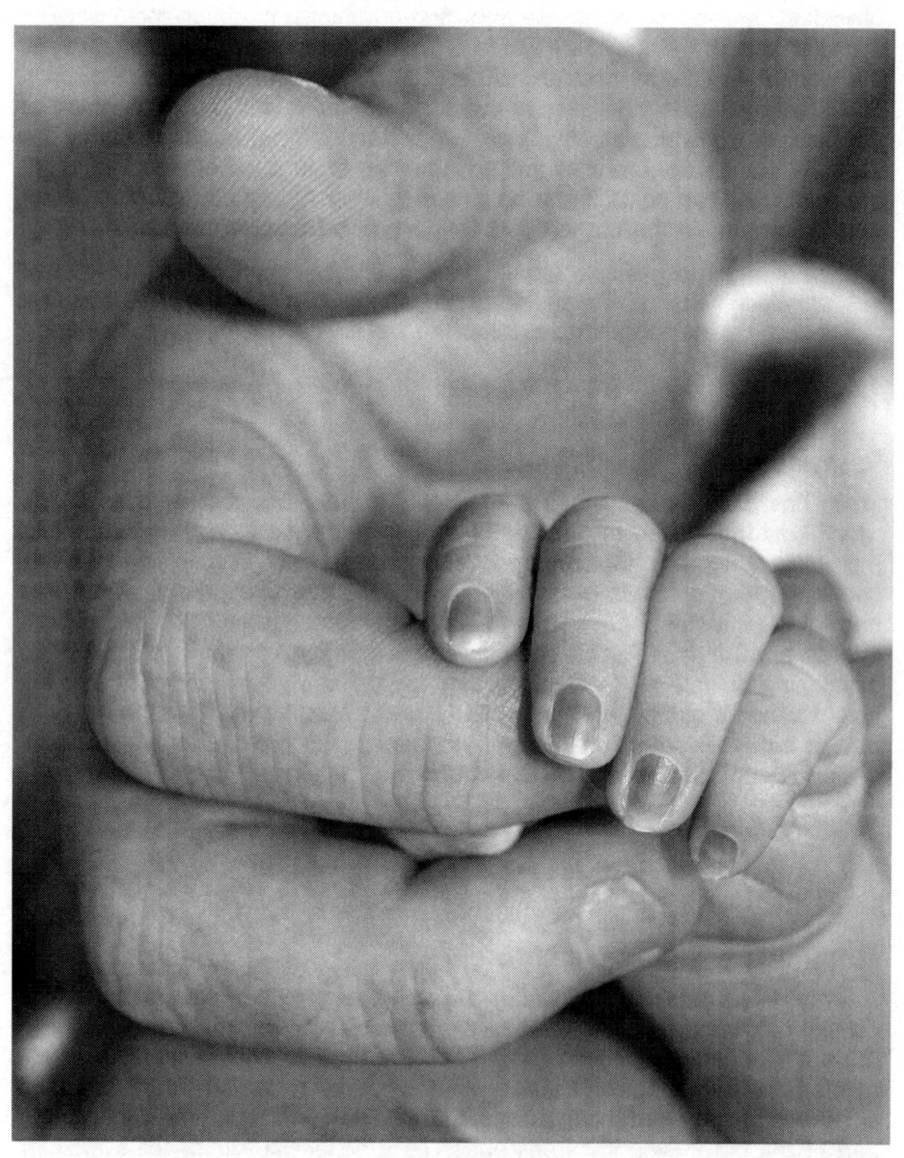

Afterword

Suzanne Arms

Promoting normal, natural birth–that is, without any outside intervention, just adequate preparation, having the woman in as good health as possible at the start of labour, and providing whatever emotional and physical support she needs–is not merely valuable for women and babies. Protecting and promoting normal birth is fundamental to the health and resiliency of our species. It is necessary that as many people as possible are born, and give birth, the way biology and their bodies intended.

Birth is a critical developmental process for *both* the mother and the baby. It affects their neurological and psychological development and the quality of the bond. A baby literally depends upon others, especially its mother, to protect and nurture it. Without her it will not survive or, if it does, it will likely never reach its potential as a human being. For the mother, achieving the most normal possible birth–and healing any trauma that might occur–is essential to her level of trust and confidence as a woman with an ability to mother.

Current scientific evidence proves what ancient wisdom and the mystics have always understood: that whether we approach life with an implicit trust and curiosity or react in fear, defensiveness, mistrust and doubt directly depends upon the experiences we have at conception, in the womb, during our birth and in the time right afterward. Those experiences, and the sense that our body makes of them, shape our cells, our brain, our immune system, everything. This is what primal health research is revealing.

Clearly, birth matters profoundly, especially at this time in human history when we and this planet are faced with a multitude of challenges that require our full human attention and involvement. That's what normal birth offers. When we meet a mother and her baby's dependency and developmental needs, which we are best able to do when birth proceeds normally, we start the family off on the best possible footing.

Suzanne Arms graduated from the University of Rochester (NY, USA) with honours in literature and a minor in cross-cultural studies and anthropology. Author of seven books related to the 'primal' period–*Immaculate Deception*, was named Best Book of the Year by the New York Times. She co-founded one of the first birth centres and the first resource centre for pregnancy, birth and early parenting (in 1978) and founded and directs a Colorado-based international charity, Birthing The Future. An international speaker and film producer, Suzanne is an advocate for the mother-baby and father-family bond, full breastfeeding, home birth and birthing centres, doulas, fully paid maternity leave for all women and paternity leave for fathers, the 'midwife model of care', and transforming consciousness across the world, as the surest way to empower women and help families and the world to thrive. Website: www.BirthingTheFuture.org

Useful websites

- AIMS (Association for Improvements in the Maternity Services)–www.aims.org.uk
- Active Birth Centre–www.activebirthcentre.com
- Association of Breastfeeding Mothers–www.abm.me.uk
- Association of Radical Midwives–www.radmid.demon.co.uk
- BLISS (premature babies–support for parents)–www.bliss.org.uk
- Caesarean Support Network–www.ukselfhelp.info/caesarean
- Care for the Family–www.careforthefamily.org.uk
- Down's Syndrome Association–www.downs-syndrome.org.uk
- Doula UK–www.doula.org.uk
- HIFA 2015 (Health Information For All by 2015)–www.hifa2015.org
- Independent Midwives Association–www.independentmidwives.org.uk
- La Leche League Great Britain–www.laleche.org.uk
- Meet-a-Mum Association (MAMA)–www.mama.co.uk
- Miscarriage Association–www.miscarriageassociation.org.uk
- NCT (The National Childbirth Trust)–www.nct.org.uk
- Parentalk–support for parents–www.parentalk.co.uk
- Patients' Association–www.patients-association.org.uk
- Primal Health Research Centre–www.birthworks.org/primalhealth
- Pubmed (US National Library of Medicine)–www.ncbi.nlm.nih.gov/pubmed/
- Society for Teachers of the Alexander Technique (STAT)–www.stat.org.uk
- Stillbirth and Neonatal Death Society (SANDS)–www.uk-sands.org
- Twins and Multiples Births Association (TAMBA)–www.tamba.org.uk
- Women Deliver (safe motherhood worldwide)–www.womendeliver.org
- Working Families–www.workingfamilies.org.uk

Index

How did this book come about?

Sylvie Donna

It's rather an unusual story... It all started with a comment an obstetrician made when I was pregnant with my first baby, 14 years ago. I'd had to arrange an appointment with him because the obstetrician I'd finally found to attend me in labour mentioned to me during my appointment at around 34 weeks: "Oh, by the way, I'm afraid I won't be in the country in the two weeks leading up to your due date. I'm attending a conference in Germany." (This was the only obstetrician I could find who would 'allow' me to have a birth with no unnecessary intervention. I'd only succeeded in finding him, with great difficulty, when I was 30 weeks pregnant and even then I'd had to beg the hospital secretary to give me just a 'five-minute' appointment.) At my next appointment he'd suggested that his teacher—who was, by then, quite elderly and retired—might be willing to attend me, should I go into labour during those two weeks he was away.

Armed with a letter of introduction and rehearsing in my mind how I was going to persuade this man to attend me *without* EFM on admission, without any drugs for pain relief, without a routine episiotomy, and with a physiological third stage, I found my way to this gentleman's house. The appointment went relatively well, until he told me he would insist on induction if I went even one day beyond my due date. I was just about to begin explaining my preference not to be induced and arguing my case (yet again) when I realised that my own obstetrician would be back in charge by then—so I merely smiled serenely and climbed off the couch. Then I heard a comment which amazed and worried me: "You'll want to write a book about this after you've had the baby." Why would he think that? It seemed such an absurd thing to say. After all, I was just planning to have a normal birth...

Two days after I gave birth (normally) the inevitable happened: I found myself typing away at my computer, my new baby breastfeeding on my lap as I worked. The book that eventually ensued (a decade and two normal births later) was *Birth: Countdown to Optimal.* Two days after it came out I gave a copy to someone heading up a well-respected organisation of caregivers—because I *happened* to get talking to her (she started it!) at an ICM conference which I *happened* to attend. (This was after a strange sequence of events which led me in unexpected directions.) Six weeks after the conference I received a wonderful email—she loved the book!—and very soon I found I was being encouraged to adapt the book for caregivers. There was a conference called 'Optimal Childbirth' six weeks after that so I took up the rather crazy challenge of completing the book in time. I did manage to do that, but was not terribly happy with the result because I hadn't managed to properly reference my work in those six weeks.

Within a year I had referenced the book completely—and it had grown from 132 pages to 684 pages—and I was just about to publish it as *Promoting Normal Birth: Research, Reflections & Guidelines* when I suddenly thought: "Why am I changing the title of a book which is selling well?" (*Optimal Birth: What, Why & How* has had almost exclusively positive feedback—and action was taken to redress anything less positive—and it soon became a resounding success.) So—you guessed it—I stuck with the original title and thought I'd better do something with this other interesting title... and it seemed a good idea to ask *other* people to write most of the content . Along the line, I published several other books too...

Also available...

Books to help your clients prepare for a normal birth...

Birth: Countdown to Optimal: information and inspiration for pregnant women—by Sylvie Donna

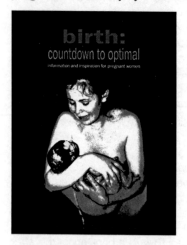

Birth Your Way: choosing birth at home or in a birth centre by Sheila Kitzinger

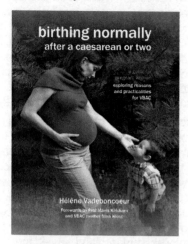

Birthing Normally After a Caesarean or Two: exploring reasons and practicalities for VBAC—by Hélène Vadeboncoeur

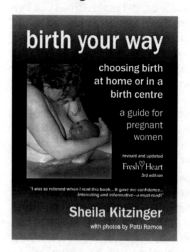

Birth Pain: Power to Transform: a guide for pregnant women—by Verena Schmid

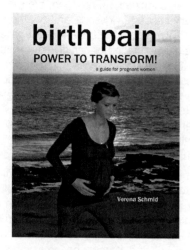

Books you yourself may find useful...

Optimal Birth: What, Why & How—a reflective narrative approach based on research evidence—by Sylvie Donna

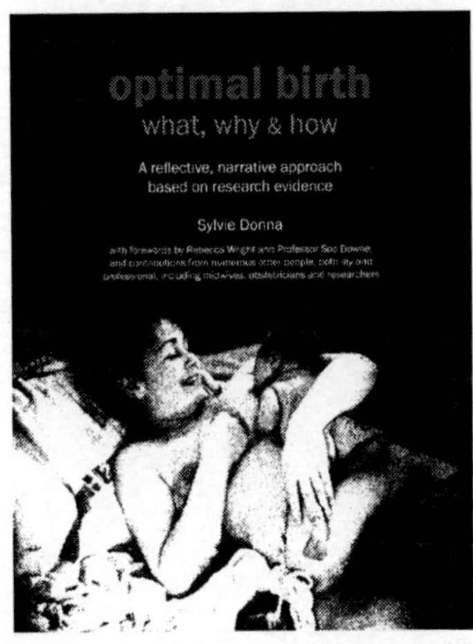

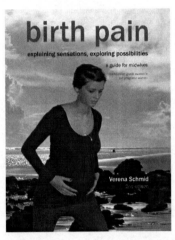

Birth Pain: Explaining sensations, exploring possibilities—by Verena Schmid

Surprising, Inspiring Birth: accounts of birth to inform, amuse and reassure—by Sylvie Donna (ed)

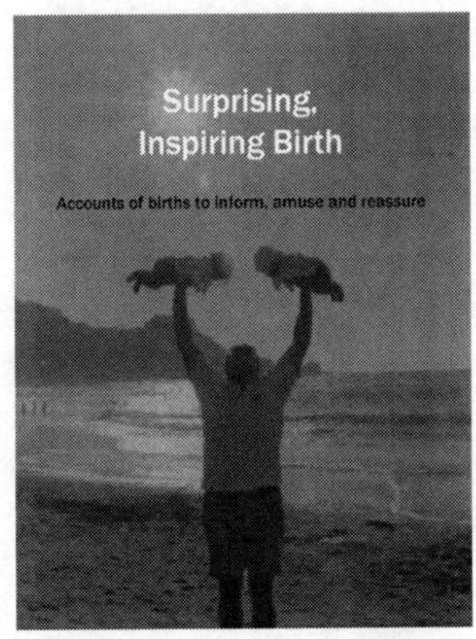

Welcoming Baby: a reflective guide for midwives [on neonatal care]—by Debby Gould

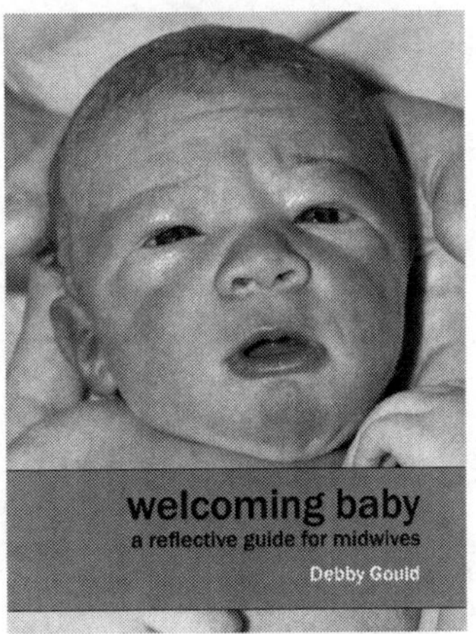

See the website for info and prices. All books are also available from Amazon.

www.freshheartpublishing.co.uk

Lightning Source UK Ltd.
Milton Keynes UK
UKOW010648230412

191281UK00001B/1/P